COMPARATIVE FEDERALISM AND COVID-19

This comprehensive scholarly book on comparative federalism and the Covid-19 pandemic is written by some of the world's leading federal scholars and national experts.

The Covid-19 pandemic presented an unprecedented emergency for countries worldwide, including all those with a federal or hybrid-federal system of government, which account for more than 40 per cent of the world's population. With case studies from 19 federal countries, this book explores the core elements of federalism that came to the fore in combatting the pandemic: the division of responsibilities (disaster management, health care, social welfare, and education), the need for centralisation, and intergovernmental relations and cooperation. As the pandemic struck federal countries at roughly the same time, it provided a unique opportunity for comparative research on the question of how the various federal systems responded. The authors adopt a multidisciplinary approach to question whether federalism has been a help or a hindrance in tackling the pandemic. The value of the book lies in understanding how the Covid-19 pandemic affected federal dynamics and how it may have changed them, as well as providing useful lessons for how to combat such pandemics in federal countries in the future.

This book will be of great interest to students and scholars of politics and international relations, comparative federalism, health care, and disaster management.

Nico Steytler is Professor of Public Law at the Dullah Omar Institute for Constitutional Law, Governance and Human Rights at the University of the Western Cape, South Africa, and the South African Research Chair in Multilevel Government, Law and Development. He is a former Commissioner of the Financial and Fiscal Commission, and former President of the International Association of Centres for Federal Studies. He has published widely on federalism, including *The Value of Comparative Federalism: The Legacy of Ronald L. Watts* (2021, co-edited), *Decentralization and Constitutionalism in Africa* (2019, co-edited); *Concurrent Powers in Federal Systems: Meaning, Making, Managing* (2017, edited); *Kenyan-South African Dialogue on Devolution* (2016, co-edited); and *Local Government Law of South Africa* (2007, co-authored).

Routledge Studies in Federalism and Decentralization

The series publishes outstanding scholarship on federalism and decentralization, defined broadly, and is open to theoretical, empirical, philosophical, and historical works. The series includes two types of work: first, it features research monographs that are substantially based on primary research and make a significant original contribution to their field. Second, it contains works that address key issues of policy-relevant interest or summarise the research literature and provide a broad comparative coverage.

Series Editors: *Paolo Dardanelli, Centre for Federal Studies, University of Kent, UK, and John Kincaid, Lafayette College, USA.*

Formerly Routledge Series in Federal Studies, edited by Michael Burgess and Paolo Dardanelli, Centre for Federal Studies, University of Kent, UK:

Emerging Practices in Intergovernmental Functional Assignment
Gabriele Ferrazzi and Rainer Rohdewohld

Swiss Federalism
The Transformation of a Federal Model
Adrian Vatter

Federalism in Asia
India, Pakistan, Malaysia, Nepal and Myanmar
Harihar Bhattacharyya

Non-Territorial Autonomy and Decentralization
Ethno-Cultural Diversity Governance
Edited by Tove H. Malloy and Levente Salat

COMPARATIVE FEDERALISM AND COVID-19

Combating the Pandemic

Edited by Nico Steytler

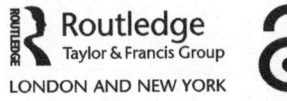

Routledge
Taylor & Francis Group

LONDON AND NEW YORK

First published 2022
by Routledge
2 Park Square, Milton Park, Abingdon, Oxon OX14 4RN

and by Routledge
605 Third Avenue, New York, NY 10158

Routledge is an imprint of the Taylor & Francis Group, an informa business

British Library Cataloguing-in-Publication Data
A catalogue record for this book is available from the British Library

Library of Congress Cataloging-in-Publication Data
A catalog record has been requested for this book

ISBN: 978-0-367-76397-8 (hbk)
ISBN: 978-0-367-76396-1 (pbk)
ISBN: 978-1-003-16677-1 (ebk)

DOI: 10.4324/9781003166771

Typeset in Bembo
by KnowledgeWorks Global Ltd.

For my mother, who, like so many others, succumbed to Covid-19 during lockdown, isolated from her loved ones.

CONTENTS

LIST OF TABLES AND FIGURES

Tables

Figures

CONTRIBUTORS

Lukman Abdulrauf is Senior Lecturer in Constitutional Law, Digital Rights, and Data Protection Law in the Department of Public Law at the University of Ilorin, Nigeria, and Fellow at the Institute for International and Comparative Law in Africa at the University of Pretoria, South Africa.

Elisabeth Alber is Senior Researcher at the Institute for Comparative Federalism at Eurac Research, Italy.

Cristian Altavilla is Director of the School of Law at University Siglo 21, and Professor of Constitutional and Public Law at University Siglo 21 and University Nacional de Córdoba, Argentina.

Paul Anderson is Lecturer in Politics and International Relations at Canterbury Christ Church University, United Kingdom.

Erika Arban is a Postdoctoral Fellow in the Laureate Program in Comparative Constitutional Law at the University of Melbourne, Australia, and Lecturer in Comparative Federalism at the University of Antwerp, Belgium.

Nicholas Aroney is Professor of Constitutional Law in the TC Beirne School of Law at the University of Queensland, Australia.

Zemelak Ayitenew Ayele is Director of the Center for Federal and Governance Studies at Addis Ababa University, Ethiopia, and extra-ordinary Associate Professor at Dullah Omar Institute for Constitutional Law, Governance and Human Rights at the University of the Western Cape, South Africa.

Simone Barbareschi is a Postdoctoral Researcher in Public Law at Roma Tre University, Italy.

Eva Maria Belser is Full Professor, Chair of Administrative and Constitutional Law, and Co-Director of the Institute of Federalism at the University of Fribourg, Switzerland.

Michael Boyce is a Law Student in the TC Beirne School of Law at the University of Queensland, Australia.

Peter Bursens is Full Professor of Political and Social Sciences and senior member of the GOVTRUST Centre of Excellence at the University of Antwerp, Belgium.

Beniamino Caravita is Professor of Public Law in the Department of Political Science at the University of Rome, Italy, and Director of *Associazione Osservatorio Sul Federalismo e i Processi Di Governo*, Italy.

Tinashe Chigwata is Associate Professor at the Dullah Omar Institute for Constitutional Law, Governance and Human Rights at the University of the Western Cape, South Africa.

Paolo Colasante is a Researcher in Constitutional Law at the Institute for the Study of Regionalism, Federalism and Self-Government (ISSiRFA) at the Italian National Research Council (CNR), Italy.

Marcelo Labanca Corrêa de Araújo is Professor of Constitutional Law in the Graduate Program in Law at the Catholic University of Pernambuco (UNICAP), Brazil.

Mireia Grau Creus is Head of Research at the Institute of Self-Government Studies at the Government of Catalonia, Spain.

Jaap de Visser is Professor of Law and Director of the Dullah Omar Institute for Constitutional Law, Governance and Human Rights at the University of the Western Cape, South Africa.

Adriano Dirri is a Lecturer in Public Law at the University of Rome, La Sapienza, Italy.

Mikel Erkoreka is a Lecturer of Public Policy and Economic History and Researcher at the Ituna Center for Basque Economic Agreement and Fiscal Federalism Studies at the University of the Basque Country, Spain.

Gisela Färber is Senior Fellow at the German Research Institute for Public Administration and held the Chair for Public Finance at the German University of Administrative Sciences, Germany.

Sérgio Ferrari is Professor of Constitutional Law at Rio de Janeiro State University, Brazil.

Yonatan Tesfaye Fessha is Professor of Public Law and Jurisprudence at the University of the Western Cape, South Africa.

Antonio María Hernández is Director of the Institute of Federalism of the National Academy of Law and Social Sciences of Cordoba; Professor of Constitutional Law and State Constitutional and Municipal Law at the National University of Córdoba, Argentina; and Postdoctoral Senior Fellow of the State University of New York at Buffalo Law School, USA.

John Kincaid is Robert B. and Helen S. Meyner Professor of Government and Public Service and Director of the Meyner Center for the Study of State and Local Government at Lafayette College, USA.

Vladimir Klistorin is Professor of Economics, and Leading Research Fellow at the Institute of Economics and Industrial Engineering in the Siberian Branch of the Russian Academy of Sciences at Novosibirsk State University, Russia.

Mario Kölling is Professor of Political Science at the Spanish National Distance University (UNED) and Senior Researcher at the Manuel Giménez Abad Foundation, Spain.

Karl Kössler is Senior Researcher at the Institute for Comparative Federalism at Eurac Research, Italy.

Nataliya Kravchenko is Professor of Economics, and Acting Head of Department, in the Department of Industrial Enterprises Management at the Institute of Economics and Industrial Engineering in the Siberian Branch of the Russian Academy of Sciences at Novosibirsk State University, Russia.

J. Wesley Leckrone is Professor of Political Science and Department Chair at Widener University, USA.

Ivan Leksin is Professor of Law, and Head of Department of Legal Foundations of Administration, in the School of Public Administration at Lomonosov Moscow State University, Russia.

Jessica Michelin graduated with a degree in Law from McGill University, Canada, and is Clerk to the Québec Court of Appeal, Canada.

Vanessa Elias de Oliveira is Associate Professor and Head of the Graduate Program in Public Policies at the Federal University of ABC (UFABC), Brazil.

Francesco Palermo is Professor of Comparative Public Law in the Faculty of Law at the University of Verona, and Director of the Institute for Comparative Federalism at Eurac Research, Italy.

Johanne Poirier is Full Professor of Law and holder of the Peter MacKell Chair in Federalism at McGill University, Canada.

Patricia Popelier is Full Professor of Law at the University of Antwerp; Director of the Research Group on Government and Law at the University of Antwerp, Belgium; Senior Research Fellow at the Centre for Federal Studies at the University of Kent, UK; and co-promoter of the GOVTRUST Centre of Excellence at the University of Antwerp, Belgium.

Gilberto M. A. Rodrigues is Associate Professor and Head of the Graduate Program in International Relations at the Federal University of ABC (UFABC), Brazil.

Cheryl Saunders AO is Laureate Professor Emeritus of the Centre for Comparative Constitutional Law at the University of Melbourne, Australia.

Viacheslav Seliverstov is Professor of Economics and Head of the Centre for Strategic Analysis and Planning, at the Institute of Economics and Industrial Engineering, and Director of the International Research Centre for Cross-Border Interactions in North and North-East Asia, in the Siberian Branch of the Russian Academy of Sciences at Novosibirsk State University, Russia.

José María Serna de la Garza is a Researcher at the Institute of Legal Research at the National Autonomous University of Mexico (UNAM), Mexico.

Francesco Severa is a PhD Candidate in Public, Comparative and International Law at Sapienza University of Rome, Italy.

Ajay Kumar Singh is Professor and Director at the Centre for Federal Studies at Hamdard University, India.

Sergio Spatola is a PhD Candidate in Public, Comparative and International Law at Sapienza University of Rome, Italy.

Nico Steytler is Professor of Public Law and the South African Research Chair in Multilevel Government, Law and Development at the Dullah Omar Institute for Constitutional Law, Governance and Human Rights, at the University of the Western Cape, South Africa.

Almira Yusupova is Professor of Economics and Leading Researcher at the Institute of Economics and Industrial Engineering in the Siberian Branch of the Russian Academy of Sciences at Novosibirsk State University, Russia.

FOREWORD

One of the areas more severely affected by emergencies in general, and by the Covid-19 pandemic in particular, is that of the vertical division of powers and the idea of federalism more broadly. Fighting a pandemic requires quick and coordinated action, for which national governments are better suited. The consequence is often both a horizontal (from parliaments to governments) and a vertical centralisation of powers, from subnational (and local) to the central level. However, the way this happens deeply differs from country to country and is most likely one of the indicators for the rootedness of the federal principle in societies and institutions.

Federalism has no doubt been subject to a stress test by the Covid-19 pandemic. Criticism has been voiced not only in countries where the 'federal spirit' (Burgess) is lacking, that is, a rooted culture, tradition, and acceptance of federalism, but also where this is undoubtedly present. The existence of separate health-care systems with different authorities introducing potentially different regulations is easy to be seen as an obstacle rather than an asset. Similarly, potential differences in solutions that might impact on the very fundamental right to life are likely to be met with scepticism. And the very essence of federalism – negotiation and dialogue – is often portrayed as a factor slowing the adoption of decisions rather than improving their quality.

A closer look at the comparative practice, however, shows a different picture. This is what this book is doing. By analysing in depth a wide range of multi-tiered systems in managing the pandemic, highlighting the different responses, their different effectiveness, and their different reasons, it provides a unique opportunity to learn and reflect on the very essence of federalism and what it is for: a better, more nuanced, more pondered, and more democratic way to make decisions. Not infrequently, a multi-level structure helps correct fatal mistakes made by national governments and as a matter of fact, during the Covid-19 pandemic, federal countries resorted to states of emergency and derogations from the constitutional order less frequently than non-federal states did, which could provide evidence of more resilience of federal structures. Importantly, federal decision-making does not mean that decisions must be different. It means that they might be different when and where this proves meaningful: tailoring solutions to the different needs of different territories might be conducive to more efficient responses.

Be that as it may, this book offers a nuanced, informed, and data-based insight on what the virus did to federalism and what federalism did and can do to tackle emergencies such as a pandemic. It is not by chance that the idea of the book has originated within the framework of the worldwide network of federal scholars, most of whom are members of the International Association of Centres for Federal Studies (IACFS), and is edited by one of its most distinguished members and former president, Professor Nico Steytler. The book is not only a valuable academic exercise. It also testifies of the possible contribution that a community of experts can offer to decision-makers and opinion leaders when addressing dramatic challenges: the provision of informed analysis.

Francesco Palermo, *President of the IACFS*

PREFACE

In mid-March 2020 as the Covid-19 pandemic rapidly swallowed the world, universities, like other public institutions, closed and we, members of the International Association of Centres for Federal Studies (IACFS), stayed at home, trying to work. We all watched how the pandemic spread throughout our respective federal countries. It then struck me that we should take a collective look at how the governments in federal systems were dealing with the pandemic. It provided a unique opportunity for true comparative research to analyse how very different types of federal systems dealt with exactly the same issue at the same time, and in real time as the pandemic unfolded in each country. It also compelled us to make sense, not only of how governments have responded to the pandemic but also of our daily lives in isolation. The planned research would give us an insight into the workings of federal systems under stress and how they could/should respond to similar disasters in the future.

The project received an overwhelmingly favourable response and academics from 19 IACFS member centres participated. It was a truly collective effort, and in this regard the contributions of Cheryl Saunders and John Kincaid to the development of the template are gratefully acknowledged.

To cover all the major federations in the world, 19 case studies were commissioned. As the country studies covered the many aspects of federalism, teams of researchers were assembled and 45 persons eventually participated in the production of the text. The collaboration of experienced professors with young researchers is a gratifying feature of this volume. The assembled 19 case studies provided us with a truly global picture of the working of federalism in times of stress.

The first milestone was the presentation of draft papers at IACFS's annual conference, which was virtually hosted from 14 to 16 October 2020; the conference scheduled to be held in Ethiopia on that date being another casualty of the pandemic.

This book would not have been possible without the strong support of the IACFS Executive Committee, and, in particular, of Francesco Palermo, the IACFS president, and the enthusiastic participation of the IACFS family. The contributors responded readily to endless requests to keep to the template in presenting the material. To them I owe a great debt of gratitude.

I would also like to acknowledge the support provided by the South African Research Chairs Initiative of the Department of Science and Technology and the National Research Foundation through the South African Research Chair in Multilevel Government, Law and Development (SARChI Chair). As part of the SARChI Chair Team at the Dullah Omar Institute, University of the Western Cape, I thank Curtly Stevens and Dr Shehaam Johnstone for their research assistance and Mandy Cupido for administrative support. A particular word of thanks goes to Dr Michelle Maziwisa, a SARChI post-doctoral fellow for acting as the managing editor – ensuring in her efficient and gracious manner that the manuscript met all the requirements of Routledge. I would also like to mention the support staff at the Dullah Omar Institute – Virginia Brookes, Kirsty Wakefield, and Kay Sapto – for their assistance in the project. Andre Wiesner is thanked for his excellent editing which was done mostly over the festive season.

The book is published in Open Access, thanks to the 'crowd funding' by the financial contributions of the following persons and institutions: IACFS, Eva Maria Belser (Institute of Federalism, University of Fribourg), Mikel Erkoreka (Ituna Center for Basque Economic Agreement and Fiscal Federalism Studies), Mario Kölling (Manuel Giménez Abad Foundation), Francesco Palermo (Institute for Comparative Federalism, Eurac Research), Patricia Popelier (Research Group on Government and Law, University of Antwerp), and the SARChI Chair in Multilevel Government, Law and Development.

Lastly, I owe a word of gratitude to John Kincaid, one of the series editors of the Routledge Studies on Federalism and Decentralisation who brought me in contact with Emily Ross, senior editor at Routledge. With great expedition she ensured the timely contracting and publication of this volume. I thank you for that.

Nico Steytler
March 2021
Cape Town

INTRODUCTION

How federations combat Covid-19[1]

Nico Steytler

1 The pandemic

On 31 December 2019, the first cases of the coronavirus, Covid-19, were identified in Wuhan City, China. Its dramatic rate of transmission and deadly effects
soon led to the city's shutdown, but not before it took wing and, borne by travellers, began alighting in other countries. Very quickly it spread throughout Asia
and Europe and then further afield to North America, South America, Africa,
and Australasia. By the beginning of March 2020, nearly every country in the
world had recorded cases of infection, and on 11 March 2020 the World Health
Organization (WHO) declared Covid-19 a pandemic.

Major initiatives were taken globally to treat the infected and curb further
infection. After a first wave of infections and mortalities during March and
April, infection rates eased off as well as containment measures. However, in the
latter half of the year, the 'second wave' of infections grew in size to exceed in
most cases the numbers of the first wave. By the end of October 2020, the number of infections reached 44 million, with more than 1 million deaths attributed
to Covid-19 (WHO 2020c).

To prevent the spread of the virus, most countries imposed lockdown measures, including the cessation of international travel and, with that, tourism;
domestically, stay-at-home orders resulted in the closure of factories, shops, and
offices. As a result, all economies showed a dramatic downturn, leading to a
world recession – the World Bank (2020) forecasted a 5.2 per cent contraction in
global gross domestic product (GDP) in 2020.

As a pandemic, the Covid-19 outbreak of 2020 differed both in nature from
other national disasters typically experienced over the past decades, such as
flooding, earthquakes and tsunamis, and in magnitude from previous pandemics:
the SARS coronavirus (2002–2003) and the swine flu (H1N1) (2009–2010) were

DOI: 10.4324/9781003166771-1

contained effectively internationally and locally (Hassan et al. 2020). It was both a threat of a disaster, requiring preventative measures, and a disaster in actuality, requiring emergency health care. Moreover, due to the preventative measures taken, innumerable people were indirectly affected by the virus through the curtailment of social and economic activity and limitations on rights to movement, education, religion, democratic governance, and so forth.

Governments thus battled on several fronts. First, preventative measures were put in place to prevent or minimise the spread of the virus – limiting or cancelling international travel, testing, tracing and quarantining suspected carriers of the virus, and eventually imposing internal movement restrictions, the so-called lockdowns. Secondly, emergency curative measures were instituted to treat the seriously ill, many of whom required hospitalisation. Accepting the spread of the disease as inevitable, governments aimed to slow down the infection rate in order not to overburden their health-care systems to a point of collapse. Thirdly, governments instituted ameliorative economic measures to shield businesses and the population from the worst effects of the lockdown measures. In developing countries, the latter had a devastating effect on a large sector of the population already living below the poverty line. Governments had to juggle two competing concerns: containing the virus through preventative lockdown measures, while at the same time easing restrictions to bring economic activity back to life. The early lifting of restrictions inevitably led to renewed escalation of the pandemic.

Small in number, but home to 40 per cent of the world's population, the federations or hybrid federations of the world (in this volume, referred to collectively as federations) were also impacted on by the pandemic. By 31 October 2020 (the end date of the period covered in this study), the Covid-19 pandemic had hit hard the federations selected for this study; among the top 15 countries ranked according to mortalities recorded, are 11 federations, and when mortality rates are compared the numbers are the same (WHO 2020a). However, the selected federations exhibited very different trends in the spread of infection and mortality associated with the virus (see Table 0.1).

Plotting the infection and death trends in Table 0.1 reveals the wide variation in extent of infections officially reported, and also in associated deaths recorded (see Figure 0.1). Furthermore, the relationship between recorded infections and deaths shows that the number of known Covid-19 infections does not perfectly predict the number of known Covid-19 deaths – the more infections the more death – suggesting other factors are at play. While some of the variation in the trends in the data can be ascribed to factors such as the age and health structure of the population, the timing of the arrival of the epidemic, and the nature and extent of recording of infections and deaths, a government's response may also have played a role in the observed trends.

The management of the pandemic in federations brought to the fore key elements of their federal systems: federal governments' responsibility over national emergencies and coordination; the autonomy of states over critical areas such as disaster management and health-care services; and at grassroots

TABLE 0.1 Population and Covid-19 infections and deaths (31 October 2020), selected federations, ranked by cumulative deaths per 100,000[2]

Rank	Country	Population (millions) (2020)	Per cent population >65 (2019)	Infections	Deaths	Fatality rate (%)	Infections per 100,000	Deaths per 100,000
1	Belgium	11.590	19	442,508	11,716	2.6	3,818	101
2	Spain	46.755	20	1,243,052	38,648	3.1	2,659	83
3	Brazil	212.559	9	5,494,376	158,969	2.9	2,585	75
4	Mexico	128.933	7	912,811	90,773	9.9	708	70
5	United States	331.003	16	8,852,730	227,178	2.6	2,675	69
6	United Kingdom	67.886	19	989,749	46,229	4.7	1,458	68
7	Argentina	45.196	11	1,143,800	30,442	2.7	2,531	67
8	Italy	60.462	23	647,674	38,321	5.9	1,071	63
9	South Africa	59.309	5	723,682	19,230	2.7	1,220	32
10	Canada	37.742	18	228,542	10,074	4.4	606	27
11	Switzerland	8.655	19	171,116	2,236	1.3	1,977	26
12	Russia	145.934	15	1,618,116	27,990	1.7	1,109	19
13	Germany	83.784	22	518,753	10,452	2.0	619	12
14	Austria	9.006	19	101,443	1,079	1.1	1,126	12
15	India	1,380.004	6	813,7119	121,641	1.5	590	9
16	Australia	25.500	16	27,582	907	3.3	108	4
17	Ethiopia	114.964	4	95,789	1,464	1.5	83	1
18	Nigeria	206.140	3	62,691	1,144	2	30	1

Source: WHO (2020a, 2020b), World Bank (2019), UN Population Dynamics (2019).

level, municipalities' responsibilities for public hygiene and the provision of certain health-care services, as well as for the continued delivery of public utilities such as water, sanitation, waste removal, and control of public spaces. The multilevel structure of government also places emphasis both on coordination and cooperation between governments vertically and horizontally and on the democratic accountability of each of them individually. Finally, the intergovernmental fiscal system became critical: how is the cost caused by the pandemic covered?

While the role of subnational governments – that is, the collective of states and local governments – is, of course, much dependent on the character of a specific federal system, there may be common patterns in and approaches to managing pandemics. The literature on comparative federalism has, however, given scant attention to this form of disaster or the impact it can have on the functioning of federal systems.

The situation was thus: at the beginning of 2020, the federations were functioning according to their own dynamics, which are forever changing. Out of the blue came a virus with no cure, one which spreads rapidly and has deadly consequences, and suddenly federations – unsuspecting and mostly unprepared – found

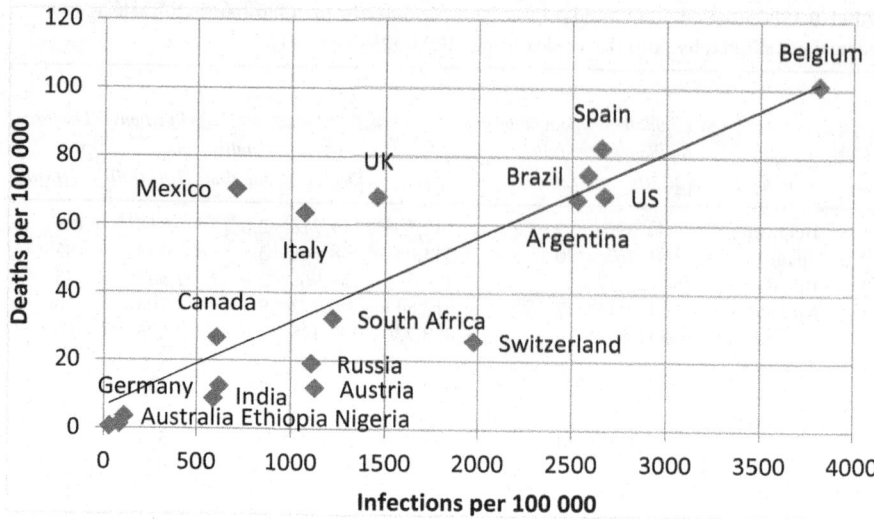

FIGURE 0.1 Relationship between recorded infections and deaths per 100,000 (31 October 2020) selected federations

Source: Table 0.1

themselves confronting a major crisis. This gave rise to critical questions of how federal systems, with decentralised decision-making at their core, responded.

2 Research questions

The immediate question is: how did federal systems respond to the Covid-19 pandemic during the first critical period of 2020, when quick, concerted, and effective action was required to limit and eliminate the virus and the dire socio-economic consequences it caused? What were the modalities of action of each level of government? How did they affect the constitutional distribution of powers – did they lead to an increase in centralisation or decentralisation? Did intergovernmental relations (IGR), the lifeblood of federal systems, work efficiently or at all? What happened to intergovernmental fiscal relations?

A second, more evaluative question then follows: how well (or badly) did federal systems perform in combating a pandemic of this scale? What do the individual experiences tell us generally about how federalism fared as a system of governance in the modern age, when confronted unexpectedly with such a global crisis? Were the federal systems resilient governance systems that could manage the fight against Covid-19? Were good health results attributable to a well-functioning federal system and poor results to failures in another one? For example, with the dispersal of powers between the levels of government, were there sufficient and effective coordination and cooperation?

Having answered these two questions, a third question arises: are the particular federal dynamics – a movement towards decentralisation or centralisation – that may have emerged in each country likely to have long-term consequences for the federal system itself? Will the system return to its old pattern of functioning, or did the management of the pandemic trigger longer-lasting reform? Will the pandemic provide a policy window where more fundamental change may be forthcoming?

It is also important to point out the issues that the study does *not* engage with, as intriguing as they may be. This is not a comparison between federal and unitary systems to see which of them did better. The study is not designed for such a purpose, and at any rate, it would be extremely difficult to tease out the explanatory value that the 'federalism factor' may have had. Moreover, 'federations' is an umbrella term encompassing many variations of federalism: for example, some in effect are close to unitary states for the purpose of combating the pandemic, while many unitary states exhibit strong features of decentralisation.

Our interest is in what combating the pandemic in federal systems revealed about the nature of federalism in a particular country in a particular period. The aim is to reflect on how the federal system functioned between the time in early 2020 that the coronavirus first broke out in a country and the latter part of the year (October). It covers the period prior to the introduction of vaccines and the dynamics that that triggered. Although the full significance of the pandemic and its management will become apparent only in years to come, the first 10 months of 2020 were highly revealing.

In most countries, the first wave of Covid-19 came and went during that period, with many of the preventative measures being eased; a second wave emerged in the second half of the year, putting a new set of dynamics in motion and typically seeing federations adopt a more differentiated response to the pandemic that brought subnational governments to the fore. During the window of time under review, the essential federal dynamics of each country manifested themselves and became visible for analysis and comparison.

During this pre-vaccine period, the studies revealed a number of failures in federal systems that had dire consequences in the battle against Covid-19. Without having to wait for closure of the pandemic, remedial action could be taken to address these failures.

3 Research methodology

3.1 Selecting federal systems for case study

These questions above have been addressed in 19 case studies that cover 6 continents and represent all the main federations in the world. While 'federations' is used as a term of convenience to refer to the group collectively, not many call themselves federations. What they have in common, and what is critical for this study, is the decentralisation (in a broad sense) of decision-making between two or more levels of government.

In the case of Europe, all the major federations and hybrids are included in this study: Austria, Belgium, Germany, Italy, and Spain. They are members of the European Union (EU), a supranational governance structure labelled as a 'confederation' and, as such, an object of study here in its own right. Falling outside the EU are Switzerland, the United Kingdom, and Russia. Turning to North America, all three federal countries are examined: Canada, the United States, and Mexico. In South America, Argentina and Brazil come under review, in Africa, Ethiopia, Nigeria, and South Africa, and in Asia, India. Australia is also covered in the study.

Grouped together in this volume is thus a range from highly decentralised federations to federal-type (quasi-federal, hybrid-federal) systems exhibiting strong centralised tendencies. The response to the Covid-19 pandemic would be much influenced by both the constitutional framework and importantly by the practice guided by the presence or absence of a 'federal spirit'. Painting with a very broad brush, the majority of countries can be grouped under the category of centralised federations: Italy, Spain, Austria, Russia, Mexico, Argentina, India, Ethiopia, South Africa, and Nigeria. Clear cases of decentralised federations are Belgium, Switzerland, the United Kingdom, the United States, Canada, Brazil, and Australia. Somewhere in between lies Germany with its system of executive federalism.

The case studies are presented in groups according to continent: Europe/ Eurasia, North America, South America, Asia/Australia, and Africa. In some respects, the geographical grouping may have also been a factor in how a particular country responded to the crisis. For example, EU countries were influenced by what their neighbours were doing (or not doing) and by the EU structures themselves. In North America, the US president's approach to the pandemic enjoyed no traction north of the border, but it bore uncanny similarities to Mexico's approach. The two South American federations – Brazil and Argentina – showed similarities to each other as well as with Mexico and the United States. Whereas the EU may have played some role in a common approach to the pandemic through its economic packages, the African Union, lacking the EU's integrative structures, may have had only very limited influence on a common approach to health care in the context of Covid-19.

3.2 Giving the case studies a consistent structure

The aim of the book is to get the story of countries told cogently and analytically. To facilitate comparative perspectives, the case studies are structured according to a detailed template. The template seeks to guide and structure that story. It begins with the geophysical, demographic, economic, social, and political background: how did these features of the country and society play out in the fight against the pandemic? What constitutional and legal framework was in place when governments had to spring into action to combat the virus? What were the institutional arrangements for dealing with a pandemic of such a magnitude? What was the state of preparedness?

Then, when Covid-19 arrived, which of the levels of government reacted first and took the initiative? How did the different levels – federal, state, and local – play their allocated roles? Since combating the pandemic inevitably fell in the jurisdiction of all three levels in one way or another, what was the nature of the ensuing intergovernmental relations? In most countries, the levels are bound together in an intergovernmental fiscal system – how, then, did the pandemic impact on it? Finally, could the way the federal system functioned under the stress of the pandemic have long-term consequences for the system itself?

3.2.1 The federal constitutional and legislative framework

In many federations, matters of health care and disaster management are subnational or concurrent functions, while the federal government has emergency powers allowing it extraordinary powers, inter alia, over subnational governments. The first substantive section of each country study looks at the legal situation prior to the pandemic by sketching the constitutional framework for the division of powers and functions between different levels of government, in particular powers and functions concerned with health care and disaster management.

Furthermore, given the exceptional circumstances caused by a pandemic, most federal governments are vested with emergency constitutional powers to override subnational powers. Also, without having to resort to a declaration of a national state of emergency, federal governments can use ordinary legislation to declare a public health emergency. In some federations, such powers can also be exercised by the states. Thus, what was the legal arsenal available to governments at the outbreak of the pandemic?

3.2.2 Preparedness for a national disaster: The institutional framework

In learning from past disasters, most federal countries have developed institutions and processes – political and technical – to deal with such emergencies. These institutions and processes are sometimes of an intergovernmental nature because health care and disaster management are in the main concurrent responsibilities – for example, a national coordinating body is established with representation from federal and state governments. The second section thus outlines the state of preparedness that existed prior to the first wave of the coronavirus. Of importance is the question of whether they played their intended role or were replaced by other, newly created bodies.

3.2.3 Rolling out measures to contain the pandemic

As countries were alerted to the outbreak of the virus in China, governments across the globe started to take measures, some more quickly than others, in the form of travel bans, testing for the virus, and tracing and quarantining infected individuals. Soon, more severe measures were proclaimed, including the social and economic lockdown of cities and towns, while health services were ramped up to cater for the seriously ill. With the announcement of the lockdown strategy, governments formulated plans on how to cope with the strategy's social and economic consequences. When countries reached peaks in infections during the first wave, governments took the difficult decision of easing restrictions, only to be confronted by the same question during the second wave of infections.

Before detailing the measures taken, two important factors relevant to such measures are discussed. First, how did political parties respond to the crisis and how did that response affect each country's federal system, and vice versa? Secondly, in countries with a diversity of communities (some marginalised), were there any indications of marginalisation (or further marginalisation) of any communities in the government responses to the pandemic?

3.2.3.1 Taking the initiative

With decision-making on health care and disaster management dispersed across the levels of government, a critical question in a federal system is who the first responders were to the looming crisis – the federal or subnational governments. Was there effective coordination and cooperation from the start, and did pre-existing (intergovernmental) institutions spring effectively to life? After the initial response, the focus shifts to the actions of the different levels of governments.

3.2.3.2 Federal action

In most countries, the federal government moved to centre stage with a raft of measures to contain the spread of the pandemic. At its disposal were an array of emergency powers, the military, and its superior financial resources. In the measures it took, did the federal government intrude into state domains, and if so, to what extent? Were the usual accountability structures maintained, or was there a shift to executive rule marginalising parliament? How did the courts deal with challenges relating to measures taken?

3.2.3.3 State action

As states usually have jurisdiction over health care, disaster management, and a host of other related functions such as education, questions arise about how they used their powers and performed their functions. Did states assert their autonomy with regard to their responsibilities, or did they readily follow the directions of the federal government and become primarily implementers of federal measures? Did federal measures obliterate the ordinary constitutional division of powers and thus override the relative autonomy of subnational governments?

Also of interest is whether states used their constitutional space to devise innovative measures to deal with aspects of the pandemic. Were they the proverbial laboratories for managing the pandemic more effectively? Conversely, were there instances where states were an obstacle to implementing much-needed preventative measures? Did some, in the name of autonomy, engage in counterproductive measures? Did states cooperate horizontally with each other in joint efforts and measures? Were internal border controls imposed? Were the usual accountability structures maintained? Did state legislatures meet and have a say, or were they suspended? What role did the courts play in scrutinising the measures taken?

3.2.3.4 Local government action

The role of local governments varies considerably according to their size and place within the federal system. Were large metropolitan municipalities with powerful mayors active in leading the way with preventative measures? Were local authorities – large and small – a crucial cog in the wheel in implementing federal and state measures as well as providing basic services? Did organised local government facilitate cooperation and mutual assistance among local authorities?

3.2.3.5 Intergovernmental relations

In view of the measures taken by the different levels of government, a key variable with regard to the success or otherwise of pandemic management was both vertical and horizontal coordination and cooperation between governments. Such coordination may have been embedded in pre-existing disaster management systems, or, in general, cooperative government forums and procedures. It may also be the case that such institutions and processes were ignored due to the exigencies of the pandemic.

Questions addressed include the following: Did intergovernmental relations become irrelevant where the federal government dominated? What role did intergovernmental relations play other than coordination? Did it also facilitate understanding of differences around the country, dissemination of innovative measures, or the harmonisation of responses, without (necessarily) effecting uniformity? Did horizontal cooperation among states and local authorities blossom, or did it degenerate into competition for resources?

3.2.3.6 Intergovernmental fiscal relations

Managing the Covid-19 pandemic was a costly business. The need for healthcare budget items – hospitals, equipment, medical staff, and medicines – grew exponentially. Furthermore, the consequences of lockdown measures for individuals and the economy as a whole were dire, necessitating huge economic stimulus packages and social relief payments for persons slipping into unemployment and poverty. As providers of health-care services and social assistance, subnational governments experienced extraordinary pressures on their revenue.

In most federations, financial transfers of one kind or another are made from the federal government to states and local governments, and from states to local governments, usually through fiscal equalisation systems. In the case of national disasters, the federal government has access to contingency funds for distribution to states and local governments in distress. Subnational governments also experienced a dramatic decline in their own revenues due to the economic downturn.

Key questions include the following: Did federal aid to state and/or local governments take the form of enhanced equalisation payments, block grants, or conditional/tied grants? What mechanisms of accountability were built into pandemic expenditure? Did corruption flourish?

3.2.4 Findings and policy implications

In the light of their findings, the chapters conclude by probing the possible long-term impact the pandemic governance may have on each federal system. Although it may be too early to tell, could the way in which the pandemic was managed lead to fundamental changes in how the system may function in the future? It has been said that 'the world *before Coronavirus* and the world *after Coronavirus* cannot be the same'. Can the same be said about each federal system?

4 Conclusion

This volume seeks to understand how the Covid-19 pandemic affected federal dynamics during the first but crucial period of pandemic governance. It provides an early slice of analysis when federal systems experienced a major shock; the need for quick, concerted, and effective central action placed the principle of decentralised decision-making under severe pressure. As the Covid-19 pandemic has, contrary to early hopes and expectations, persisted in 2021 and is bound to continue in 2022, this volume might provide some useful lessons on how to correct current systemic failures. Since Covid-19 is unlikely to be the last pandemic or disaster to engulf the world on such a massive scale, this volume may too, provide useful lessons on how to combat pandemics in federal countries in the future.

Notes

1 I wish to acknowledge the research assistance of Dr Michelle Maziwisa, the SARChI Chair postdoctoral fellow at the Dullah Omar Institute of the University of the Western Cape. Dr Jean Redpath's (Dullah Omar Institute) assistance with the statistical analysis is much appreciated.
2 There are small variations between the figures drawn from international organisations (WHO, UN, World Bank) and those provided in the country chapters, due to different data sets used.

References

Hassan, T. A. et al. 2020. 'Firm-Level Exposure to Epidemic Diseases: Covid-19, SARS, and H1N1', NBER Working Paper Series No. 26971.

UN Population Dynamics. 2019. 'Total Population (Both Sexes Combined) by Region, Subregion and Country, Annually for 1950–2020 (Thousands), Estimates, 1995–2020', https://population.un.org/wpp/Download/Standard/Population/ (accessed on 8 April 2021).

WHO. 2020a. 'Covid-19 Explorer', https://covid19.who.int/explorer (accessed on 8 April 2021).

WHO. 2020b. 'Coronavirus Disease (COVID-19) Dashboard 2020', https://covid19.who.int/ (accessed on 8 April 2021).

WHO. 2020c. 'Weekly Operational Update on COVID-19, 30 October 2020', https://www.who.int/publications/m/item/weekly-operational-update—30-october-2020 (accessed on 20 November 2020).

World Bank. 2019. Data Portal 'Population Ages 65 and Above (% of total population)', https://data.worldbank.org/indicator/SP.POP.65UP.TO.ZS (accessed on 8 April 2021).

World Bank. 2020. *Global Economic Prospects*. Washington DC: International Bank for Reconstruction and Development/The World Bank.

PART I
Europe and Eurasia

1

FACING THE PANDEMIC

Italy's functional 'health federalism' and dysfunctional cooperation

Elisabeth Alber, Erika Arban, Paolo Colasante, Adriano Dirri and Francesco Palermo[1]

1.1 Introduction

Italy was severely affected by the Covid-19 pandemic, with a disproportionately high number of infections and an even higher mortality rate (due to the large number of elderly people who died). As of 31 October 2020, 709,335 people in a population of about 60 million had been infected, with 38,826 fatalities. The impact of the first wave of infection was extremely uneven across Italy's territories, with most of the cases concentrated in a handful of urbanised and industrialised regions in the north of the country. In the second wave, in autumn 2020, the prevalence of the virus was instead more evenly distributed among the territories.

When the pandemic reached the country in January 2020, Italy's hybrid territorial set-up, falling in between a fully fledged federal system and a unitary state, was undergoing reforms aimed at strengthening its regional and local system. Although reforms were put on hold as a result of the emergency, they succeeded in raising concerns and generating proposals for counter-reform, not least because the country's pandemic management laid three issues bare.

First, cooperation mechanisms across and within governmental levels are deficient and underutilised; secondly, while Italy's 20 regions have a wide range of powers, including over health matters, in many cases they lack the capacity to face a major crisis; and thirdly, issues of insufficient capacity also afflict the country's highly diverse and fragmented system of local government.

This chapter assesses the legal framework put in place at the national (state), the subnational (regional), and the municipal levels to face the Covid-19 emergency. It seeks to identify how different measures and actors in the management of the pandemic relate to each other and points out inconsistencies and synergies as well as their impact on Italy's asymmetric regionalism. The different responses

DOI: 10.4324/9781003166771-3

by the territories revealed both the potential of the country's asymmetric territorial governance and the weaknesses of its incomplete, quasi-federal system, especially as far as the unclear division of powers and inadequacy of intergovernmental relations (IGR) are concerned.

1.2 The constitutional and legal framework

1.2.1 Distribution of powers

Italy is a regional state blending together unitary and federal features, with 20 regions being the main, though not the only, players at the subnational level. Article 5 of the Constitution promotes autonomy and decentralisation, while article 114(1) provides that, in addition to the state, Italy is composed of municipalities, provinces, metropolitan cities, and regions, all of which are 'autonomous entities having their own statutes, powers and functions'.

The regional model is asymmetrical, in reflection of the numerous socioeconomic, cultural, geographical, and other cleavages that characterise the country. Of the 20 regions, five – Friuli-Venezia Giulia, Sardinia, Sicily, Trentino-Alto Adige/Südtirol, and Valle d'Aosta/Vallée d'Aoste – have special forms of autonomy in terms of their form of government, distribution of legislative and administrative powers, and financial arrangements. These features are entrenched in their statutes of autonomy, which were bilaterally negotiated with the national government and have the rank of constitutional law (unlike the case with ordinary regions). Article 116(2) of the Constitution mandates, furthermore, that Trentino-Alto Adige/Südtirol (Trentino-South Tyrol) 'is composed of the autonomous provinces of Trento and Bolzano/Bozen'. Unlike other regions, in Trentino-South Tyrol, most powers are vested with the two autonomous provinces, and not with the region (which results in two health-care systems in one region).

A constitutional reform in 2001 sought to reduce the gap between special and ordinary regions. Article 116(3) of the Constitution, introduced in 2001, allows ordinary regions to negotiate 'additional special forms and conditions of autonomy' with the national government, something which three regions – Lombardy, Veneto, and Emilia-Romagna – have been doing. This process, known as 'differentiated regionalism', entails further regionalising powers in health matters, as a result allowing, for instance, for the possibility to tailor training courses to local needs, and for the creation and management of complementary health insurance schemes (Grazzini et al. 2019).

The division of legislative powers between the national government and ordinary regions is enshrined in article 117(2) of the Constitution, which lists powers falling within the exclusive competence of the state. Article 117(3) enumerates powers shared by the state and the regions. In shared areas, legislative powers are vested in the regions, while the fundamental principles governing these powers are laid down in national legislation. Regions enjoy residual powers by virtue of article 117(4) of the Constitution. This division of legislative powers applies only to ordinary regions, since the powers of autonomous regions are spelled out in their statutes of autonomy.

In practice, regional autonomy is conditioned by the financial relations that each region or entity has with the centre. Special regions are financed differently to ordinary regions: each special region enjoys a bilaterally negotiated financial regime based on a share of state taxes referable to the territory (from 25 to 90 per cent), while ordinary regions depend largely on the centre. Such asymmetry is also reflected in how the local government level is financed: special regions in the north run local finance, whereas in Sicily and Sardinia local finance remains with the centre.

1.2.2 Distribution of powers in health matters

Article 32 of the Constitution protects the right to health, mandating that '[t]he Republic safeguards health as a fundamental right of the individual and as a collective interest ....' Law No. 833/1978 introduced universal health coverage, providing uniform and equal access to the National Healthcare Service (NHS) (Cicchetti and Gasbarrini 2016).

The NHS is organised at national, regional, and local levels and comprises an intricate web of responsibilities. Health protection is a competence shared between the state and the regions in an arrangement in which the national government 'sets the fundamental principles and goals of the health system, determines the core benefit package of health services guaranteed across the country ... and allocates national funds to the regions' (Scaccia and D'Orazio 2020: 109). Regions, in turn, 'are responsible for organising and delivering health care' (Cicchetti and Gasbarrini 2016: 1). At the local level, local health authorities deliver community health services and primary care directly, while secondary and specialist care is delivered directly or through public hospitals and accredited private providers.

This arrangement has given rise to 21 regional health-care systems, all quite different in their effectiveness in service delivery and the efficiency with which they operate. In this regard, there is high patient mobility between regions along the north-south divide; at the same time, the national government acts as a (financial) watchdog imposing corrective policies based on a set of indicators for all those regions that are not able to guarantee the core benefit package of health services. In recent times, regions in the centre-south in particular (though not exclusively) have been subject to recovery plans that include actions to address the structural determinants of costs (Toth 2014).

Since 2001, different regions have made different choices as to their governance models in health care, models that range from the heavily centralised, such as in Tuscany, to the heavily privatised, such as in Lombardy. The latter opted for a so-called choice and competition model (Nuti et al. 2016: 18–19), while Tuscany (followed by other regions such as Emilia-Romagna, Friuli-Venezia Giulia, and Veneto) adopted a model that combines hierarchy and targets, transparent public ranking, and pay for performance (ibid: 21–2). From a substantive viewpoint, it has thus been argued that in the last 10–15 years, the NHS has been strongly decentralised even though this evolution is not yet recognised formally (Neri 2019: 166).

1.2.3 Declaration of emergencies or disasters

Italy's Constitution does not include any specific emergency provision. Article 77 allows the national government to legislate, without previous delegation by Parliament, in cases of 'necessity and urgency'. In such event, it can adopt, under its own responsibility, a temporary measure (law decree), one which needs to be converted into law by the national parliament within 60 days, otherwise it loses its validity from the outset.

The declaration of a state of emergency for public-health reasons is regulated in ordinary legislation in article 24 of the Code of Civil Protection. The Code, however, does not define the powers that the national government may exercise under a state of emergency, nor does it authorise to limit fundamental freedoms. It indicates simply the type of emergency events that can activate civil protection powers at local, regional, or state level.

In the case of Covid-19, the nature of the threat required the use of national civil protection powers. The head of the Civil Protection Department (CPD) was vested with the power to issue special orders in derogation of any current provision and in compliance with the general principles of the legal system (extraordinary ordinances of necessity and urgency) (Raffiotta 2020). While administrative in nature, these acts can derogate legislative provisions: in this way, the legal machinery was equipped to intervene at any given moment.

1.3 Preparedness for a national disaster: The institutional framework

In Italy, civil protection responsibilities are not assigned to a single level of government but involve the entire territorial organisation. Although the country is frequently exposed to natural hazards, the civil protection system currently in place was established only in the early 1990s. In 1992, Law No. 225 established the civil protection system, dividing its actions into three categories (article 3): forecasting and prevention, relief and assistance, and management of state of emergency and recovery programmes.

Since its inception, the civil protection system has been an integrated one based on the principles of vertical and horizontal subsidiarity and thus entailing the involvement of all governmental levels and many actors across, within and beyond levels (with a highly mobile force of volunteers). Within the civil protection system, regions and local governments, acting in terms of national framework regulations, formulate and implement their own emergency programmes and transmit data to the CPD as the operative arm of the national government. In 2010, the Organisation for Economic Co-operation and Development

(OECD) gave this decentralised system a positive evaluation, especially in regard to monitoring risks and providing efficient first-on-site response actions in case of earthquakes. However, in terms of health-related emergencies, in the absence of any major emergency in the past five decades prior to Covid-19, Italy has not been put to the test and its authorities have neglected to update their pandemic plans.

At a national level, the CPD was consequently forced to implement the 2006 national plan against pandemics when Covid-19 entered the scene. Unlike other European Union (EU) member states, Italy's authorities failed to update their pandemic plan in 2017 when the World Health Organization (WHO) and European Centre for Disease Prevention and Control issued new guidelines. Regional health authorities were forced to apply outdated regional pandemic plans to the best of their knowledge.

Though it differed in extent from one region to another, this lack of preparedness – rather than decentralisation – compromised the effectiveness of responses to the emergency in the first half of 2020. Resources to face the pandemic were missing (for instance, personal protective equipment), as were risk-prevention protocols in care facilities and the capacity for mass testing and contact tracing. Intergovernmental data-sharing was, and remained, deficient; different territorial systems were, and remained, poorly interconnected and coordinated. All of these issues triggered off various quarrels between the north and south and eventually turned into an intense political battle, one in which the weak coalition government became entrammelled and which cast its shadow over regional politics.

1.4 Rolling out measures to contain the pandemic

1.4.1 Taking the initiative

Caught unprepared, Italy followed an incremental 'mitigation path' rather than a 'containment path' in its pandemic management. It tried to dampen the pandemic's impact on the health system and the resultant mortalities within a territorial system that, thanks to political gamesmanship, typically does not benefit much from intergovernmental institutional learning capabilities. Overall, Italy's pandemic response was impaired chiefly by three issues: first, the national government's moderate to low capacity to implement its decisions collaboratively and launch relief and recovery packages speedily; secondly, incoherent policy-making tenuously based on evidence; and thirdly, deficient IGR structures (Capano 2020: 327–30).

Although experts had been warning of the severity of the coronavirus outbreak since the beginning of the year in 2020, the national government was unable to contain the virus whilst it was still in its infancy. It was only from early March 2020 – following the recommendations of the National Health Institute (NHI) and an ad hoc expert committee formed on 5 February including the president of the NHI – that a flood of measures were adopted at the national level. The expert committee was to be supplemented several times with further experts, in addition to which its gender representation was improved (initially it was male-only). Numerous other taskforces were also established in individual ministries and at the subnational level.

From 18 March 2020, a special commissioner appointed by the national government coordinated all actions. For instance, until the end of April, the expert committee had been setting the standard for how tests were administered (for instance, only to persons with symptoms). This was considered controversial. The policy of the Veneto region at that point was to opt against such an approach in favour of mass testing and tracing (Lavezzo et al. 2020). In hindsight, Veneto is an example of how regional organisational autonomy in health care played out well in comparison to other regions such as Lombardy (even though the latter was under the same regional party-political leadership). Generally, pandemic management was, from the outset, caught up in a blame game between the national government and the opposition, one that unfolded in the context of an already volatile political situation.

Following the 2018 general elections, the anti-establishment party, the Five Star Movement (M5S), and the populist League (*Lega per Salvini Premier*, headed by Matteo Salvini), agreed on a government programme led by the independent Giuseppe Conte, who had never before held political office. After months of internal bickering, the ill-fated coalition government broke down when Salvini, in early August 2019, withdrew the League from the alliance and called for a snap election with the aim of becoming Prime Minister. The M5S, however, teamed up with the Democratic Party (PD), and in less than a month the new coalition government, again under the prime ministership of Giuseppe Conte, was sworn in.

It fell to this alliance, composed by traditionally staunch rivals, to navigate through the 2020 pandemic year, with polls showing an increase in popular support for centre-right parties. The second half of 2019 had suggested how fractious this alliance was – as part of the coalition government, former Prime Minister Matteo Renzi, elected in 2018 with the PD, left the PD in mid-September 2019 to form his own party, *Italia Viva*. Throughout autumn 2020, dissenting opinions on how to manage the pandemic and the resources connected to the EU Recovery Fund continued to weaken the coalition government, one which, in essence, managed the pandemic by decree while stressing that all measures taken were based on the recommendations of experts – a reading of the expert committee's protocols shows, however, that many of its recommendations were disregarded. At the beginning of the new year, a new crisis within the government arose, whose consequences have been the end of the second Government of Giuseppe Conte, succeeded by Mario Draghi, supported by almost all political parties in the Parliament.

Policy responses at regional level were likewise informed by volatile political dynamics. Some regions took the lead in clearly voicing their strategies to contain the pandemic and its impact; however, party allegiances alone were not an indicator or predictor of how effective (or ineffective) the strategies adopted were. Generally, many factors determine to what extent regional (and local) governing practices are dependent on and affected by the political situation at the national level. The most important are differences in fiscal capacity; differences in health-care models and the capacities of regional administration (in the case of the pandemic in 2020); and differences in personality and character of regional political leaders (all except two presidents are directly elected).

After the regional elections in 2020 (Emilia-Romagna and Calabria voted on 26 January and Aosta Valley, Veneto, Liguria, Tuscany, Marche, Campania, and Puglia on 20–21 September), the centre-left held on to five regions, while the centre-right retained 14 regions (among them the autonomous province of Trento, led by the League). Aosta Valley and the autonomous province of Bolzano/Bozen are led by autonomist political parties. In brief, the September elections saw victories for those presidents who performed well during the first wave of Covid-19 infections, such as Luca Zaia in Veneto from the League.

1.4.2 National action

On 31 January 2020, one day after the WHO declared the Covid-19 outbreak a public emergency of international concern, the Italian government declared a state of emergency. The country's first cases of infection were reported on 17 February in two small towns in Lombardy and Veneto. At that time, the national strategy was to contain the pandemic by local ordinances. Likewise, a regional ordinance introducing quarantine measures was issued on 21 February regarding the outbreak of the coronavirus in some municipalities in Lombardy.

As the coronavirus rapidly began to spread, the national government issued Law Decree No. 6 of 23 February 2020 which vested subnational authorities with the power to 'adopt all containment and management measures that are adequate and proportionate to the evolution of the epidemiological situation' (article 1(1)). Thereafter, further decrees and ordinances by the Prime Minister, CPD and Minister of Health provided detail as to who the 'competent authorities' were and what their margin of action was.

Regarding lockdowns, a series of Prime Minister's Decrees (DPCM) were issued from 23 February to 4 March 2020 with the aim of gradually tightening restrictive measures for the containment of the pandemic and providing for the isolation of the affected areas ('red zones'). These containment measures, initially limited to some municipalities, were also imposed on the residents of Lombardy and of 14 provinces in other northern regions. The nationwide lockdown was regulated by the DPCM issued on 8 and 9 March (and subsequently extended until May). It included severe travel restrictions (with exceptions for work or health-related grounds, or any exigency, always to be stated in a self-certification), a ban on outdoor gatherings, the closure of educational facilities (and transition to online learning), smart work procedures for the public and private sectors, and the suspension of all public events (including religious ceremonies).

The DPCM of 11 March 2020 tightened the lockdown measures, closing restaurants and the like (except for home deliveries) and retail commercial activities (except for essential ones such as grocery stores and pharmacies). As for local public transport, the decree left it to the presidents of regions to determine how they would maintain minimum essential services. On 20 and 22 March 2020, ordinances by the Minister of Health closed parks and public gardens as well as restricted exercise and sports activities (to be done individually and in proximity to one's home). The DPCM of 22 March 2020 suspended all non-essential industrial and commercial activities, while several DPCMs in March and April extended the duration of the lockdown measures until 17 May 2020, when a further DPCM lifted some of the restrictions and allowed for an incremental reopening of businesses and resumption of activities.

In regard to economic aid and relief, a first small package was adopted at the beginning of the pandemic. On 28 February 2020, the national government enacted a law decree supporting families and commercial activities with EUR 5.7 billion. Much more important was the second package, the Law Decree 'Cure Italy' of 16 March 2020, the purpose of which was to strengthen the health system and grant economic relief to families and commercial enterprises (especially in sectors such as tourism, logistics, and transportation). During the first hard lockdown, an additional law decree was issued on 6 April 2020 that supported businesses by providing loan guarantees, tax relief, and government assumption of non-market risks. Law Decree No. 19/2020 ('Relaunch Decree') of 19 May 2020 injected EUR 55 billion in support of health care, employment and the economy, and social policies. The last major act in support of the economy before autumn was Law Decree No. 104/2020 of 14 August 2020.

In autumn 2020, the national government found itself in political deadlock in deliberations over the national plans for recovery and resilience that Italy, like all EU members, had to submit to the European Commission by April 2021 as part of the requirements of the EU Recovery Fund. The national government continued to rule by decree, doing so in terms of calculations linked to a catalogue of 21 indicators, and imposed a phased lockdown policy on subnational entities that involved a shift from stricter to softer measures. The focus was on supporting the economy, with the regions given greater latitude in combating the pandemic.

1.4.3 Regional action

In declaring a state of emergency, the national government seized a significant extent of power from the regions or at least was formally entitled to do so. In the first half of 2020, a long list of national measures were enacted regarding the rules of the strict lockdown (from 8 March 2020) and its gradual easing (from 4 May 2020, with the lifting of the inter-regional travel ban as first measure). The roll-out of various measures at the national, regional, and local levels made it difficult to distinguish between the measures taken at different levels of government, not least because of the lack of coordination among all the various actors.

During an initial series of vague national measures and a proliferation of regional ordinances, the first half of 2020 was characterised by acrimony between the national government and the presidents of the regions. Many of the regional presidents issued regional ordinances aimed at imposing restrictive measures beyond those adopted at the national level, such as the clearly unconstitutional closure of regional borders in Campania, obligatory flu vaccinations in Lazio, and the closure of all educational institutions in Marche. Other examples of regional ordinances in the first phase include the identification and delimitation of red zones that were to be isolated from the rest of the regional territory for a limited period (e.g., in Emilia-Romagna, Lazio, and Abruzzo). A similar trend re-emerged in October 2020 during Italy's second wave of infections.

Both article 32 of Law No. 833/1978 (the one introducing the NHS) and articles 6, 11, and 25 of the Code of Civil Protection vest regional presidents with the power to issue ordinances in the field of civil protection whenever a health-related emergency occurs. The mayors have the same powers for their respective municipal territories under the law on local authorities (Legislative Decree No. 267/2000). The multiple powers assigned to the regions in the field of civil protection, especially in the event of health emergencies, and the proliferation of 'insufficiently coordinated' (Baldini 2020: 985) national and regional measures, made it very difficult to ascertain who was responsible for which measures. While some regional ordinances were suspended, others with the same content were not.

The tug of war between the national government and the regions continued, increasing in April and May 2020 with the relaxation of the lockdown. Regions governed by centre-right coalitions (thus opposing the centre-left national government in Rome) and those less affected by the pandemic were especially eager to put their own spin on the rules specifying the exact timetable for easing measures (e.g., in regard to reopening bars and restaurants, or allowing visitors to access public beaches).

Calabria serves as an example: on 29 April, its president signed a regional ordinance easing the lockdown by reopening bars, restaurants, and pizzerias with outdoor-table service. The national government challenged these measures and, on 9 May, the administrative court of Calabria found in its favour, on the ground that it is the responsibility of the central authorities to identify measures to limit the spread of Covid-19, whereas regions are entitled to intervene only within the limits outlined in these national measures.

Likewise, the autonomous province of Bolzano/Bozen (South Tyrol) is noteworthy for its individuality of style. The national government intended to be the one to ease the lockdown and to allow regions to do so from 18 May 2020, but – uniquely among the regions – South Tyrol jumped the gun by passing its own law on the resumption of activities (Law No. 4 of 8 May 2020) several days before then. In doing so, its provincial authorities clearly intended to demonstrate the political autonomy that their region enjoys. In November 2020, Aosta Valley followed suit by adopting its own regional law, which was however struck down by the Constitutional Court in February 2021, while other regions kept intervening by way of administrative measures (ordinances) rather than by passing their own laws.

Another example of dysfunctional intergovernmental cooperation is provided by the unilateral decision of a regional health authority that, in September 2020, decided to ban a professional football team of the first division from travelling to another region to play a match because a few players had tested positive for Covid-19; it thereby flouted a special protocol negotiated by the national government and the football league which regulates such cases in the interests of regular championship matches.

1.4.4 Municipal action

The evolution of the pandemic shows that regional and municipal ordinances are critical to tailoring containment measures to the needs of different territories (Boggero 2020: 362). After the state of emergency was declared, the national government set a centralist tone at the outset when its first law decree, No. 6 of 23 February 2020, essentially appropriated the power of local authorities to issue ordinances and attempted to regulate local government's scope of action in managing the pandemic (Cerchi and Deffenu 2020: 671). Thereafter, in March, the national government sought to introduce clarity to the regulatory chaos that had reigned since the pandemic began and individual local authorities had acted independently of the national government.

Law Decree No. 9 of 2 March 2020 established that municipal ordinances that stood in contrast with national measures were to be considered unlawful, while Law Decree No. 19 of 25 March 2020 stressed the relevance of measures issued at the central level. It also explicitly defined the area of competence of local and regional authorities. In the absence of any DPCM on the same matter and only in case of aggravated health conditions, the presidents of the regions and the mayors were granted the power to introduce additional and more restrictive measures. However, any action by local and regional authorities that could limit activities strategic to the national economy, such as the production of medicines or health-related equipment, along with any action that could compromise civil and social rights, or any action in health preventive measures at the international level, were unlawful and remained the sole prerogative of the state.

Within this regulatory framework, local authorities had little room for manoeuvre during the hard lockdown of March to May 2020, though it began to expand again as the lockdown was relaxed. Local authorities in Italy were thus insufficiently involved in pandemic management. Several scholars claimed that, in keeping with the law on local authorities (Legislative Decree No. 267/2000), local government should have been granted the power to issue ordinances 'as a matter of principle' during the emergency (Luciani 2020: 22). In terms of articles 50(5) and 54 of Legislative Decree No. 267/2000, in the event of local health emergencies, mayors can enact urgent and necessary ordinances. The same law also grants the mayor the power to enact ordinances acting as officer of the national government in situations when public safety and urban security are under threat (Sabbioni 2019: 304). Furthermore, article 32(3) of Law No. 833/1978 also raises the possibility for mayors to adopt urgent emergency ordinances in areas that normally fall under the jurisdiction of the Minister of Health.

Examples abound of how the tug of war between local authorities and the national government unfolded. On 23 February 2020, the municipalities of the island of Ischia restricted access to the island for specific categories of citizens. On that same day, the ordinance was nullified by the prefect (De Siano 2020: 3–4) on the ground that municipal ordinances cannot contradict national legislation: in the absence of any specific health risk, local authorities cannot limit freedom of movement.

Another example was the ordinance of the Sicilian municipality of Messina (5 April 2020), which restricted access to the city harbour that connects the island to continental Italy – a vital route. The provision required any boat to register online 48 hours before its departure and await the municipality's authorisation to enter the harbour. The national government challenged the ordinance in the administrative court, which nullified it (Pignatelli 2020a) for violating several constitutional provisions, among them the principle of equality (article 3), personal liberty (article 13), freedom of movement (article 16), and state jurisdiction over public order, security, and disease prevention (article 117(h)–(q)). The court observed that a national emergency demands unitary management of the crisis and thus regional or local measures cannot undermine the national strategy.

In general, local actions in the first half of 2020 mainly concerned the issuance of ordinances aimed at closing public areas and ensuring social distancing. Despite centralisation, the power of municipalities was not seized entirely and, indeed, proved to be an essential part of the engine of Italy's emergency legislation (Pignatelli 2020b).

In regard to social-economic action, (in)activity at the local level showcased how unprepared local authorities were but also how much potential they hold as institutions. Solidarity and socio-economic relief measures were implemented through public-private partnerships and territorial networks that mobilised informal relationships among communities, often so in cooperation with volunteers from the Red Cross and the civil protection system. Several municipalities organised volunteers to provide basic services for persons and families hard hit by the pandemic or its consequences. Italian local government demonstrated innovativeness and cost-effectiveness in drawing on active citizenship and community volunteerism in the contribution it made to the country's pandemic response.

1.4.5 Intergovernmental relations

The management of the first wave of the pandemic in early 2020 was strongly centralised, mainly due to two reasons. First, capacity was often lacking at the regional and local levels of government. Secondly, the national government was unable to make effective use of the extant but deficient IGR mechanisms. Consultation and cooperation initiatives with regional and local authorities were rare and implemented only half-heartedly, with the lack of transparency in managing the pandemic being ill-received by the authorities of subnational governments as well as by experts and the public.

More generally, dysfunctional cooperation between levels of government is the reason that many of Italy's federalising reforms since the late 1990s remain little implemented. Given that the 1948 Constitution was silent on mechanisms of collaboration between the regions and the state, it fell to the Italian Constitutional Court (ItCC) to introduce a few such mechanisms judicially, among them the principle of loyal cooperation between state and regions (Caretti and Tarli Barbieri 2012: 384). For the ItCC, loyal cooperation should apply in areas of shared powers but also, more broadly, to all institutional relations between regions and the state (Judgment No. 242/1997), the aim being to limit conflict and solve complex governance issues collaboratively both in ordinary and extraordinary times. Decisions taken by the national government that are based on a merely formal consultation with the regions are illegitimate (Judgment No. 246/2019).

The principle of loyal cooperation, eventually entrenched in article 120(2) of the Constitution in 2001 and confirmed as a core principle by the ItCC in many rulings, is embodied in a system of intergovernmental conferences. These are consultative bodies for meetings of the regional presidents, the presidents of the autonomous provinces of Trento and Bolzano, and the Prime Minister (who chairs it), or competent regional and national ministers. The conferences were introduced to compensate for the fact that the Italian Constitution does not provide for a federal second chamber: the national parliament is bicameral (Chamber of Deputies and Senate), but the Senate does not function as a typical 'federal' upper chamber, since it does not represent regions or other territorial autonomies. Over the past few decades, a number of proposals have been advanced to change the Senate into a 'regional' chamber, but to no avail.

During the first wave of the pandemic, the 'Permanent Conference for the relations among state, regions and autonomous provinces' (Permanent Conference), created in 1983 and regulated by law in 1988, met even less frequently than usual and could not serve as a viable body for negotiating policies (Cortese 2020: 5). Empirical evidence shows that in the first half of 2020 neither the state nor the regions adhered properly to the principle of loyal cooperation. They did not make the best use of the Permanent Conference to coordinate responses to the pandemic. Regulatory chaos and court litigation were the consequences. Wisely, however, the national government never appealed to article 120 of the Constitution which enables it to 'act for bodies of the regions, metropolitan cities, provinces and municipalities ... in the case of grave danger for public safety and security'.

During the second wave of the pandemic, the use of the Permanent Conference became much more frequent, even though the regions preferred to resort as far and often as they could to bilateral relationships with the national government while, for its part, the national government continued to rule by decree. Regional presidents maintained a stance in favour or against the central government mainly on the basis of their financial dependence from Rome and their leadership capacity within the region. This in part explains why even those regions governed by the same political leadership approached both IGR and regional management of the pandemic so very differently.

1.4.6 Intergovernmental fiscal relations

Although the full impact of the pandemic is yet to be reckoned, the dangerous 'scissors effect' of rising expenditure and falling revenues in subnational financing is significant. What is more, when the pandemic struck Italy, the south of the country had not yet recovered from the effects of the 2008 financial crisis: the gross domestic product (GDP) was still substantially lower than before the financial crisis, given that since 2008 the economy had entered a recession with plummeting productive capacity, employment levels, and consumer demand.

Thus, although the south experienced a less severe health emergency in early 2020 than the north, the impact of the pandemic on household incomes, factoring out government support, was larger there than in the north. In addition, unemployment in 2020 grew more in the south than in any other part, with disastrous consequences for all those unable to profit from governmental relief packages because they were engaged in the informal economy that is typical of Italy's south (Banca d'Italia 2020). When the second wave of infection hit the south, the economic impact was even more devastating than in the first wave.

The Association of Italian Municipalities developed three scenarios for the loss of revenue among municipalities, with the high-risk scenario entailing a projected drop of almost 21 per cent compared to 2019 and consequences that cause severe recovery difficulties for all economic sectors (ANCI 2020). The low-risk scenario with a drop of 9 per cent compared to 2019 was projected in case of a relatively rapid exit from the emergency starting in May 2020, while the medium-risk scenario was associated with a drop of 14 per cent. Regional governments faced significant financial difficulties too, as most of their expenditure was concentrated on health (85 per cent on average) while at the same time they lost much of their income from the regional tax on productive output (IRAP), the regional surtax on personal income tax, and the regional tax on vehicles. In health matters, concerted policy-making between central and regional governments has decreased significantly in recent years, as a result of which health systems have been under-financed compared to those in central and northern European countries (Neri 2019: 158).

The case of the health-care system in Calabria, which has been subject to a recovery plan for more than a decade, is an example of the deficiency of intergovernmental fiscal relations in health governance. The special commissioner nominated by the national government failed to implement basic aspects of the centrally directed regional Covid-19 mitigation strategy (such as collecting accurate data on hospital beds, one of 21 indicators on which the national government based its regionally differentiated lockdown policy in autumn 2020). The pandemic could not but worsen Calabria's financial dependency on the state, with the situation clearly showing how dysfunctional cooperation was between different levels of government.

Under these kinds of circumstances, most subnational governments were unable to fulfil costly responsibilities in pandemic management on their own and became more dependent on the state. The national government set up technical committees to monitor the pandemic's effects on the adequacy of revenue to cover the expenditure needs of subnational governments. These committees assisted the national government in deciding how best to provide additional funds to subnational governments – such funds had no conditions attached to them other than the requirement of extra accountability and transparency in their management.

More generally, it is important to stress that in Italian intergovernmental fiscal relations, central authorities retain considerable control over financial resources. In health matters, complex negotiations between the national government and regional authorities normally determine financial allocations to the regionalised health-care systems, with the allocations channelled through the National Health Fund (NHF) and the national government discussing its proposal in the Permanent Conference. Basically, the national government annually allocates to the regions a budget for the provision of health-care services by calculating the essential assistance levels in the budget law on the basis of a population-based formula only partially weighted by demographic factors and the health status of the population.

The total amount of resources to be allotted to the NHF is calculated initially, then split up among the regions after they have been heard. On average, the capitation rate represents 97 per cent of the total health-care resources available to regions, while the remaining 3 per cent of resources are made up by the regional systems through own-source funding, including fees paid by patients and co-payments for specialised treatments. Local health units are funded mainly through capitated budgets, albeit in the absence of clear guidelines applicable throughout the country. Funding schemes for special regions differ to a certain extent from these arrangements (Balduzzi and Paris 2018).

No systematic datasets are available yet to shed light on how effective the 2020 relief and aid packages were. Evidence based on observation and scattered (ministerial) documentation, however, suggests they were so only to a very limited extent. The main reasons for this are, first, that bureaucratic obstacles hindered speedy processing of applications and provision of aid, with these obstacles compounded by corruption scandals and the lengthy court proceedings to which they gave rise; secondly, the national government tried to navigate the crisis in a short-term, ad hoc way by adopting small relief packages rather than bigger ones that would support Italy's subnational authorities and their very different economies in a more holistic manner.

By and large, the effects of the pandemic on subnational financing and fiscal relations were shaped by five factors (OECD 2020: 16). First, the degree of decentralisation and spending responsibilities: intergovernmental fiscal relations in Italy are characterised by a centralised tax system and a significant decentralisation of spending responsibilities. This gives rise to a noteworthy vertical fiscal gap that applies to both the local and, above all, the regional level. Resources in 'health federalism' are channelled to regions through their own tax revenues, shares of national taxes and national equalisation transfers sustained by central value-added tax (VAT) revenue. Given that the regions have markedly different fiscal capacities, and that health care varies widely across the country, equalisation is crucial. Secondly, the characteristics of subnational government revenue: subnational governments in Italy rely heavily on grants and subsidies.

The remaining three factors to which the OECD points when addressing the territorial impact of the pandemic are the ability of subnational governments to absorb exceptional stress ('fiscal flexibility'); the fiscal health conditions of subnational governments; and the scope and efficiency of support policies. Empirical evidence shows that all these factors were highly compromised in Italy, a state which for the past 10 years had suffered from severe fiscal consolidation measures and in which the debt burden (reaching 134.8 per cent of GDP in 2019) has been posing serious constraints on government public spending and on the implementation of expansionary fiscal reforms.

1.5 Findings and policy implications

When the Covid-19 pandemic hit Italy, the country was about to celebrate the 50th anniversary of the establishment of ordinary regions – special ones having been in place since 1948. With the powers of the regions having been enhanced by reforms over the course of more than seven decades, the time was ripe for reconsidering Italy's territorial structure. In this regard, three sizeable and politically and economically strong regions in the north – Lombardy, Veneto, and Emilia-Romagna – were about to conclude agreements with the national government on the transfer of additional legislative powers (and related funds) in a long and significant list of areas, one ranging from environmental protection to education, from airports to labour security and protection, and from foreign trade to disaster management, among other things. The process was stalled by the pandemic – but, ironically, these regions were the worst affected by it, which raised the question of whether greater regional autonomy is indeed desirable or not (Malo 2020).

Finally, in September 2020 a national referendum endorsed a constitutional reform that reduces the size of both chambers of the national parliament by one-third, thereby further limiting the already feeble link between the Senate and the regions and making it politically more difficult to table a reform that transforms the Senate into a chamber of regional representation – a proposal that, as noted above, has been on the agenda unsuccessfully for decades.

The pandemic is likely to impact strongly on these ongoing reform processes. It is too soon to tell what its institutional consequences will be, particularly given that at the time of this writing Italy was still in the midst of an unfolding health and economic emergency. Nor is it possible to say whether a more centralised or more decentralised structure of the country would have led overall to better or worse management of the pandemic, since performance varied markedly among the regions. It is certainly the case, however, that the emergency revealed the main weaknesses of the Italian regional system: the unclear division of powers between the centre and the regions; weak intergovernmental relations; and the high degree of asymmetry in powers, administrative capacity, and political strength among the regions (Clementi 2020).

As regards the division of powers, the constitutional reform adopted in 2001 increased the role of the regions but also created a number of overlaps and potential conflicts; above all, it by no means enhanced the 'federal spirit' (Burgess 2012). Rather, in the political and academic debates, sentiments against regional autonomy are generally on the rise. As happened after the global financial crisis of 2009/10, the pandemic confirmed that the division of powers in Italy is not sound enough to resist a moment of crisis – indeed, Covid-19 has amplified the debate between those advocating greater centralisation and those supporting greater regional autonomy.

With regard to IGR, the absence of a territorial chamber and the structural weakness of the existing bodies for intergovernmental cooperation, notably the Permanent Conference, reduced regional involvement to a mere formality, with the state having appropriated all powers at the height of the emergency. At times like these when strong coordination is needed, the role of mechanisms that are effective in representing the voice of subnational entities becomes crucial. If the mechanisms are ineffective, as in the case of Italy, joint decisions simply become top-down impositions and the involvement of regions, a sham. The inefficiency of multilateral IGR mechanisms encourages the more powerful regions to engage in bilateral negotiations, thus accentuating the asymmetry inherent in the design of the territorial set-up and arousing jealousy among the regions.

Strong pre-existing de jure and de facto asymmetries among the Italian regions became ever more acute during the pandemic. Regional performance in tackling the emergency, especially in the area of health care, was mixed. Some regions fared extraordinarily well despite severe cuts over the past decade due to the debt-cutting policies, while others made serious mistakes, such as placing Covid-19 patients in elderly homes. Differences in performance were reflected in the political sphere, with some regional presidents increasing their popular support and others losing it in elections held in September 2020.

In sum, Covid-19 has placed the tensions between calls for further decentralisation and for re-centralisation under the spotlight. At the same time, ongoing reform processes stand to be significantly impacted, and their trajectory will not be the same as it would have been without the pandemic. The main pressure is no doubt for public health care to undergo a certain degree of re-centralisation. Even though most regions reacted well, the dominant discourse focuses on their large differences in terms of services, resources, and performance, and it is not unlikely that the opportunity will be seized to introduce stronger national control (Ciardo 2020). For some reason, the predominant sentiment in both politics and academia is the fear that regional differentiation might impair the equal protection of social rights.

Some reforms in the Italian regional system are indeed necessary, and the pandemic has made this all the more evident. As to the content of the reforms, however, opinions that were all but unanimous before the pandemic became ever more divided during it. These divisions of opinion will probably slow down, rather than speed up the necessary reforms and intensify, rather than subdue, conflicts between the centre and the territories.

Note

1 Sections 1.2.1, 1.2.2, 1.4.3, and 1.4.5 were written by Elisabeth Alber and Erika Arban; Section 1.2.3 by Paolo Colasante; Section 1.4.2 by Paolo Colasante and Adriano Dirri; Section 1.4.4 by Adriano Dirri; and Sections 1.3, 1.4.1, and 1.4.6 by Elisabeth Alber. The Introduction and section 1.5 were written by Francesco Palermo.

References

ANCI. 2020. *Audizione informale presso le Commissioni Bilancio riunite*, 28 maggio 2020.

Baldini, V. 2020. 'Riflessioni sparse sul caso (o sul caos) normativo al tempo dell'emergenza costituzionale', *Dirittifondamentali.it*, 2(1): 979–85.

Balduzzi, R. and D. Paris. 2018. 'La specialità che c'è, ma non si vede: la sanità nelle Regioni a statuto speciale', in F. Palermo and S. Parolari (eds), *Le variabili della specialità: evidenze e riscontri tra soluzioni istituzionali e politiche settoriali*, pp. 453–85, Napoli: Edizioni Scientifiche Italiane.

Banca d'Italia. 2020. *Economie regionali*, numero 22 – novembre 2020.

Boggero, G. 2020. 'Le "more" dell'adozione dei DPCM sono "ghiotte" per le Regioni: prime osservazioni sull'intreccio di poteri normativi tra Stato e Regioni in tema di Covid-19', *Diritti Regionali*, 21 March, 1: 362–7.

Burgess, Michael. 2012. *In Search of the Federal Spirit*. Oxford: Oxford University Press.

Capano, G. 2020. 'Policy design and state capacity in the COVID-19 emergency in Italy: if you are not prepared for the (un)expected, you can be only what you already are', *Policy and Society*, 39(3): 326–44.

Caretti, P. and G. Tarli Barbieri. 2012. *Diritto Regionale*, 3rd ed. Torino: Giappichelli.

Cerchi, R. and A. Deffenu. 2020. 'Fonti e provvedimenti dell'emergenza sanitaria Covid-19: prime riflessioni', *Diritti Regionali*, 23 April, 1: 648–78.

Clementi, F. 2020. 'Il lascito della gestione normativa dell'emergenza: tre riforme ormai ineludibili', *Osservatorio Costituzionale* 3: 33–47.

Ciardo, C. 2020. 'Il servizio sanitario nazionale alla prova dell'emergenza Covid-19: il rischio di una sanità diseguale', *BioLaw Journal* 2(Special Issue): 227–38.

Cicchetti, A. and A. Gasbarrini. 2016. 'The healthcare service in Italy: regional variability', *European Review for Medical and Pharmacological Sciences*, 20(1 Suppl.): 1–3.

Cortese, F. 2020. 'Stato e Regioni alla prova del coronavirus', *Le Regioni* XLVIII(1): 3–10.

De Siano, A. 2020. 'Ordinanze sindacali e annullamento prefettizio ai tempi del Covid-19', *Federalismi.it* (Osservatorio emergenza Covid-19, no. 1), 15 April, https://www.federalismi.it/nv14/articolo-documento.cfm?Artid=41992.

Grazzini, L. et al. 2019. 'Asymmetric decentralization: some insights for the Italian case', *Osservatorio Regionale sul Federalismo*, Istituto Regionale Programmazione Economica Toscana, March, Nota 4.

Lavezzo, E. et al. 2020. 'Suppression of a SARS-CoV-2 outbreak in the Italian municipality of Vo', *Nature*, 584: 425–9.

Luciani, M. 2020. 'Il sistema delle fonti del diritto alla prova dell'emergenza', *Rivista AIC*, 2: 109–41.

Malo, M. 2020. 'Le Regioni e la pandemia: variazioni sul tema', *Le Regioni* XLVIII(1): 231–4.

Neri, S. 2019. 'The Italian National Health Service after the Economic Crisis: From Decentralization to Differentiated Federalism', *E-Cadernos CES Online*, 31/2019.

Nuti, S. et al. 2016. 'Making governance work in the health care sector: evidence from a "natural experiment" in Italy', *Health Economics, Policy and Law*, 11(1): 17–38.

OECD. 2010. *Reviews of Risk Management Policies: Italy – Review of the Italian National Civil Protection System*. Paris: OECD.

OECD. 2020. 'The Territorial Impact of COVID-19: Managing the Crisis across Levels of Government', 10 November.

Pignatelli N. 2020a. 'Il potere di annullamento straordinario *ex* art. 138 TUEL di un'ordinanza comunale: il Covid-19 non 'chiude' lo stretto di Messina', *Diritti Regionali, September 1*, 5: 68–82.

Pignatelli, N. 2020b. 'La specialità delle ordinanze dei sindaci nell'emergenza sanitaria nazionale: un potere 'inesauribile', *Diritti Regionali*, 2/2020 (Special Issue): 69–85.

Raffiotta, E.C. 2020. *Norme d'ordinanza: contributo a una teoria delle ordinanze emergenziali come fonti normative*. Bologna: Bononia University Press.

Sabbioni, P. 2019. 'Art. 50 e 54 TUEL', in C. Napoli and N. Pignatelli (eds), *Codice degli enti locali*. Roma: Feltrinelli, 304 ff.

Scaccia, G. and C. D'Orazio. 2020. 'La concorrenza fra Stato e autonomie territoriali nella gestione della crisi sanitaria fra unitarietà e differenziazione', *Forum di Quaderni Costituzionali*, 3: 108–20.

Toth, F. 2014. 'How health care regionalisation in Italy is widening the North-South gap', *Health Economics, Policy and Law*, 9(3): 231–49.

2

DECENTRALISATION AND COVID-19

Stress-testing the Spanish territorial system

Mikel Erkoreka, Mireia Grau Creus and Mario Kölling

2.1 Introduction

In mid-March 2020, the Spanish government triggered the constitutional mechanisms that were necessary for it to declare a state of alarm and embark on drastic measures to combat the spread of Covid-19, measures that involved curtailing fundamental rights. This was the first time the country had faced a deadly nationwide pandemic. It took the institutional and political system by surprise, deprived as it was of any experience of reacting to crises of this kind as a decentralised entity; moreover, Spain was far from placid when the virus struck, finding itself amidst turbulence blowing in from different social and political fronts.

This chapter sets out to examine how the country's governance system and territorial model responded to the stress test forced on it by the Covid-19 pandemic. The analysis covers the period from March to October 2020, which allows us to consider how institutional responses and intergovernmental relations (IGR) evolved between the domestic outbreak of the coronavirus and the start of a second declared state of alarm.

To set the scene, Spain has an area of 506,000 km^2 and a population of 46.3 million, making it the second-largest country by size in the European Union (EU) and the fifth largest by population. A high proportion of the population lives in urban areas, and the country has a number of sizeable cities – the two largest are Madrid and Barcelona, which have populations of 6.2 million and 5.2 million, respectively. Spain's population density is lower than that of most other Western European countries.

The 1978 Constitution introduced a form of political organisation that saw the country shift from a highly centralised system to, according to some, a quasi-federal arrangement. At present, Spain is divided into 17 autonomous communities

DOI: 10.4324/9781003166771-4

(ACs) and the autonomous cities of Ceuta and Melilla. Decentralisation has been moderately successful, although for years experts have been calling for the Constitution to be revised in order to reflect the current reality of the territorial model and establish a federal framework ensuring an equilibrium between unity and diversity, shared rule and self-rule.

Spain is credited with one of the best-performing health systems in the world, having been ranked 15th in the Global Health Security Index in 2019 (Johns Hopkins Bloomberg School of Public Health 2019). Life expectancy in Spain is the highest in the EU, and social inequalities in health are less pronounced than in many other countries. However, an ageing population and the associated increase in chronic diseases pose some risks to the system's sustainability.

After the global financial crisis of 2008 and the prolonged recession that ensued, public spending on health decreased for several years before beginning to increase again recently. Since 2014 the trend has been towards an increase in expenditure per capita in all ACs. However, the differences between the ACs are important. There is in 2019, on the one hand, a group of ACs with expenditure of about EUR 1,200 per inhabitant (Andalusia, Madrid, Catalonia, and Murcia) and, on the other, a group where it is about EUR 1,700 (Basque Country, Navarre, and Asturias). In general terms, in 2019 health spending per capita in Spain was more than 15 per cent lower than the EU average (OECD and European Observatory on Health Systems and Policies 2019).

As regards the political landscape, Spain has been in crisis mode for a decade. The economic and financial crisis has led to the so-called crisis of representative institutions in which there has been a huge loss of popular confidence in aspects of the democratic system. At the same time, the secessionist conflict in Catalonia intensified in 2012, culminating in 2017 in a unilateral declaration of independence. This was followed by the application of article 155 of the Constitution, which empowered the central government to remove the Catalan government, impose direct rule, dissolve the parliament, and call for snap elections that took place on 21 December 2017.[1] In parallel, the leaders of the independence movement were prosecuted and jailed.

The conflict in Catalonia has hindered reforms of the territorial model, for example, of the Senate or the territorial funding system. More widely, reform initiatives in general have not been successful, due to, among other things, party politics. From the mid-1980s to the mid-2010s, Spain's party system was dominated by a straightforward competition between the social-democratic Spanish Socialist Workers Party (PSOE) and the conservative People's Party (PP). Since 2014, however, the leftist *Podemos* party and the centre-right liberal *Ciudadanos* have entered the national arena, the moderate nationalist Catalan forces have collapsed, and a radical-right populist party, *Vox*, has emerged with strength. Due to the fragmentation and polarisation of the party system, since 2015 no party has been able to form a stable governmental majority after elections.

The fragmentation of the party system intensified after the 2019 general elections, when 22 parties obtained representatives in the Congress of Deputies, the lower house of the Spanish parliament. In January 2020, a minority left-wing coalition government consisting of the PSOE and *Unidas Podemos* ('United We Can') came to power. This first Spanish-wide coalition government since the Second Republic (1931–1939) had a long to-do list. After years of austerity policies, the new government wanted to increase public spending; it was also ready to start a dialogue with political parties in Catalonia on how to resolve the crisis in the region.

In contrast to the turbulent political panorama, economic growth remained solid before the outbreak of the 2020 pandemic. Nevertheless, in November 2019, the European Commission decreased its gross domestic product (GDP) growth forecast for Spain from 2.6 per cent to 1.9 per cent. Growth rates were expected to slow down even further in 2020 to 1.5 per cent, which was already worrisome given the size of the country's public debt burden.

The coronavirus's entry into Spain was confirmed on 31 January 2020, when a German tourist on the Canary Islands became the country's first case of Covid-19. Community transmission had begun by mid-February; at the beginning of March, Spain recorded its first Covid-19 fatality, and by 13 March, cases had been confirmed in all the ACs, with the death toll rocketing. At the start of June, there were no reported fatalities, but afterwards the number of cases again increased. In September, health authorities were detecting greater numbers of new infections than they had witnessed in April and May.

Nevertheless, July had marked a turning point. The situation in that month was very different than in the months before it. During the first wave of infections – only serious cases were recorded; from July onwards, many of those who tested positive had but minor symptoms or were asymptomatic, a shift that pointed to the onset of a second, and more expansive wave of the pandemic. As at the end of October, health authorities had detected more than 1.2 million cases, and there were more than 36,500 confirmed deaths (Centro de Coordinación de Alertas y Emergencias Sanitarias 2020). These statistics placed Spain among the worst-affected countries in the world.

2.2 The federal constitutional and legislative framework

Since the 1980s, Spain developed from a unitary state with a long-standing centralist tradition into a highly decentralised state. However, the Constitution does not clearly establish a decentralised system; instead, it contains rules and procedures to be followed in order to achieve self-government. Some competences are expressly attributed to the central state (Constitution, article 149), whereas all matters not allocated to it may be assumed by the AC (Tudela and Kölling 2020).

In 2020, the ACs had assumed most of the competences available to them, such as health, disaster management, education, and regional economic development. Nevertheless, the central state continued to maintain, as it does generally, the responsibility of coordinating state-wide policy-making.

In regard to the health-care system, it is based on the principles of universality, free access, and equity. Coverage is funded mainly by taxes, and care is provided predominantly within the public sector (Bernal-Delgado, et al. 2018).

Responses to the Covid-19 crisis were based largely on the constitutional provisions regulating one of the three types of states of exceptionality: that of the state of alarm. Of the three exceptional regimes provided for in article 116 of the Constitution and in Organic Law 4/1981 – the states of alarm, emergency,[2] and siege[3] – only the state of alarm expressly provides that it may be declared in the event of health crises such as epidemics and situations of serious pollution (Organic Law 4/1981, article 4(b)). However, the Constitution establishes several limits (article 116(2)): measures taken under a state of alarm must be temporary, confined to a specific area, and restricted to what is necessary to contain the emergency.

Furthermore, if the emergency is limited to a specific AC, the latter can request that the central government declare a state of alarm in its territory. The central government or the government of the affected ACs may serve, in case of a state of alarm, as the competent authority. Accordingly, the authorities have a wide margin of discretion to determine measures under a state of alarm – for example, the first state of alarm was decreed in 2010 solely to maintain control of Spanish airports following a strike by air-traffic controllers.

The Organic Law 3/86 on Special Measures in Matters of Public Health lists the conditions under which the central or AC health authorities may, within their jurisdictions, adopt public health measures in times of emergencies. According to article 3, health authorities may, in addition to general preventative actions, take appropriate measures for the control of persons who are or have been in contact with infected persons or their immediate environment, as well as take measures necessary to prevent the risk of transmission.

2.3 Preparedness for a national disaster: The institutional framework

As mentioned, Spain had no experience of dealing with a disaster like Covid-19. For instance, unlike the rest of Europe, it had not been affected by either SARS (Severe Acute Respiratory Syndrome) or MERS (Middle East Respiratory Syndrome). The country has, however, been embroiled in a long-term conflict with the terrorist organisation ETA (Basque Homeland and Liberty) and, since the early 2000s, with international jihadism. The Madrid terrorist bombings of 11 March 2004 led (temporarily) to improved coordination among the National Intelligence Agency, the armed forces, and the police and security forces of the ACs.

In 2013, the National Early Warning and Rapid Response System, or *Sistema Nacional de Alerta Precoz y Respuesta Rápida* (SIAPR), was created. Within this system, the Coordination Centre for Health Alerts and Emergencies – a Spanish health ministry department – assumes the functions of coordination, notification, and evaluation of epidemiological or pandemic crisis. SIARP was favourably evaluated in the Global Health Security Index 2019, although it was ranked low for its ability to prevent and react to pandemic challenges – in particular, because the only intergovernmental relations for which it provides involve meetings at the lower administrative level rather than engagement between the central government and ACs (Arteaga 2020). As it proved, the Coordination Centre for Health Alerts and Emergencies was quickly overwhelmed by the Covid-19 crisis at its outset in March 2020 and unable to collect data in a timely, orderly way.

2.4 Rolling out measures to contain the pandemic

In analysing the evolution of the framework of action at federal and state level, it is necessary to differentiate between four consecutive stages of pandemic response, as shown in Figure 2.1:

1. the period of the appearance and spread of the virus prior to the declaration of the first nationwide state of alarm (late January–13 March);
2. the period in which the first state of alarm was in force and was then de-escalated (14 March–21 June);
3. the period of the 'new normality' (22 June–24 October); and
4. the period of the second nationwide state of alarm (25 October–9 May 2021).

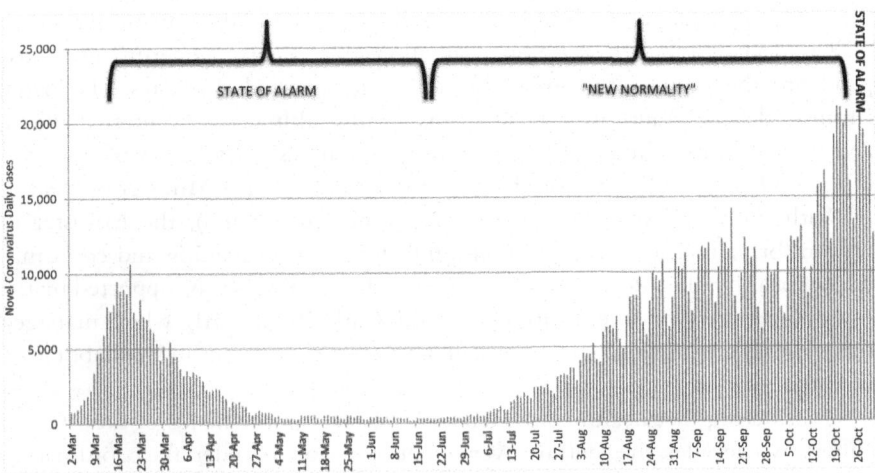

FIGURE 2.1   New Covid-19 cases in Spain per week, March–October 2020

Source: Spanish Ministry of Health (2020).

2.4.1 Taking the initiative

The virus began to spread erratically and unevenly across Spain and its ACs at the end of January 2020. In this first stage, the ACs played a leading role in taking measures to contain it, albeit in an uncoordinated, under-planned fashion, with each AC applying measures of its own depending on the prevalence of the virus in its territory. The measures failed to curb the increase and spread of cases in the country as a whole.

On 9 March, by which point there were already more than 1,500 confirmed cases, the central government issued initial warnings and countrywide recommendations; on 13 March, when the figure had exceeded 7,500, Prime Minister Sánchez (in office since June 2018) announced a nationwide state of alarm. In a comparative perspective, Spain was a notable laggard in raising the level of response, given that other countries had done so when they reached 1,000 confirmed cases (Timoner 2020).

2.4.2 Federal action

Spain's state of alarm was declared under Royal Decree 463/2020, which came into force on 14 March 2020 and conferred full responsibility on the national government to manage and implement measures for addressing the Covid-19 crisis. Such measures included placing the country under a lockdown compelling people to stay at home, as well as ensuring the supply of goods and services needed for health, food, and power. On 29 March, under *Real Decreto-ley* 10/2020, all non-essential workers were ordered to remain at home for 14 days. In addition, the central government adopted legislative measures addressing health matters and the economy at large, with the focus on small and medium-sized enterprises, the self-employed, persons affected by the lockdown, and the tourism industry.

The declaration of the state of alarm allowed the central government to suspend, and then assume, the powers of the ACs for a period of 15 days. The Prime Minister delegated authority to the ministers of health, defence, internal affairs, and transport, mobility, and urban affairs in their respective areas of responsibility, with any residual responsibility being assumed by the Minister of Health.

With the creation of the *mando único* (single command), the Minister of Health formally assumed the responsibility for decision-making and coordination of health policy decisions in the 17 ACs. The ministry was supported by the research organisation, the Institute of Health Carlos III (ISCIII), which managed the country's epidemiological surveillance in coordination and collaboration with the ACs.

Considering that health competences have been in the hands of the ACs for almost two decades, the central government's position to undertake coordination was weak. During the first weeks, the Ministry of Health could not obtain and provide operational data, let alone coordinate joint actions with the ACs in, for example, the procurement of protective clothing and masks (Kölling 2020).

The economic and social costs of the lockdown were very high. To address this situation, the central government approved the mobilisation of nearly EUR 200 billion, an amount to account for about 20 per cent of the Spanish GDP (see section 2.4.6 for a fuller discussion). The pandemic also caused serious interference with the Congress of Deputies, as the latter's parliamentary activity was reduced to a minimum – basically, to voting several times to extend the state of alarm. This reinforced the traditionally weak position of the Spanish parliament vis-à-vis the executive, all the more so given that the proclamation of the state of alarm further strengthened the executive. Nevertheless, the Congress retained important leverage by virtue of its role in approving the state of alarm and its extensions (Kölling 2020).

At the request of the government, the Congress authorised six extensions of the state of alarm, which ended on 21 June 2020 (see Table 2.1). The first extension, from 25 March to 11 April, was passed with the support of 269 of the 350 members of the Congress; only the members of *Vox* abstained. However, in subsequent votes the level of criticism increased, with the PP, which abstained in the votes for the third and fourth extensions, voting against the fifth and sixth extensions. In addition, the pro-Catalan independence parties, the left-wing *Esquerra Republicana de Catalunya* (ERC) and conservative *Junts per Catalunya* (JxC), voted against the fourth extension after unsuccessfully trying to get the central government to agree to convene a 'negotiation table' with the Catalan government in exchange for a vote for another extension.

The increasing polarisation in Parliament was also reflected in major demonstrations against the Spanish government in April and May 2020. These were organised mainly by *Vox* and partly by the PP; however, neither party was able to benefit significantly from the crisis.

On 28 April 2020, the Spanish government presented a four-phase 'Plan for the transition to a new normality'. The first phase – entailing reopening small shops and allowing café terraces to operate at 50 per cent capacity and places of worship, at one-third – came into force in some provinces on 4 May. The restrictions were thus gradually lifted by 21 June. Although the ACs did not participate in the declaration of the state of alarm, the plan to move from the state of alarm

TABLE 2.1 Spain: Congressional voting on extensions of the state of alarm

Extensions and dates	Votes in favour	Votes against	Abstentions
1. 25/03/2020	321	0	28
2. 09/04/2020	270	54	25
3. 22/04/2020	269	60	16
4. 06/05/2020	178	75	97
5. 20/05/2020	177	162	11
6. 03/06/2020	177	155	18

Source: Congress of Deputies (2020).

to the 'new normality' in late June was developed in close collaboration between the central government and the governments of the ACs (Marcos 2020a).

In May, the central government announced new legal mechanisms that would facilitate the implementation of measures in 'co-governance' with the ACs without having to impose another state of alarm, albeit that at the time of this writing in October, the government had not submitted any legislative proposals to Parliament. During the 'new normality', it thus decided to coordinate decisions with ACs and clarify the ways in which they could adopt the state of alarm in their territories. For example, after an emergency meeting with health officials from the ACs, the government on 17 August announced new social-distancing measures across Spain, but it was in the hands of the ACs to implement them. Similarly, until mid-September, central government efforts were directed largely towards engaging with ACs to coordinate minimum standards for reopening schools.

However, some of the measures by the autonomous and local administrations were annulled in the courts, especially those restricting fundamental rights (mobility and social gatherings, for example), as it was ruled that they could be valid only in a constitutionally provided state of alarm. From August to October 2020, the number of new infections increased sharply, marking the second wave of the pandemic, and during this period, the government reached agreement with most of the ACs on thresholds for local lockdowns. The Community of Madrid, one of the ACs with the highest rates of infection early in the second wave, imposed local lockdowns in terms of these criteria, but the Madrid High Court ruled that the central government could not limit fundamental rights without resorting to a state of alarm. As a consequence, the central government imposed a selective state of alarm of 15 days in parts of the AC Madrid – this was a 'surgical' intervention that restricted entry and exit only in the concerned municipalities.

By mid-October, the second-wave pattern of spiked rates of infection had spread throughout the country. Faced with this situation, 11 ACs – including Catalonia and the Basque Country – asked that the central government declare a new general state of alarm to avert the need for court approval of their measures and thereby improve their speed of response and ability to take further action, such as imposing nightlife curfews and additional mobility restrictions.

On 25 October 2020, the central government declared a second nationwide state of alarm in Spain, doing so with the approval of the Congress (194 votes in favour, 53 against, and 99 abstentions), and, controversially, ordering it until 9 May 2021. The measures attendant on the declaration were set out in Royal Decree 926/2020 of the same date and included perimetral lockdowns, restrictions on social and religious gatherings, and a mandatory nationwide curfew between 23:00 and 6:00. In contrast to the first state of alarm in March, the second was implemented in a decentralised manner and managed primarily by AC governments. Measures taken under it were less severe than those under the first, as no lockdown was involved.

2.4.3 *State action*

Before the declaration of the state of alarm, the ACs played a leading role in adopting preventative measures. In the most affected ACs, measures were decreed that closed educational centres (for example in Madrid and the Basque Country), placed restrictions on social gatherings, and introduced the first perimetral lockdowns (in La Rioja and Catalonia). On 13 March 2020, merely a few hours before the declaration of the state of alarm, the Basque government decreed a state of health emergency that enabled it to take drastic measures at the subnational level. The least affected ACs, by contrast, delayed taking measures to contain the pandemic and, when they did, imposed relatively lax restrictions.

The situation changed dramatically when the first state of alarm came into effect on 14 March. Finding themselves under the sole command of the central government, the autonomous administrations lost their decision-making capacity albeit that they remained responsible for the management of centrally issued instructions. In other words, this intervention in self-government did not bring the activities of autonomous administrations to a halt at either the parliamentary or executive level but instead placed them at the service of the central government.

Working as they did within the limits established by the central government, the autonomous governments still had a certain margin of discretion in planning and implementing their public policies. This led to, among other things, competition between ACs in acquiring medical resources on the international market, an uneven ratio of detection tests per inhabitant and territory, heterogeneity in the statistical data provided by ACs, differences among the ACs in models of cooperation between the public and private health-care sector, and obstacles to transferring patients and resources between ACs.

In addition to the improvement of the health indicators, the transition plan to the 'new normality' referred above was driven largely by pressure from the AC governments in the face of wishes by Congress to extend the state of alarm. The plan, agreed with the ACs, involved a gradual de-escalation in four phases. The transition from one phase to the next was decided by the central government on the basis of public health indicators such as an AC's number of cases and the capacity of its health-care system. In this fashion, restrictions were lifted phase by phase, territory by territory.

Having met the requirements, Galicia was, on 15 June 2020, the first AC to obtain central government authorisation to move to the 'new normality'. On 19 June, the Basque Country and Cantabria also made this transition, and free movement between these neighbouring ACs was re-established. On 21 June, after 98 days, the state of alarm ended throughout the country. In the new normality, free movement between ACs was restored.

During the transition to the new normality, the ACs gradually recovered the competences and functions that had been centralised under the single command of the central government, giving way to a scenario of co-governance of the pandemic between the central government institutions and the ACs. After the end of the state of alarm, the AC executives exercised their powers in managing their health-care systems, in organising Covid-19 tracking mechanisms, in developing and implementing containment measures, and in applying policies on social protection and economic reactivation. For example, ACs could decide on the use of masks, restrictions on gatherings, and certain social distancing requirements. They also developed their individual procedures for managing the start of the academic year and, in cases, imposed restrictions on mobility or selective confinements. Although there were differences among them, especially with respect to efficiency and periods of implementation, the ACs all applied similar measures and restrictions.

The second countrywide state of alarm, decreed at the end of October 2020, provided the ACs with the legal instruments to enforce more severe measures in fighting the pandemic. Furthermore, the ACs preserved the power to approve and implement measures at the regional level within the general framework set by the state of alarm. After the declaration of the second state of alarm, the ACs introduced new restrictions on mobility – including perimetral lockdowns – and social life, for example by limiting social gatherings to six people or closing bars and restaurants.

2.4.4 Local government action

Local governments in general kept a low political profile. The pandemic did not significantly alter the framework of either their functional or administrative competences, and as a result, they continued to take responsibility for providing basic everyday services and goods.

Given that local governments do not have relevant competences in health matters, their role in containing the pandemic focused on implementing and enforcing restrictive and preventative measures – notably, municipal police forces were central in this undertaking – and in regulating economic activity within the scope of their competences, for example in matters related to the customer capacity and opening hours of bars and restaurants.

Similarly, depending on the needs and characteristics of each municipality, local governments adopted and funded social measures to help especially vulnerable groups and facilitate social cohesion, for instance through assistance in paying for housing or support to poor families. They also promoted plans and policies to aid economic recovery at the local level, for example through local tax incentives and reductions or by subsidising bonds to stimulate local commerce. Finally, it is worth noting the work of local governments in supporting cultural activity and cultural agents, a sector that was severely affected by the lockdown restrictions.

Local governments, mainly from the de-escalation onwards, had to adapt to the decisions of the respective AC executives. Nonetheless, with the exception of some isolated episodes, relations between local and autonomous administrations were generally collaborative. During the pandemic in 2020, no additional or extraordinary mechanisms of horizontal municipal cooperation were developed that exceeded the autonomous sphere; one way or another, organised local government did not play any significant role in this regard.

2.4.5 Intergovernmental relations

In the absence of any constitutional provision of shared rule involving the ACs, Spanish intergovernmental relations (IGR) were developed at the initiative of the central government authorities. IGR was envisaged initially in terms of inter-administrative interaction (and was contained in legislation on administrative cooperation) and it developed a strong administrative profile and functioning. Actually, most of the intergovernmental political interaction took place within parliamentary and intraparty arenas. In 2004, the central government established an intergovernmental forum of premiers, the Premiers' Conference (*Conferencia de Presidentes*), in order to promote an IGR institution that potentially could absorb some of the intergovernmental interaction usually debated in other arenas.

Spain's IGR system has at least six characteristics: hierarchical structure and functioning; a strong bilateral approach (central government and each individual AC); a lack of horizontal interaction; a deeply sectoral approach; a focus on administrative implementation; and large diversity (Arbós et al. 2009; Pérez-Medina 2020). Over the past decades, two mechanisms have fostered IGR: intergovernmental sectoral and multilateral forums, which are meant to bring the central government and AC ministries together to discuss and agree on policy issues, and the compacts (*convenios*), that is, administrative mechanisms for financing the implementation of central government policies in the ACs.

Intergovernmental sectoral forums accord central government authorities a commanding role (for instance, they set the agenda and call meetings) and, in some cases of fundamental importance, such as the forum on financing ACs, a casting vote that overrules the others. As for *convenios*, they are always welcome in that they provide ACs with external financing, but they reveal the influence of central government spending-power in policy areas that do not usually receive media attention. These features explain, at least in part, the very limited impact that Spain's IGR system has made in building solid political and institutional trust. Shared rule has never developed in its strict sense of involving subnational governments within nationwide decision-making processes.

In a decentralised country like Spain, where implementation powers in health matters fall exclusively under the ACs, it was clearly impossible to manage the Covid-19 crisis without intergovernmental cooperation (León 2020). However, as Capano (2020) said in remarks on Italy's management of the pandemic, 'If you are not prepared for the (un)expected, you can be only what you already are'. This meant that the first response was a hierarchical one that centralised all powers in a single decision-making unit by declaring the state of alarm. The ACs were left on the sidelines because, leaving political considerations aside, there are no legal or institutional provisions for them to play any role at all.

The IGR system came into play right after the declaration of the state of alarm and the publication in the Official Gazette of all measures that were adopted, when the Prime Minister called for a meeting with the AC premiers. As said, meetings of the Prime Minister and AC premiers were institutionalised in 2004, but prior to Covid-19, only six of these had been held, with the meetings rarely attended by all of the AC leaders – facts which reflect the weakness of Spain's federal culture and the problems of trust that have beset IGR for many years.

In a videoconference on 15 March 2020, two days after the declaration of alarm, the Prime Minister informed the AC premiers (17 out of 17 ACs) of the measures and asked them to commit to 'unity of action' and loyalty. An institutional manifesto confirming their commitment was released after the meeting, a benchmark in the history of this high-profile IGR mechanism. All the premiers signed it except the Catalan leader, who voiced his disagreement with the unitary command structure and what he regarded as an encroachment on subnational powers (Marcos 2020b). Although the premier of the Basque Country signed the manifesto, he too expressed strong opposition to what he saw as Spain's hierarchical and centralised approach to the crisis, declaring that 'cooperation and collaboration do not mean [acceptance of or entitlement to] imposition' (Vega and Segura 2020).

As the extensions of the state of alarm were approved one after another by the Congress, the perception that the central government's idea of cooperation was entirely top-down in orientation started to spread, in the process sparking criticism by other premiers. Given that these criticisms arose across the political spectrum and that the central government – a minority coalition – was in need of support in parliament on issues other than Covid-19, the federal-level approach to cooperation was reappraised, with the central government opening the door to some degree of participation by ACs in decision-making on the pandemic.

The wording used to describe this new approach was itself a novelty in the Spanish context. In view of the hierarchical connotations that the phrase 'intergovernmental cooperation' had acquired over the decades, the new word – 'co-governance' – was chosen to stress the sense of an equalising or levelling of the status of the participants. In early May, the Spanish Ministry of Health issued a ministerial order (Order SND/387/2020 of 3 May 2020) aimed at regulating the role of the ACs in decision-making on the de-escalation phase. Although for some it was far too much, and for others far too little, the point is that it was acknowledged that the lack of institutional instruments for enabling the ACs to participate in state-wide decision-making processes was a problem linked to an unfit decentralised setting and not just to an 'incomplete' institutional setting, as it used to be defined.

In any case, and in spite of all the ups and downs, during the 98 days of the state of alarm, the Prime Minister and AC premiers' meetings stood out as the main forum for coordination, consultation, and reaching agreement on managing the pandemic. Virtually inoperative until the onset of Covid-19, this forum met on 16 occasions (15 of them online) while the state of alarm was in effect. In addition, the Inter-Territorial Council for the Health System had a prominent role. Throughout the state of alarm, it met online twice a week to exchange information and reach agreement on, for example, common standards for tests for Covid-19, closing bars, restricting smoking in public spaces, and measures in residences for the elderly.

Other lower-profile intergovernmental mechanisms also saw a revival – more than a hundred sectoral meetings were held between March and September 2020, whereas in the whole of 2019 there had been less than 50 (Marcos 2020a). Nevertheless, due to their entrenched sectoral perspectives and traditionally compartmentalised vision of public administration, these mechanisms did not contribute to providing the breadth of perspective the pandemic response required.

As regards the views of the actors on the functioning of the IGR mechanisms, most of the AC premiers stressed the usefulness of the Premiers' Conference despite its purely informative nature and their passive, subordinate role in pandemic management. The regularity of the meetings and the need for a problem-solving approach probably had its benefits, one of which seems to have been to re-humanise political adversaries after years of polarisation. In a television interview with the premier of Castilla La Mancha, a PSOE leader, the presenter asked him to rate the behaviour of the Catalan premier at these meetings on a scale of 'bad, very bad, worse', a question intended to elicit the antagonism the PSOE customarily has towards leaders of the Catalan government. To the surprise of the TV presenter (and no doubt the audience), he replied that the atmosphere of the meetings was actually always constructive and that many of the Catalan premier's proposals were sensible (Costas 2020).

Even allowing that this is a single anecdote without empirical data to support it, what should not be underestimated, in a context as polarised as Spain's, is the potential importance of high-profile IGR mechanisms as a means to pave the road towards de-polarisation by bringing tough adversarial politics into a space of fair play. In this regard, relationships between ACs traditionally have been poor; however, during the pandemic no additional or extraordinary instruments of horizontal cooperation among them were established. Horizontal cooperation was limited mainly to bilateral agreements between neighbouring ACs.

2.4.6 Intergovernmental fiscal relations

The system of financing the ACs in Spain has an asymmetrical character and is regulated under two differentiated regimes: the so-called common regime and the foral regime. The common regime is applied uniformly to all the ACs on the Spanish peninsula,[4] except for the Basque Autonomous Community and Navarre, which are ruled under the foral regime. Based on their historical and political circumstances, the Basque Country and Navarre preserve a singular and privative foral system of financing and self-government, which provides them with broad fiscal and financial power in contrast with the common regimen ACs. Questions related to the system of financing the ACs occupy a large part of the debates on the territorial organisation of power in Spain. With regard to social security, its economic management falls under the exclusive powers of the central government, which finances the pension system and unemployment benefits, among other things.

Following the declaration of a state of alarm, the central government played a prominent role in initiating measures on social protection, economic recovery, and employment. The range of measures was extensive and includes instituting the mechanism, Temporary Employment Regulation Dossiers (*Expedientes de Regulación Temporal de Empleo*); the creation of a minimum living wage (safety-net income of between EUR 462 and 1,015 for the neediest of families); the mobilisation of more than EUR 150 billion in public guarantees to ensure the liquidity and solvency of the business sector; and various plans for reactivating consumption (De la Fuente 2021; KPMG 2020).

Pending the arrival of European funds and fiscal reforms that might be implemented in the 2021 budgets, these measures were funded mainly through the deficit and public debt. The Spanish central bank, *Banco de España*, predicted that the deficit would be above 10 per cent of GDP and that public debt would rise by more than 20 points to greater than 115 per cent of GDP in 2020 (Banco de España 2020). The ACs and local governments also formed their own plans of action to confront the health crisis, strengthen the health and social protection systems, and apply measures to support the revival of economic activity and consumption. The tax authorities of the Basque Country and Navarre, like those of the central government, also used fiscal policy to introduce flexibility into tax obligations and establish fiscal incentives to boost economic recovery.

The budgetary policies of the public administrations were conditioned by the Budgetary Stability Law, which was passed in 2012 in the context of the European rescue in Spain and sets strict targets for deficit, public debt, and expenditure. The deficit targets set for 2020 were 1.8 per cent for the public administration as a whole (0.5 per cent, the central administration; 0.2 per cent, the ACs; 0 per cent, local governments; and 1.1 per cent, social security). However, in March 2020 the EU activated the 'general escape clause', which allows member states facing severe economic shock not to meet the deficit and debt objectives required by the Stability and Growth Pact.[5]

Due to the ACs' limited financial autonomy, the central government had to provide financial assistance to them through advances on accounts, down payments from the liquidated 2018 fiscal year, and other extraordinary funds and resources. These transfers made it possible to reduce the margin of deviation in the deficit and debt targets of the ACs of the common regime. In summer, the Basque Country and Navarre, whose regime of financing is independent of the pattern of flows described above and is ruled by the principle of unilateral risk, bilaterally negotiated the adjustment of their deficit (which increased to 2.6 per cent) and debt targets for 2020 with the central government. Later, at the end of September 2020, the government suspended the application of the tax rules in 2020 and 2021 for all public administrations (La Moncloa 2020a). This decision authorised public administrations to relax their budgetary policies, allowing them to increase public spending. However, the central government urged the common regime ACs to limit their deficit in 2021 to 2.2 per cent; of this, the centre would assume 1.1 per cent through an extraordinary transfer of funds.

Aside from the regular system of financing, the central government approved a non-repayable fund of EUR 16 billion so that ACs could confront the impact of the pandemic (Ministry of Finance 2020). The Covid-19 Fund, made up of four sections of unconditional transfers, created tensions among the governments of ACs due to the criteria for revenue-sharing established by the central government. The distribution to ACs of the first and third sections (EUR 9 billion in total) was based on health variables. The second section, of EUR 2 billion and associated with education, was shared out according to the youth population ratios of each AC. The fourth section of the fund, to which EUR 5 billion was assigned and which excludes the Basque Country and Navarre, was aimed at compensating for the drop in tax revenues.

With the precedent of the Covid-19 Fund on the table, the sharing of EU recovery funds led to a new debate among ACs and the central government about determining the distribution criteria. Spain was to receive close to EUR 140 billion from the EUR 750 billion Next Generation EU recovery plan. On 7 October 2020, the central government presented the Recovery, Transformation and Resilience of [the] Spanish Economy Plan to guide the deployment of EUR 72 billion from EU recovery funds between 2021 and 2023 (La Moncloa 2020b). The plan is structured around four priority areas: the ecological transition, digital transformation, gender equality, and social and territorial cohesion. It does not, however, determine the territorial distribution of funds.

2.5 Findings and policy implications

The Covid-19 pandemic was an unprecedented challenge and severely tested both the Spanish territorial model and the national health system. The delayed reaction by the central and AC governments, poor coordination among governments, and the variance in measures and test frequency may help to explain the strong impact Covid-19 had on the country. However, many other endogenous and exogenous factors were crucial in their effect on crisis management, among them a tendency towards physical proximity and greetings, or the urban environment – Spain has one of the largest urban population concentrations in West Europe.

In such a context, the Spanish government opted for an initial response based on a centralised control, one that rapidly unveiled the institutional weaknesses of the IGR system. The political and institutional management of the first wave of infections alerted the central authorities to the logistical as well as legitimacy problems of exercising sole, unitary command; as a result, there was a switch-over to integrating the ACs in decision-making processes. Thus, managing the crisis brought into relief the tension between, on the one hand, the constitutionally determined framework legislation of the central government and, on the other, the reality of a country consisting of heterogeneous regional health systems. Due to a combination of party politics, territorial cleavages and long-standing institutional deficits, such as poor coordination among governments and an unclear division of competences, decisions were taken very late and slowly. However, the crisis may have been a turning point in regard to these deficits in Spain's territorial model.

In relation to funding the pandemic, as happened in earlier crises, exposed the cracks in the system for financing the ACs of the common regime and underscored their dependence on central government transfers when there is a budgetary emergency. In analogous terms, the principles of fiscal co-responsibility and unilateral risk continued to guide the framework of bilateral fiscal and financial relations between the foral ACs and the central government, once again revealing the deep differences that exist in the asymmetrical Spanish funding model.

In debates about Spain's management of the pandemic, there were calls for reform of the national health system and the strengthening of the Ministry of Health. According to these demands, the Ministry should improve its constitutionally determined coordination function and ensure national standards in health-care delivery. However, this debate should also be seen in the context of balancing institutional trust and the demand for institutionalised co-governance between the ACs and the central government, and the demand of preserving the self-government margin of the ACs, as well as the future role of the EU in crisis management. A future European Health Union may improve preparedness and resilience for cross-border health threats, but it would also affect the territorial distribution of responsibilities at the national level.

As a general conclusion, the Covid-19 crisis has made evident the structural deficits in the institutional design framing decentralisation in Spain and has changed the central government's perception on IGR. For long, the system had been analysed in terms of its assumed progressive adaptation towards federalism, as if institutions could evolve on their own. The Covid-19 crisis, by unveiling the weakness of shared rule, has brought about the questioning of traditional IGR approaches. The promotion of shared rule, at least in health matters, seems to be the most relevant institutional output. Time will tell whether this new institutional output would generate new policy dynamics and would expand to other policy areas and institutions or would stay encapsulated within the management of the pandemics.

Notes

1 Article 155 allows the central government to take measures in exceptional cases to restore constitutional order or prevent major harm to Spain's interests. In 2017 the Senate granted the government these powers to enable it to impose direct rule on Catalonia. The interpretation and application of article 155 have been widely debated.

2 A state of emergency may be declared by the government when 'the free exercise of the citizens' rights and freedoms, the normal operation of the democratic institutions, that of the public services that are essential to the community, or any other aspect of law and order, are so seriously altered that the use of ordinary authorities is insufficient to establish it and maintain it' (Organic Law 4/1981, article 13).

3 A state of siege may be declared by the Government 'when an uprising or act of force occurs against the sovereignty or independence of Spain, its territorial integrity or the constitutional system that cannot be solved by other means' (Organic Law 4/1981, article 32).

4 The Canary Islands and the two North African enclaves of Ceuta and Melilla have a special tax regime.

5 In this volume, see Chapter 6 on the European Union.

References

Arbós, X. *et al.* 2009. *Las Relaciones Intergubernamentales en el Estado Autonómico. La Posición de los Actores*. Barcelona: Institut d'Estudis Autonòmics.

Arteaga, F. 2020. '*La Gestión de Pandemias Como el COVID-19 en España: ¿Enfoque de Salud o de Seguridad?*', *RIE*, 2020–42.

Banco de España. 2020. 'Macroeconomic Projections Report', https://www.bde.es/bde/en/secciones/prensa/notas/Briefing_notes/ (accessed on 19 October 2020).

Bernal-Delgado, E. (et al.). 2018. 'Spain Health System Review', *Health Systems in Transition Profile*, 20(2): 1–179.

Capano, G. 2020. 'Policy Design and State Capacity in the COVID-19 Emergency in Italy: If You Are Not Prepared for the (Un)Expected, You Can Be Only What You Already Are', *Policy and Society*, 39(3): 326–44.

Centro de Coordinación de Alertas y Emergencias Sanitarias. 2020. '*Enfermedad por el Coronavirus (COVID-19)*', https://www.mscbs.gob.es/en/profesionales/saludPublica/ccayes/alertasActual/nCov-China/documentos/Actualizacion_177_COVID-19.pdf (accessed on 19 October 2020).

Congress of Deputies, Spain. 2020. 'Congressional Voting on Extensions of the State of Alarm', www.congreso.es (accessed on 12 March 2021).

Costas, N. 2020. '*Zasca de García Page a Cristina Pardo tras incitarle a cargar contra Quim Torra de forma sibilina*', *El Confidencial*, 23 March.

De la Fuente, Angel. 2021. 'The Economic Consequences of Covid in Spain and How to Deal with Them', *Applied Economic Analysis*, 29(85): 90–104.

Johns Hopkins Bloomberg School of Public Health. 2019. *Global Health Security Index: Building Collective Action and Accountability*. Washington DC: Nuclear Threat Initiative.

Kölling, M. 2020. 'Federalism and the COVID-19 Crisis: A Perspective from Spain', *Forum of Federations Working Paper*.

KPMG. 2020. 'Spain: Tax Developments in Response to Covid-19', https://home.kpmg/xx/en/home/insights/2020/04/spain-tax-developments-in-response-to-covid-19.html (accessed on 19 October 2020).

La Moncloa. 2020a. '*El Gobierno suspende la aplicación de las reglas fiscales en 2020 y 2021*', 30 September, https://www.lamoncloa.gob.es/serviciosdeprensa/notasprensa/hacienda/Paginas/2020/300920-reglas_fiscales.aspx (accessed on 19 October 2020).

La Moncloa. 2020b. 'Pedro Sánchez Presents Recovery Plan to Guide Implementation of 72 Billion Euros from European Funds to 2023', 7 October, https://www.lamoncloa.gob.es/lang/en/presidente/news/Paginas/2020/20201007recovery-plan.aspx (accessed on 19 October 2020).

León, S. 2020. '*De Gestión Centralizada a Gestión Autonómica de la Pandemia: Desafíos y Oportunidades*', EsadeEcPol Insight #14.

Marcos, J. 2020a. '*Todos los Presidentes Autonómicos Cierran Filas con el Gobierno Pese a las Críticas de Torra*', El País, 15 March.

Marcos, J. 2020b. 'La Crisis del Coronavirus Reactiva los Engranajes del Estado Autonómico', El País, 2 August.

Ministry of Finance. 2020. '*Fondo COVID*', https://www.hacienda.gob.es/en-GB/CDI/Paginas/SistemasFinanciacionDeuda/InformacionCCAAs/Fondo_COVID.aspx (accessed on 8 November 2020).

OECD and European Observatory on Health Systems and Policies. 2019. *Spain: Country Health Profile 2019, State of Health in the EU*. Paris: OECD Publishing.

Pérez-Medina, J. M. 2020. 'Dinámica de las Conferencias Sectoriales. Entre la Intergubernamentalidad y la Cooperación Administrativa', *Revista d'Estudis Autònòmics i Federal – Journal of Self-Government*, 31: 17–64.

Spanish Ministry of Health. 2020. 'Covid-19', https://cnecovid.isciii.es/covid19/#ccaa (accessed on 8 November 2020).

Timoner, A. 2020. 'Policy Responsiveness to Coronavirus: An Autopsy', *Agenda Pública – El País*, 8 June.

Tudela, J. and Kölling, M. 2020. 'The Kingdom of Spain', in A. Griffiths, R. Chattopadhyay, J. Light and C. Stieren (eds.), *Handbook of Federal Countries*. London: Palgrave – Forum of Federations.

Vega, N. and Segura, F. 2020. '*El Lehendakari critica que el Estado asuma el mando, pero acatará el Decreto*', El Diario Vasco, 15 March.

3

GERMANY'S FIGHT AGAINST COVID-19

The tension between central regulation and decentralised management

Gisela Färber

3.1 Introduction

As happened throughout the world, Germany's society and economy suffered as a result of restrictions that were imposed to combat the Covid-19 pandemic. Although infection and fatality rates in Germany in 2020 were relatively low in international comparison and its economic crisis less grievous than in other countries, the burdens of the pandemic weighed heavily on those who fell ill or lost income and livelihoods due to lockdown measures. The question at issue in this chapter, then, is whether Germany's federal multilevel system of government was a help or hindrance in managing the pandemic. In particular, it examines the country's efforts not only to cure the ill, prevent infections, and control the spread of the virus but also to provide compensation for economic damages and avoid a deeper depression.

To begin with, Germany is a federal country with a population that stood at 83.2 million at the end of 2019: 18.3 per cent of people were younger than 20 years, 53.3 per cent were between 20 and 60 years, and 28.4 per cent were older than 60. The fastest-growing age group – which increased by 33 per cent in the last decade – were people of age 80 years and older. Seventy-seven per cent of Germany's inhabitants live in areas of high-to-medium population density; overall, the country has 107 free cities, 1,951 cities, and 8,056 villages, all of which are located within 294 counties.

In the German federal system, local governments are the lowest level of governance and lie within 16 states (*Länder*), of which three are city states. In terms of the Basic Law, the federation (*Bund*) and the *Länder* have full constitutional powers and their own institutions; accordingly, local governments have the right of self-administration in all local matters. The federal government in office during the pandemic was a 'grand coalition' led by Chancellor Angela Merkel and

DOI: 10.4324/9781003166771-5

bringing together the Christian Democratic and Social Democratic parties. At the state level, the governments were likewise coalitions made up of the country's various parties with the exception of the right-wing group, Alternative for Germany.

As regards health care, medical services are split between, on the one hand, private-sector medical practices and hospitals – either commercial or owned by non-profit organisations – and pharmacies, and, on the other, local-government-owned hospitals and state-owned university hospitals. Patients may choose where they receive medical treatment. The majority of the population has health cover through either the country's Social Health Insurance or private insurance.

The first case of Covid-19 in Germany was recorded on 27 January 2020. At this early stage, given that there were so few patients and that they and the people they had been in contact with were soon isolated, the public was not overly worried; but at the beginning of March, the rate of infection grew as infected persons took part in mass events and there were increasing numbers of people returning from skiing trips to Ischgl in Austria (see Chapter 4, in this volume). On 25 March, the federal parliament declared an 'epidemic situation of national importance' and, two days later, specified the Law for Protection against Infection by passing the Law to Protect the Population during an Epidemic Situation of National Importance, thereby imposing a nationwide lockdown.

By the end of May, infection rates had declined and Germany began to relax its restrictions incrementally, with inner-European frontiers being reopened to spare the domestic tourism sector and revive trade and industry. However, in late summer, when more and more people returned from holidaying abroad in countries with significant levels of infection, the number of new infections again increased – indeed, at the beginning of October, the number exploded within only a few days to more than 19,000 a day and the seven-day incidence to 130 per 100,000 inhabitants. Berlin, Bremen, and several cities and counties surpassed the critical number of 50 cases per 100,000 inhabitants; many cities and counties even experienced a seven-day incidence of more than 200 new infections per 100,000 inhabitants.

As at 1 November 2020, Germany's total number of infections had reached 532,930 (or 649 per 100,000 inhabitants), with 356,410 recoveries in that figure and 10,481 deaths (or 13 per 100,000 inhabitants). Infection rates varied substantially among the states, although, in general, during the first wave of infection they were higher in Western Germany than in East Germany, whereas in the second wave that emerged in October they were at their highest in some East German counties.

Although the Covid-19 pandemic caused the sharpest recession in the history of the Federal Republic of Germany, the economy recovered quite well until the beginning of October. This stabilisation was in good part the result of the numerous support programmes rolled out at all levels of government, as well as the use of a Keynesian-style fiscal policy accepting of the fact of a decline in tax revenue and willing to fund additional expenditure by means of public debt.

3.2 The federal constitutional and legislative framework

Multilevel governance in Germany takes the form of an executive federal system in which the federal level is generally responsible for legislation (both exclusive and concurrent) and the state and local levels are responsible for administration and the execution of laws (Huegelin and Fenna 2015; Färber 2015). That is to say, the *Länder* regulate only some policy fields as their own competence – these mainly involve the police, some aspects of environmental law, and education in schools and universities; however, the *Länder* decide on the way in which to execute federal law and on the institutions through which this is accomplished.

Government actions against infectious diseases are among the concurrent competences set out in the Basic Law (article 74(19)); in terms of these provisions, the federation can pass legal regulations if and insofar as they are necessary either for the unity of the law or economy or for the provision of equivalence of living conditions in Germany. The *Länder* convert federal law into regulations for implementation and then often transfer the associated administrative responsibilities to their local governments. If federal law does not furnish details about its administration, the *Länder* are free to determine this within their broad scope of action. Cities and counties are usually responsible for civil protection and emergency management. Municipalities have to follow the regulations laid down in federal and *Land* laws and decrees; conversely, they can act freely only if what they want to do is not (yet) regulated.

In the event of pandemics, a high degree of centralisation obtains, given that they invariably impact on economic development and that the *Bund* has the competences relevant in taking ameliorative measures, including competences in taxation and expenditure management, the regulation of social insurance (in regard to pensions, health and long-term care, and unemployment), and in covering state- and local-level deficits if necessary. In all cases in which the details of administration are regulated or the states are obliged to pay for measures, the approval of the *Bundesrat* – the federal second chamber representing state governments – is compulsory.

Not least because of the strong position of the *Länder* governments in *the Bundesrat*, a coordinated decision-making process among the federal chancellor and all 16 minister-presidents is a common occurrence in many areas. These parties decide on political measures that would apply more or less uniformly across Germany. Particularly in cases where the issues are thorny – such as imposing lockdowns on citizens and enterprises – this coordinated process is advantageous in building consensus and facilitating unified communication about the measures decided upon; the disadvantage is that this tends to leave the federal and state parliaments, in particular its non-governing parties, partly excluded from decision-making.

Finally, as all measures are part of administrative law, they fall under the jurisdiction of the administrative courts. Given that pandemic restrictions very often conflict with basic rights, the courts have to decide whether the actions are proportionate to the goal of protecting the population and whether the constraints on basic rights are necessary for achieving this goal. In practice, the courts often check whether the explanatory statements provided in regulatory documents warrant limitations on the individual's rights to freedom of action.

3.3 Preparedness for a national disaster: The institutional framework

In Germany, institutions that manage natural disasters are separated from those dealing with epidemics or pandemics, albeit that disasters often include medical problems and vice versa. The relevant regulations and institutions can nevertheless be orchestrated in cooperation with each other and across all levels of government if necessary. Since 2001, the Law to Protect against Infections – a merger of several pre-existing laws – has regulated measures to prevent and curb infectious diseases. To achieve these goals, it empowers the responsible ministries and agencies to pass decrees to restrict basic rights such as freedom of assembly, freedom of movement, and the inviolability of the home.

The central actor at the federal level – besides the Ministry of Health – is the Robert Koch Institute (RKI), which is one of three administrative successors of the former Federal Health Agency. The RKI cooperates with the other responsible federal and *Land* agencies and scientific institutions, as well as with foreign institutions, particularly so the World Health Organisation. It produces Germany's official epidemiological statistics, publishes them, and advises political institutions. It undertakes its own research and provides technical assistance to *Land* health agencies.

The 2001 Law to Protect against Infections also regulates compensation where people are forced into quarantine due to contact with an infected person or to entry from a country with high epidemic risks. Such persons receive the same financial compensation as they would have if they were ill, namely six weeks of full payment, followed by 90 per cent of net income; however, their employers are refunded by the responsible *Land* administration. The same compensation is paid if schools and kindergartens are closed in terms of pandemic regulations and parents have to stay home from work to take care of their children.

Land governments usually include ministries (often those for social affairs) which are – among other fields of action – responsible for health matters. They coordinate their policies, if necessary, in a Conference of Ministers of Health. As the *Länder* have to transfer federal regulation into *Land* law that often affects several *Land* ministries, the state chancelleries have a central role not only in regulation but in their 'public relations' function of declaring and explaining the special *Land* regulations.

The local level is the most important in administering a pandemic; some local governments may be even more deeply involved than others because they own a local hospital. In the implementation and administration of pandemic measures, local health agencies and local regulatory offices are the decisive actors. The former collect data and produce local disease statistics, trace the contacts of infected persons, place them under quarantine, and determine whether they stay at home; they also receive information about travellers from countries with high infection rates and control their observance of quarantine measures. In turn, the local regulatory offices monitor compliance with pandemic regulations.

All the necessary functions and responsibilities existed prior to the Covid-19 pandemic. However, whereas all levels of governments routinely undertake exercises to stay prepared for natural disasters, the health authorities did not undertake comparable exercises for the eventuality of an infectious disease like Covid-19.

This pandemic, in particular the lockdown that was imposed to curb it, not only affected public health but also impacted, severely, on the economy. In this regard, the key institutional actors were the Federal Ministry of Finance and Federal Ministry of Economic Affairs, both of which drew on their experience of managing the global financial crisis of 2008.

3.4 Rolling out measures to contain the pandemic

3.4.1 Taking the initiative

Local governments, particularly the affected counties, were the first to react when the virus began to spread in February following an increase in infections due to large public events such as carnivals and beer festivals. The *Länder* governments requested quarantines in the municipalities concerned. Although the head of the county authority was responsible, the regional boards of the *Land* administration were involved in all measures at the local level to combat epidemics.

When infections escalated in late February both in number and rate, it was time for the *Bund* to take action. On 27 February 2020, a crisis management group, including medical experts and the RKI, was established by the Federal Ministry of Health and Federal Ministry of the Interior. All of the country's governments nevertheless attempted for a long time to convince the public that infections in Germany could remain purely localised incidents, but this strategy failed when holidaymakers returned ill from skiing in Ischgl in Austria and the rate and spread of infections escalated again.

Given that the measures contemplated in the Law to Protect the Population during an Epidemic Situation of National Importance need the approval of the *Bundesrat*, the *Länder* were directly involved in the decision-making process. Being part of the 'grand coalition' government, the heads of the governing factions of the *Bundestag* and the heads of the Social Democratic Party participated in developing the measures. The final decision to impose a nationwide lockdown under common rules was taken in a meeting between Chancellor Merkel and the minister-presidents of the *Länder*. Public life was severely restricted: all shops not necessary for essential supplies had to close, as did schools, universities, restaurants, theatres, opera houses, and the like. Face masks were made compulsory in all places where people were in close proximity to each other, as was social distancing of least 1.5 m; and people were allowed to work from home if their employers agreed to it.

The debate in the *Bundestag* took place under extreme time pressure. At that point, only the right-wing party Alternative for Germany was critical of the lockdown regulations. By law, the Ministry of Health was authorised to regulate by decree, inter alia, the requirements for entry to the country; rules for public transport; data gathering for the identification and early registration of infected persons; measures in special institutions, such as long-term nursing homes; the provision of medicines; and health care for outpatients. The Ministry's powers were limited until 31 March 2021 but could be extended for another year.

3.4.2 Federal action

The actions of the *Bund* had two main goals: combating Covid-19 infections and stabilising the economy. In regard to the first, the Federal Ministry of Health (*Bundesgesundheitsministerium* 2020) not only passed the necessary decrees for the lockdown but also arranged additional medical equipment for all hospitals, long-term nursing homes, and medical practices. In March 2020, Germany ran out of masks and protective clothing because the federal government had not built up reserves of the necessary equipment in case of a pandemic. Consequently, the Ministry bought 1.7 billion FFP2, KN95, and FFP3 masks, along with about 4.2 billion simpler medical masks.

The Ministry also coordinated a nationwide database on intensive-care beds with ventilators and offered subsidies for hospitals that converted normal hospital beds into ones for intensive care. By July 2020, 32,400 beds had been registered, with the Federation paying for 39,700 more (RBB Online 2020). The RKI took 'normal' measures of health protection and regularly reported to the public. The head of the RKI and its experts advised federal and state governments to prepare for the near future and consider the necessary measures to take. In addition, the Ministry organised digital information systems – by the end of October, its Covid-19 cell phone app had been downloaded by 40 million people.

As people hesitated to consult their medical doctors and dentists due to fear of infection, medical service providers suffered economic losses; as a result, by the end of April 2020, a programme of financial support was set up for all decentralised medical services; it included compensation to all hospitals for empty beds (Covid-19-*Krankenhausentlastungsgesetz*).

Germany introduced border controls from 16 March 2020 with several, though not all, of its neighbouring countries (e.g. not for the Netherlands); this regulation was based on the new Covid-19 Law. People who wanted to enter from high-risk countries had to stay in quarantine for 14 days. Where borders were closed, foreign commuters living across the border were de facto excluded from their workplaces unless they arranged accommodation in Germany. Couples and family members were separated from each other. Long-distance truck drivers who transported food to Germany, for example from southern Europe, had to stay in their vehicles to avoid quarantine. From early February, passengers returning by plane from high-risk regions had to provide their travel and Covid-19-related health information that was sent to their local health administration in control of quarantine.

The *Bundestag* also changed its own rules of procedure to enable it to continue operations. The quorum was lowered to one-quarter and virtual participation in committee meetings was allowed, with written votes cast during session weeks. This exemption was terminated on 30 September 2020, but then later renewed until the end of 2020 (*Deutscher Bundestag* 2020).

Because lockdown measures and later restrictions impacted on economic activity not only in Germany but in other countries from which German enterprises import materials for their production processes and to which they export their products, the economy experienced its deepest decline since the Second World War. Three federal ministries – finance, economic affairs, and labour and social affairs – took steps to help prevent businesses from going bankrupt and those who could not work, from sinking into poverty (*Bundesfinanzministerium* 2020a), among them the following:

- The regulations for prolonged short-term allowances were reactivated. The number of registered recipients boomed by 624,977 between March and June 2020 but declined afterwards. Despite the *Bund's* efforts, Germany's unemployed increased from 2.335 million in March to 2.955 million in August 2020 but has since then started to decline slightly.
- The self-employed were offered increased access to basic security benefits for jobseekers.
- People in under- or unemployment were protected from losing their accommodation if they could not afford to pay their rent for the three most burdened months (March to May).
- Small enterprises and the self-employed received subsidies to keep them financially liquid. The duty to declare insolvency was suspended until December 2020.
- Severely affected large enterprises, including Lufthansa and TUI, a leading tourism company, received substantial financial subsidies in the form of credits and/or government shareholding. The *Bund* had permission from the EU for an exemption from the latter's ban on public financial aid to such enterprises.
- A special programme to the value of EUR 1 billion was established for economically damaged cultural enterprises; the programme included subsidies for investments in providing for hygiene measures at events.

In addition, the federal government initiated an economic stabilisation programme to the cost in 2020 of EUR 103 billion. The programme focused on four areas:

- Families received an additional children allowance and a tax reduction for single parents. There was wage continuation for parents with ill children or nursing family members. The turnover tax declined from 19 per cent/7 per cent to 16 per cent/5 per cent for the second half of 2020.
- Various forms of tax relief sought to lower the tax burden and improve liquidity. Small and medium-sized enterprises (SMEs) received a bonus of EUR 2,000 if they maintained the same number of vocational training places. Subsidies of another EUR 150 million were allocated to accelerate digitalisation. A special credit programme was introduced to support non-profit organisations suffering from the Covid-19 restrictions.
- Local governments that cover a share of the accommodation costs of the basic security benefit allowances were supported by a higher federal transfer. Together the *Bund* and *Länder* provided EUR 12 billion to compensate for losses of local business tax. Additional transfers sought to mitigate the pandemic's impact on local public transport enterprises, local sport organisations, and local investments in climate protection.
- 'Investment expenditures for a better future' covered a bonus for electric cars and electric loading infrastructure, subsidies for the modernisation of automobile industries, and the purchase of low-emission vehicles. German Railway received additional government investment of EUR 6 billion. A further billion euros were spent on investments in climate change, research in general, and medical research related to Covid-19.

A special factor in federal crisis policies was that Germany presided over the EU Council of Member States in the second half of 2020. The federal government was therefore deeply involved in developing and negotiating the EUR 750 billion EU programme. For many German politicians, the fact that the EU intended for the first time to take on own debt – which is forbidden in the Treaty – is not only a political problem but a legal question. It can be expected that the German Federal Constitutional Court will again be involved in the 'interpretation' of the content of the European competences.

3.4.3 State action

As the *Länder* have competences in many fields that deal with the fight against Covid-19, particularly in the implementation of federal regulations, they had an important influence on the management of the pandemic. During the first lockdown in April and May 2020, they all applied the same restrictions, but by mid-April divergent ideas were already appearing in regard to the speed and details of reopening economic activity and social life.

When, in May, the number of infections had declined, the political initiative shifted to the *Länder*. The minister-presidents, fearing that local enterprises – particularly shuttered retail outlets, hairdressing salons, hotels, and restaurants – would not survive a longer lockdown, began to develop hygiene regulations for these enterprises. The first divergences in regulation thus appeared in an effort to safeguard regional economic sectors.

For instance, when retail outlets reopened, North Rhine-Westphalia allowed furniture stores and kitchen studios to do so too because many of their man-ufacturing suppliers operate in this state. *Länder* with a high share of tourism – such as Bavaria, Mecklenburg-Pomerania, and Schleswig-Holstein – tried to reopen hotels and restaurants as quickly as they could under strict hygiene reg-ulations. Similarly, Mecklenburg-Pomerania initially restricted hotels to longer stays in order to prevent crowds of weekend guests from entering the state. Later the states held cultural and sports events for in-person spectators – all under hygiene and social-distancing regulations that varied from state to state. Angela Merkel expressed disapproval of such risky events but was unable to coordinate the divergent state policies.

Finally, when infection rates increased again in certain regions from the end of August 2020, the minister-presidents of those states where the incidence had been below average refused to implement decisions taken in the meetings of the federal chancellor and the minister-presidents: they argued that divergent rates of infections called for differences in policy. For example, Saxony-Anhalt tried to march to the beat of its own drum and, among other things, refused to fine people for not wearing masks. Indeed, in all matters of state competence, the state governments passed regulations that differed from each other's to one extent or another, whether it be in the opening of schools and universities, guidelines for hotels and restaurants, the number of people and households allowed to meet, the size of social, cultural and sports events, and more.

The reasons for the divergence stem from several factors: differences among states in infection rates; the economic composition of a state and how the pandemic response affected its chief industries; and the federal and state elections in 2021 that were to take place in Baden-Württemberg, Rhineland-Palatinate, Thuringia, Saxony-Anhalt, Berlin, and Mecklenburg-Pomerania.

The most conspicuous public conflict was that between the minister-presidents of Bavaria and North Rhine-Westphalia, Markus Söder and Armin Laschet. Both states were among the first to witness Covid-19 infections, with Bavaria having, until October 2020, the highest number of confirmed cases (874 per 100,000 inhabitants vs. 807 in North Rhine-Westphalia) as well as the highest death rate (22 per 100,000 inhabitants vs. 12 in North Rhine-Westphalia). Söder argued for a stricter regulation, Laschet, for a liberal policy. As the two were in consideration to be the chancellor candidates of the Christian parties [Christian Social Union (CSU) in Bavaria and Christian Democratic Union (CDU) in all other states] in the federal elections in September 2021, they represented two policy styles in open competition with each other.

Generally, the divergences were minor, did little to compromise the equivalence of living conditions in Germany, and reflected the usual kinds of intergovernmental dynamics at work in federal states:

- Some states topped up the first federal enterprise support programme with their own state subsidies in administering the programme's payment process. The efficiency of these procedures varied depending on the digitalisation of the state administration concerned. False applications for support were a common problem, with some state administrations being less capable than others of identifying them.
- In April and May 2020, Mecklenburg-Pomerania 'closed' its state borders to all tourists – including Germans – who did not have reservations for seven days or more. It sought to exclude day-trippers and weekend tourists to avoid overcrowding at its beaches.
- When infection rates in counties started to rise again in October 2020, Mecklenburg-Pomerania, Schleswig-Holstein, and Bavaria initiated or maintained bans on overnight stays by travellers from high-infection counties and cities (ones with 50 infections per 100,000 inhabitants in the past seven days). Given that the autumn holidays begin at the same time in many of Germany's states, travellers who had made hotel bookings in the mentioned states protested at the measures – some went to the administrative courts, which decided that the state actions were inappropriate. After but a few such judgments, the state governments withdrew their regulations.
- Schools and kindergartens did not reopen in summer at the same time. The states decided individually on the opening date, the number of in-person and digital lessons, and the like. Later, they all agreed that, in spite of increasing infection rates, it was important to keep schools and kindergartens open and avoid repeating the experience of a total lockdown. Nevertheless, the regulations varied from state to state in their details regarding, for example, whether pupils needed to wear masks during lessons, or whether to close a whole school or only parts of it in case of infections.
- The states diverged with regard to permits for cultural and sport events, particularly in respect of the maximum number of spectators. After long discussion, they agreed on a common policy for spectators at first- and second-league soccer matches: a restricted number of spectators, with electronic tickets for special seats, were allowed as long as infections rates remained low. However, rising infection rates led again to soccer and tennis matches being played in empty stadiums.
- In spring, Mecklenburg-Pomerania paid accommodation bonuses to workers from Poland who had to reside in Germany given that the requirement that they spend a fortnight in quarantine on crossing the border meant they could no longer commute daily to their places of employment in Germany. The regulation was reintroduced in autumn after the infection rate in Poland placed it on the list of high-risk countries.

- When in August 2020 the Federal Chancellor and minister-presidents decided to introduce a fine of a minimum of EUR 150 for people not wearing a mask or refusing to do so, the minister-president of Saxony-Anhalt declared that he would not follow this agreement. By contrast, other states imposed even higher fines for so-called mask deniers (EUR 500 in Berlin). A mask denier taking a long-distance train trip thus ran the risk of a multitude of different fines on one and the same journey.

All the states endeavoured to prevent total lockdowns and instead adopt context-specific management for cities and counties with high infection rates. There were also identifiable factors behind the growing number of infections from August 2020 onwards, such as foreign labourers in large slaughterhouses working under insufficiently hygienic conditions and living together in cramped accommodation; numerous people living together in refugee homes; travellers returning from summer holidays in high-risk countries, particularly in the Balkans; wedding parties with more than 400 guests; and illegal parties where hundreds of young people would revel without masks or social distancing. Usually, it was enough to reduce local infections within a few weeks by identifying sources of infection, tracing contacts, conducting tests, and quarantining all of the identified contact persons – that is, until mid-October 2020 when Germany too was caught in the long-dreaded 'second wave' of Covid-19 infections.

This led to a unanimous agreement among the states to impose a new, partial lockdown in November. To reduce unnecessary contact between people, the states closed restaurants, gyms, cinemas, theatres, and opera houses; expanded the duty to wear masks (with a fine for mask deniers); and restricted the number of contacts in public to 10 persons from two households; in addition, hotel accommodation was available only for business purposes.

3.4.4 Local government action

Because local governments are the lowest level of administration in Germany, they played an important role in combating the pandemic. Within the legal frameworks set by federal and state laws and decrees, they gave Covid-19 restrictions further detail applicable in their respective territories:

- Local health agencies tested people for Covid-19 infection, traced their contacts, placed them under quarantine, and controlled whether these observed the restriction. They conducted testing not only by using their staff but also by acting in cooperation with non-profit organisations and private laboratories. They collected data on infections and sent them via the state health administration to the RKI.
- Local regulatory agencies, which included local auxiliary police, monitored observance of Covid-19 regulations, in particular whether restaurants and cafés complied with minimum distances and maximum numbers of visitors,

whether masks were worn and whether customers' details were recorded for contact tracing in case any of them proved to have been infected. The agencies enforced compliance with closing hours in high-infection communities and issued fines if regulations were violated.

- Local administrations authorised local events ranging from concerts and sports events to markets of various kinds, fairs, carnival parades, and political demonstrations, doing so without regard to whether the organisers were public or private actors or even the local government itself: permits could be granted only if the application complied with all the regulations. These processes held the potential for conflict given that the events in question were often of considerable importance not only for restaurants and hotels but so too for a local retail trade keen to attract spendthrift foreign guests.

Problems arose due to staff shortages in local health administrations. The federal government and *Länder* discussed a goal in terms of which local health agencies would establish groups of five staff members per 20,000 inhabitants to trace the contact persons of infected citizens. In April 2020, the federation offered to pay EUR 150,000 per agency to modernise their digital equipment, and, in September, EUR 4 billion for recruiting more personnel. The agencies, however, were unable to hire staff as quickly as necessary. Berlin, for example, had 200 vacancies in its health administration (Heim 2020), while in Covid-19 hotspots, local governments asked the military for support – as a result, by the end of October 2020, several thousand members of the military were working in local health agencies. In the same period, Rhineland-Palatinate asked state civil servants if they were willing to work temporarily in local health agencies involved in tracing contact persons.

Not everyone obeyed the restrictions. In summer, youngsters shifted their night-life activities to parks, squares, and pedestrian zones in the cities, seldom wearing face masks or adhering to minimum distances between people. The situation was difficult to control. When police in Stuttgart and Frankfurt tried to enforce the regulations, crowds of young people became aggressive and the police had to quell street violence; in Stuttgart, shops were damaged and plundered (*Stuttgarter Zeitung* 2020).

Moreover, Berlin as well as other state capitals had to contend with demonstrations by Covid-19 deniers. In the name of civil liberties, alternative groups and right-wing supporters staged protests against the restrictions. They denied the dangers of Covid-19 or even the existence of the pandemic, which was variously claimed to be a myth or biological experiment instigated by the likes of Chancellor Angela Merkel or a Bill Gates intent on world domination. During the demonstrations – allowed in principle by local governments as an exercise of basic rights – people did not practice social distancing or wear masks, never mind mounting an ideological challenge to the very foundations of pandemic governance in Germany. Although the police tried to make them comply with the regulations, success was anything but assured. It was unknown how many new infections resulted from these demonstrations.

The federal government and *Länder* decided in June 2020 to avoid nation- or state-wide lockdowns in future and rather impose restrictions on municipalities with high infection rates (initially, a high infection rate was considered to be more than 50 infections per 100,000 inhabitants in the past seven days, but the threshold was later reduced to 35 infections). Lord Mayors and county chief executives were frequently torn between imposing restrictions in order to contain infections and facilitating local economic recovery, particularly in the case of restaurants, mass events, and sports matches, which were important as sources of revenue and job creation but severely damaged by the lockdown in early 2020. The locally responsible politicians thus tried to ensure that the enterprises concerned could continue to operate at least in an alternative or reduced form. Until the *Bund* and *Länder* began a second nationwide lockdown on 2 November 2020, local governments acted autonomously in working out the details of their control measures.

3.4.5 Intergovernmental relations

The pandemic in Germany was managed by way of established modes of intergovernmental relations. The combination of a few common regulations and their implementation at state level allowed for slightly diverging measures, thereby giving regional actors space in which to respond differently from each other depending on the individual nature of the infection rates and economic concerns in their jurisdictions. Within this context, the meetings of the Conference of Ministers-President with the Federal Chancellor were an essential institution of intergovernmental coordination for ensuring that the spread of the coronavirus did not become uncontrollable and exceed the capacities of hospitals and intensive care beds. Further such coordination took place in the conferences of the education ministers, the health ministers, and the ministers of the interior. Federal and state governments established so-called CORONA cabinets where the ministers with key responsibilities discussed measures to be taken and consulted with national and regional medical experts.

The administration of the majority of restrictions and other measures took place at the local level, where it was regulated by national laws and state decrees. Important instruments at this level were weekly, or, if necessary, daily, crisis conferences where all administrators involved at the state and local level in concrete pandemic responses decided on how to manage impending problems. In larger states, the state district offices provided support or intervened in cases where local governments did not follow the state regulations.

'Physical' intergovernmental support and cooperation took several forms:

- When infections increased in spring 2020 and hospitals, medical practices and nursing homes found themselves without enough protective equipment for their staff, the federation attempted to address this as quickly as possible. However, although it was the task of the federation to have a sufficient reserve of such equipment in the case of a pandemic, it was not available. Insofar as the *Bund* had neglected its duties, it sought to rectify the situation as expeditiously as it could.

• When the number of critical infections exceeded the regional and local capacity of hospitals and intensive care beds, neighbouring jurisdictions absorbed the overflow of patients. The RKI's database of available intensive care beds facilitated coordinated efforts of this kind. For the second wave of infections, cooperation among states was formalised to serve these purposes (NDR 2020).

For many weeks after the first lockdown, it was the states rather than the federation that dominated the field of play. When it became apparent in the summer of 2020 that the return of holidaymakers had caused a spike in infection rates, the Bavarian minister-president set up test centres for returnees near borders and in airports and offered tests for free. The Minster of Health had to follow suit a day later and roll this out as a measure for the entire territory (Hickmann et al. 2020). There was similar pressure on the states to act speedily when it came to reopening society and the economy after the first lockdown in 2020, albeit that in this instance the conflict among the minister-presidents was obvious.

3.4.6 Intergovernmental fiscal relations

Intergovernmental fiscal relations were an important dimension of pandemic management in Germany. This was so not only because of the need to stabilise the locked-down economy, but because the federation compensated for its lack of competences by making various grants to state and local governments. The impact of Covid-19 on public finance was threefold: the pandemic, and particularly the lockdowns, (1) led to the country's largest-ever drop in tax revenue, (2) generated additional public expenditures at all levels of government, and (3) increased public debt as it presented, without any doubt, a case for an exception from the constitutional 'debt brake'.

The breakdown of tax revenue shows a divergence among the levels of government because their respective tax sources were affected in different ways. After years of continuing growth in tax revenue, the federation's revenue declined by 16.3 per cent in 2020 and that of local government by slightly less (9.8 per cent). The states suffered the smallest percentage of losses (5.5 per cent), while the EU received a larger share of national tax revenue (+4.5 per cent) (*Bundesfinanzministerium* 2020b). Governments and economic experts anticipated that tax revenue would increase again in 2021, albeit remaining below the level of 2019.

Additional expenditure linked to Covid-19 caused 'automatic' stabilisers built into the tax and social security system to kick in. They varied among the levels of government. At the federal level, Covid-specific expenditure was covered not only by the normal budgets but by the social insurances, for which the *Bund* has financial responsibility. In total, additional federal expenditure amounted to EUR 146.5 billion (for details, see *Bundesfinanzministerium* 2020c).

Länder governments supplemented federal programmes for SMEs and the self-employed by paying for add-ons. They compensated costs for closed kindergartens and also administered federal transfers to private enterprises and local governments. These activities, for which they were refunded, counted as additional expenditure. In total, state expenditure increased by 39 per cent in the second quarter of 2020 compared to the same period in 2019.

Local governments had to cover additional expenditure for staff in the local health agencies as well as for the local 'police' services that were needed in some communities to enforce pandemic regulations – as they were not able to employ additional staff of their own, they would often employ private security firms. In addition, local governments paid for hygiene equipment in local administration workplaces and schools. Even garbage collection generated higher expenses than usual – a great deal of refuse had to be removed, given that many people used the lockdown as an opportunity to clear out their cellars and attics, in addition to which a surge in e-commerce generated a large amount of disposable packaging. The loss of revenue from locally owned enterprises due to lockdowns and other restrictions (including from amenities such as theatres, opera houses, museums, sport stadiums, swimming pools, public transport, fairgrounds, and airports) also made its impact felt.

Overall, the financial burdens of Covid-19 were unevenly distributed among the three levels of government, conceived vertically; such unevenness also became apparent horizontally within levels of government. This reflects the fact that differing epidemiological patterns and correspondingly differing restrictions on social and economic life generated diverse impacts on regional and local economies and hence on their tax revenue.

Fiscal equalisation schemes – federal-state and state-local – stabilised public budgets. They equalised the majority of horizontal divergences in loss of tax revenue, though not the vertical effects and differences in necessary expenditure. As such, the respective superior levels of government created additional vertical grants from the federal to state tier, from the state to local tier, and from the federal to local tier, the latter despite the constitutional prohibition of direct federal intervention in local governments. To enable constitutional grants from the federation to local governments, the federation used the changes of the Basic Law in 2019. This included particular grants from federal and state budgets (50:50) for the compensation of local losses in trade tax revenues.

Vertical differences in Covid-related expenditure increases and revenue losses were most apparent in regard to public debt. Fiscal policies of a Keynesian type stabilise economic development (Auerbach 2012). They imply an acceptance of using public debt to cover deficits arising from loss of tax revenue and/or the need for additional expenditure. The *Bund* and *Länder* stated the case for an exemption from the restrictive rules of the debt brake, which usually contemplates a credit maximum of 0.35 per cent of GDP for the *Bund* and balanced budgets for the *Länder*. In addition, the *Bund* used its *Kreditanstalt für Wiederaufbau* (Credit Institute for Reconstruction) to provide additional funding through loan guarantees on behalf of endangered enterprises. The federal budget received approval from Parliament for new credit of up to EUR 218 billion, corresponding to 13 per cent of GDP. The limit for guarantees was increased to 47 per cent of GDP (*Deutsche Bundesbank* 2020). The debt finally borrowed was allocated to a special extra-budgetary fund and is to be redeemed over 50 years.

Likewise, all *Länder* had budgetary deficits, which were estimated to amount in total to about EUR 50 billion. The states administered an important share of their debt-funded programmes in special extra-budgetary accounts. They, too, decided on a long period for redemption. Local governments also wound up with high deficits, notwithstanding the transfers paid to them. 'Unhealthy' cash credit was far in excess of local borrowing for investment expenditure. The sole good news for public budgets in 2020 was that interest rates in the next few years seemed likely to remain low, meaning that additional redemptions would 'only' become payable in the years thereafter.

In summary, Covid-19 contributed to a higher degree of fiscal centralisation. It was an open question whether this would continue after the crisis or lead to new, and fundamental, reforms granting greater autonomy to lower levels of government. A majority of members of the various parliaments asserted that the enormous increase in public debt was sustainable – assuming that this Keynesian fiscal policy would succeed in preventing a deep(er) recession.

3.5 Findings and policy implications

During the first wave of the Covid-19 pandemic, the German federal system was successful in responding to its challenges and was fortunate to have a relatively low number of infections and deaths. The limited legislative powers of the central government meant that state and local governments were not inhibited in their initial response. By the end of March 2020, however, the *Bund* had initiated the common action of a nationwide lockdown, with the *Länder* passing detailed regulations in this regard and local governments administering and enforcing them. From the outset, there was a policy emphasis on focusing on local hotspots and customising tighter restrictions there to prevent the virus from spreading out of control and to limit the number of critical cases needing intensive care. With the rise in autumn of a second wave of infections, the federal system was again faced with the challenge of doubling down to contain the pandemic – and, at the time of this writing, had once more proven itself capable of containing a threat of this nature and magnitude.

Usually, citizens take little note of state-by-state differences in regulations, particularly when it is the federation that holds the legislative competence. At the end of April 2020, though, when questions about the speed and extent to which the economy and education sector should be reopened became issues of debate, it was both apparent that the state governments were dominating the political dialogue and plain to see not only that there were differences in state government actions but that these differences mattered. Citizens often expressed their lack of understanding that regulations in their home town were different to those in another *Land* where they had gone on holiday; all the same, they did not protest at the inconvenience of restrictions in local hotspots.

The intergovernmental decision-making that underlay this situation was nonetheless unusual. Conventionally, the federation passes the necessary legal regulations, the states transform them into state laws, decrees and administrative prescriptions, and then, often along with local governments, execute them. Many competences necessary for combating pandemics are located at the state level, however, and even at the level of municipalities, which can opt to tighten restrictions if necessary. In response, the central government sought to influence the states into heeding its political preferences.

It did so in two ways: first, through the public communications of the Chancellor and Minister of Health and by inviting the Conference of the Ministers-President to consultations; and, secondly, by spending taxpayers' money on a scale hitherto unknown in Germany – sometimes it was clearly apparent that it was only the *Bund's* generous transfer payments that had broken the resistance of the minister-presidents to the plan to combat Covid-19 by means of a common, nationwide action. Neither feature of the intergovernmental management of the pandemic is without problem: the extreme dominance of executive decision-making led to sharp conflict in the federal and state parliaments, while the public debt incurred will probably result in higher – perhaps much higher – taxes in future.

The upcoming election campaigns not only for the federal elections in September 2021 but also for several State Parliament elections in 2021 have already played an important role and will continue to do so in 2021 in the formation of Covid-19 policies. The prospective competing candidates for, on the one hand, the leadership of CDU/CSU (two of them Minister Presidents), and, on the other hand, the candidate of the SPD (Social Democratic Party of Germany), the incumbent Federal Minister of Finance, may try to show their own special profile in fighting against the pandemic and its economic consequences.

Finally, observers were astonished at the divergent advice provided by academic experts working for the federal and state governments, the majority of them epidemiologists. Many of them advocated a strategy of reducing interpersonal contact in the population the higher infection rates became. A minority, however, asserted that, on balance, the harm wrought by infections would not be severe enough to warrant heavy restrictions. It is unclear whether the 'opinion' of a government invited the corresponding experts, or if the experts' advice influenced the more rigid or more liberal measures that were adopted; at any rate, powerful groups no doubt employed the halo of expertise to legitimate their particular interests.

In conclusion, Germany's executive federalism emerged as an adequate model for the management of the Covid-19 pandemic. Although a framework of legal rules was necessary, the gravamen of the country's actions did not lie in federal legislative measures but in the regionally and locally specified application of regulations and controls, including information management and communication. That Germany utilised the scope for decentralised action inherent in its model of federalism is probably the most important reason for its relatively low Covid-19 mortality rate during the first wave of infection.

The German experience of the management of the first wave of the Covid-19 pandemic thus merits further research, particularly in the light of events subsequent to the period examined in this chapter and relating to the second wave and later period of vaccination. Three questions come to the fore:

- First, what is the 'ideal' mixture of central regulation, on the one hand, and decentralised execution and administration, on the other? What ratio of uniformity and diversity is needed in order to control infection rates and secure the population's compliance with restrictions?
- Secondly, what was the specific role of the civil service in managing the pandemic? What can we learn about new modes of working, particularly telework in home offices? What are the consequences of digitalisation not only for public administration but the education sector – the schools and universities – which, in Germany, fall under public sector management?
- Thirdly, what are the consequences of the pandemic's huge financial burdens for intergovernmental fiscal relations? Does Germany need greater decentralisation of tax-raising and -spending autonomy or greater central regulation, including more transfer payments? What was the role of multilevel tax-sharing and fiscal equalisation schemes in stabilising economic development and attempting to ensure the sustainability of public sector budgets?

Finally, the apparent contrast of the – relative – weakness of the federation in deciding restrictive measures, on the one hand, and its costly financial 'generosity', on the other hand, should be under further observance if that will continue after the pandemic or whether there will be decentralisation particularly of the intergovernmental financial relations in order to fund state and local governments 'sufficiently' by own (tax) sources.

References

Auerbach, Alan J. 2012. 'The Fall and Rise of Keynesian Fiscal Policy', https://eml.berkeley.edu/~auerbach/TheFallandRiseofKeynesianFiscalPolicy.1.pdf (accessed on 28 October 2020).

Bundesfinanzministerium. 2020a. 'Umsetzung des Konjunkturprogramms', BMF-Monatsbericht 6/2020, https://www.bundesfinanzministerium.de/Monatsberichte/2020/06/Inhalte/Kapitel-2b-Schlaglicht/2b-umsetzung-des-konjunkturprogramms-pdf.pdf?__blob=publicationFile&v=3 (accessed on 27 October 2020).

Bundesfinanzministerium. 2020b. '*Ergebnisse der Steuerschätzung vom 8. bis 10*', *BMF-Monatsbericht,* https://www.bundesfinanzministerium.de/Monatsberichte/2020/09/Inhalte/Kapitel-3-Analysen/3-4-ergebnisse-der-steuerschaetzung-pdf.pdf?__blob=publicationFile&v=2 (accessed on 12 October 2020).

Bundesfinanzministerium. 2020c. '*Nachtragshaushalte des Bundes 2020 (Sollbericht)*', *BMF-Monatsbericht,* https://www.bundesfinanzministerium.de/Monatsberichte/2020/08/Inhalte/Kapitel-3-Analysen/3-1-nachtragshaushalte-2020-des-bundes-sollbericht-pdf.pdf?__blob=publicationFile&v=2 (accessed on 12 October 2020).

Bundesgesundheitsministerium. 2020. '*Coronavirus SARS-CoV-2: Chronik der bisherigen Maßnahmen*', https://www.bundesgesundheitsministerium.de/coronavirus/chronik-coronavirus.html (accessed on 26 October 2020).

Deutsche Bundesbank. 2020. '*Öffentliche Finanzen*', *Monatsbericht der deutschen Bundesbank,* https://www.bundesbank.de/resource/blob/841044/8a5ca70e34510ecde9c99d-d9eaf6edd6/mL/2020-08-oeffentliche-finanzen-data.pdf (accessed on 12 October 2020).

Deutscher Bundestag. 2020. '*Parlamentsmaterialien zur Corona-Pandemie*', https://www.bundestag.de/dokumente/parlamentsdokumentation/dossier (accessed on 23 October 2020).

Färber, Gisela. 2015. 'Fiscal Equalization in Germany: Facts, Conflicts and Perspectives', in Giancarlo Pola (ed.), *Principles and Practices of Fiscal Autonomy: Experiences, Debate and Prospects,* pp. 113–34. Farnham: Ashgate.

Heim, Manuela. 2020. '*Rückstand im Gesundheitsamt*', http://taz.de/Steigende-Infektionszahlen-in-Berlin/!5717559/ (accessed on 29 October 2020).

Hickmann, Christoph et al. 2020. '*Der Getriebene*', *Der Spiegel,* 45: 34–7.

Huegelin, Thomas and Alan Fenna. 2015. *Comparative Federalism: A Systematic Inquiry,* 2nd ed. Toronto: University of Toronto Press.

NDR. 2020. '*Corona: Nord-Länder wollen bei Klinik-Kapazitäten kooperieren*', https://www.ndr.de/nachrichten/info/Corona-Nordlaender-wollen-bei-Klinik-Kapazitaeten-kooperieren,covidpatienten100.html (accessed on 20 November 2020).

RBB Online. 2020. '*Kampf gegen Corona – Viel Geld für neue Intensivbetten: Doch wo sind sie?*', https://www.rbb-online.de/kontraste/archiv/kontraste-vom-16-07-2020/viel-geld-fuer-neue-intensivbetten-doch-wo-sind-sie.html (accessed on 26 October 2020).

Robert Koch Institute. n.d. 'Covid-19 Dashboard', https://experience.arcgis.com/experience/478220a4c454480e823b17327b2bf1d4 (accessed on 01 November 2020).

Stuttgarter Zeitung. '*Polizei nennt erste Hintergründe zu den Ausschreitungen*'. 2020. *Stuttgarter Zeitung.* 21 July, https://www.stuttgarter-zeitung.de/inhalt.krawalle-in-stuttgart-polizei-nennt-erste-hintergruende-zu-den-ausschreitungen.b545276f-8621-4ed3-8908-dc346c55e494.html (accessed on 20 November 2020).

4

MANAGING THE COVID-19 PANDEMIC IN AUSTRIA

From national unity to a de facto unitary state?

Karl Kössler

4.1 Introduction

After several months into the Covid-19 pandemic, few things are certain. But one of the key insights for any government response is the importance of demographic features. As of 2020, Austria had a population of 8.9 million, with 19.3 per cent of its inhabitants between 0 and 19 years of age, 61.6 per cent between 20 and 64 years, and 19 per cent over 65 years of age. Besides age, the degree of urbanisation is another relevant factor in pandemic management, and here Austria probably benefits from being characterised mostly by villages and small towns. As of 2018, 52 per cent of its population lived in municipalities with less than 10,000 inhabitants and 48 per cent in only 86 towns and cities with larger population sizes. Apart from the capital, Vienna, which has 1.9 million inhabitants, no other city reaches a population size of 300,000.

In terms of its legal and political system, Austria is, under its Constitution of 1920, a federal country, though a highly centralised one. The federal constitutional make-up was, of course, not the only factor influencing the response to the pandemic. A relevant political factor was the composition of government both at the federal level and in the nine *Länder*. Since January 2020, shortly before the onset of the pandemic, the federal coalition brought together the conservative Austrian People's Party (ÖVP) and centre-left Green Party as a junior partner. Although the ÖVP chancellor, Sebastian Kurz, assumed a prominent role in communicating the response to Covid-19, a key cabinet member – Rudolf Anschober, the Minister of Health was from the Green Party. While the *Länder* had been ruled for decades either by the ÖVP or the Social Democratic Party (SPÖ), all but one were ruled by coalitions and thus included various smaller parties in their governments.

Another crucial factor in addressing the pandemic was the presence of a well-developed public health-care system; this holds true despite an increasing

DOI: 10.4324/9781003166771-6

number of private profit-oriented providers. With 5.1 physicians and 7.6 hospital beds per 1,000 inhabitants (OECD 2020), Austria's medical-service capacity is among the strongest in the world. In view of Covid-19, it is also important that the country has a relatively high number of beds in ICU units, that is, 28.9 per 100,000 persons.

Due to Austria's closeness to Italy, it is hardly surprising that when it reported its first ascertained cases of Covid-19 on 25 February 2020, the patients were a young couple from Lombardy living in Innsbruck in the *Land* Tyrol. However, the real epicentre of the outbreak in Austria became the Tyrolean ski resort of Ischgl. As many ski tourists from Northern European countries were tested positive upon their return from this alpine village, authorities from these countries – starting with Iceland on 5 March – began to classify it as a high-risk area. An indication of the size of the outbreak in Ischgl is that as many as 42 per cent of the village's inhabitants already had antibodies by the end of April. As a result, Tyrol was Austria's initial epicentre, with 3,352 coronavirus cases until 15 April (in a population of approximately 758,000) compared to only 2,101 in Vienna (with a population of 1.9 million).

Over time, the spread of infection tended to even out across the *Länder*, a development that prompted them to align themselves closely with the national government, at least initially. The central argument of this chapter is that – after early national unity – Austria's brand of 'pandemic federalism' oscillated between attempts towards autonomy and differentiation, on the one hand, and, on the other, the dynamics of a de facto unitary state.

4.2 The federal constitutional and legislative framework

4.2.1 Constitutional distribution of powers

Unlike subnational entities in other federal systems (Palermo and Kössler 2017), Austria's *Länder* do not have extensive legislative competences in health care. In fact, article 10(1)(12) of the 1920 Constitution stipulates that public health is in principle a federal responsibility in regard to both its legislative and executive dimension. However, the same provision also foresees certain exceptions, such as municipal sanitation and, importantly for Covid-19, hospitals and nursing homes, even if these are under federal health supervision. Article 12(1)(1) specifies that, in relation to the latter health facilities, the federal government is limited to passing basic legislation on principles, whereas the implementation of laws falls within the jurisdiction of the *Länder*.

Thus, while *Länder* authorities execute federal and own laws concerning hospitals and nursing homes autonomously, the execution of federal public health legislation, based on article 10(1)(12), falls within what is called 'indirect federal administration' (Constitution, articles 102–5). This means *Länder* officials execute federal law not as their own prerogative but as delegates of the federal government. The *Land* governor is subject to instructions from the competent federal minister, with his or her autonomy confined mainly to organisational considerations of how to achieve the goals determined by the minister (VfSlg 9507/1982). Instructions may be disregarded only for the reasons exhaustively listed in article 20(1) – that is, instructions issued by a minister without authority and infringing the criminal code (VfSlg 10510/1985) – with the result that the *Land* governor is barred from weighing up different legal interests autonomously and making his or her own decision. In case of non-compliance with instructions, he or she may even be charged before the Constitutional Court under article 142(2)(e) of the Constitution. While this is the legal situation, indirect federal administration makes the federal minister politically dependent on implementation by the *Land* governor and thus forces both government levels to cooperate and compromise.

Regarding the executive sphere, the district administrative authorities also play an important role. They comprise Austria's 15 cities, each of which has its own city statute[1] and 79 unelected district commissions (*Bezirkshauptmannschaften*) with a district commissioner appointed by the *Land* government. As subordinate units, these authorities carry out administrative tasks on behalf of their *Land* and – upon the instructions of the *Land* governor – tasks falling under indirect federal administration. Concerning health care, a district medical officer is, for example, responsible for health matters and supervision of the hygiene of hospitals located in the district. In comparison, the municipalities play a lesser administrative role, one focused mainly on health and hygiene inspections, and in view of their small size, often carry out their functions jointly with each other.

Importantly, health care is not an exclusive domain of the various government levels mentioned so far; rather, it includes other actors within a corporatist scheme of governance relations, as is typical of a Bismarckian welfare-state system based largely on mandatory health insurance through payroll contributions (Trukeschitz et al. 2013: 154). Whereas one category of employees is insured via medical aid funds based on occupation (e.g., railway workers, farmers, or civil servants), most employees are covered by the nine *Länder* medical aid funds (one fund per *Land*). This makes the medical aid funds key players, especially in corporatist negotiations regarding outpatient care. Concerning inpatient care, on the other hand, the *Länder* are, given their abovementioned responsibility for hospitals, the main actors (ibid: 158). Consequently, the Minister of Health lacks (in normal times) direct control over much of the country's health care.

In terms of policy-making, the separation of powers outlined above is complemented by intergovernmental agreements on health care based on article 15(a) of the Constitution. Since 1974, this provision has enabled both vertical as well as horizontal accords which are binding though not self-executing (VfSlg 9581/1982; 9886/1983), inasmuch as their content still needs to be adopted formally by Parliament. Agreements under article 15(a) concerning hospitals first appeared in 1978, and since the late-1980s became a primary tool for regulating an extremely complex financing system that involves contributions from the federal government, *Länder*, municipalities and medical aid funds. A key agreement in 1997 introduced a binding general hospital plan and gave rise to health funds at the federal level and in the *Länder* for the sake of better coordinating inpatient and outpatient care. Austria pressed ahead with these reforms because the separation between two areas of care is, together with the complex financing arrangements, often seen as responsible for an overly fragmented health-care system (Kostera 2013: 151).

4.2.2 Constitutional emergency powers

A key question is whether the ordinary distribution of functions, as outlined, also prevails in the extraordinary circumstances of a pandemic. In fact, even though there has been much talk of 'emergency ordinances' issued by the federal and *Länder* governments, no one has ever declared a state of emergency in Austria due to Covid-19.

Article 18(3) of the Constitution grants the Austrian President (upon proposal by the federal government) the power to issue ordinances 'necessary to prevent obvious and irreparable damage to the general public' at a time when the first chamber of Parliament is not assembled, cannot meet, or cannot act as a result of *force majeure*. Yet, during the pandemic in 2020, the chamber did actually meet and play some role, albeit a very limited one (see section 4.2). Importantly, a presidential ordinance may change ordinary law but not constitutional law; nor may it entail a 'permanent financial burden' for the federal government or a 'financial burden' for the *Länder* or municipalities (article 18(5)), which is obviously an illusion in times of a pandemic. In short, there are several reasons why the presidential emergency power is of no practical use in such circumstances.

Another avenue for ushering in a period of emergency would be article 15 of the European Convention on Human Rights, which has been incorporated into Austria's legal order constitutional rank that is above ordinary legislation. This article provides a possibility to derogate certain rights '[i]n time of war or other public emergency threatening the life of the nation'. However, the Austrian government, unlike others,[2] did not invoke this right of derogation (Lachmayer 2020), which would have required keeping the Secretary-General of the Council of Europe informed about the emergency measures taken and the reasons for them.

4.2.3 The legislative framework for addressing Covid-19

As for ordinary legislation, the Epidemic Diseases Act was most relevant at the outset of the Covid-19 pandemic. A key problem, however, was that this piece of legislation dates back to 1950 (and is based largely on an even older law passed in 1913), which makes it less than ideal for contending with an emergency in the 21st century.

Several of its anachronistic features were identified, among them the obligation to report a case of infection to the authorities only within 24 hours.[3] In today's highly mobile world, this time span is short enough for an infectious disease to spread from *Land* to *Land*, or even to another country. Naturally, this old law also fails to pay adequate attention to more contemporary issues such as data protection, a dimension that was introduced only when the Act was amended during the pandemic in 2020 (BGBl. I Nr. 16/2020). Another aspect of the law that improved in response to Covid-19 was its harsh rules on gatherings and events. An amendment made it clear that, apart from outright prohibition, there are less intrusive measures that can be taken, such as limitations applicable to specific groups of persons, or stipulations in regard to physical distancing, face masks, and sanitary requirements (BGBl. I Nr. 43/2020).

4.3 Preparedness for a national disaster: The institutional framework

Instead of specific institutions for public health emergencies, Austria has several general health-care bodies on which the Minister of Health can rely for advice. The Health Austria Company (*Gesundheit Österreich GmbH*), owned by the Austrian government, is an applied research institute in charge of, among other things, health-care capacity planning, which is a matter of vital importance in pandemic management. Another institution, the Supreme Health Board (*Oberster Sanitätsrat*), brings together more than 40 health experts and provides, as do the *Länder* health boards (*Landessanitätsräte*) at the subnational level, technical support and guidance on major medical issues. However, the Minister of Health, allegedly due to the need to focus on the pandemic, failed to re-nominate the members of the Supreme Health Board, which is an unlawful state of affairs. Instead, he relied for advice on an ad hoc 'coronavirus taskforce'. For coordination with the *Länder* and local governments, the federal government utilised general mechanisms of intergovernmental relations.

4.4 Rolling out measures to contain the pandemic

4.4.1 Taking the initiative

Although Austria recorded its first two cases of Covid-19 in Innsbruck on 25 February 2020, a comprehensive response was triggered only later on by the events in Ischgl. On 4 March, Icelandic authorities sent an e-mail to Austrian colleagues warning that eight of their positive cases had travelled to the ski resort, information which the Ministry of Health forwarded to Tyrol's health authorities. However, it was only on 12 March that tourists were informed that ski resorts would be closed, and even so, not immediately but two days hence. On 13 March, the national government placed the valley around Ischgl under quarantine.

Reconstructing these events – in particular, determining who acted first, acted at all or failed to act – takes on a legal dimension which is highly interesting from a federalism perspective. This is because more than 6,000 Ischgl tourists joined the Austrian Consumer Protection Association in its efforts to claim damages, while over a thousand of them were joined as private parties in criminal charges against the relevant authorities, charges that were ongoing at the time of this writing.

The main claim is that the authorities knew, or should have known, about the risk of mass infection but responded too slowly out of greed and the priority given to the interests of the tourism industry (Consumer Protection Association 2020). The significance of tourism becomes evident from the facts that roughly one-fourth of jobs in Tyrol are tied to this sector and that a village like Ischgl, with 1,600 inhabitants, hosts as many as 10,000 tourists in the skiing season. Article 23(1) of the Constitution stipulates that authorities are, under civil law, liable for injuries inflicted in executing laws through illegal and culpable behaviour. As the potential wrongdoing would have occurred within the scope of indirect federal administration (see section 2.1), the claim goes against the Republic of Austria for alleged mistakes made by both the national as well as Tyrolean authorities.

4.4.2 Federal action

As part of a dual strategy, the federal government amended the Epidemic Diseases Act to make it fit for the 21st century and adopted ad hoc legislation. Although measures during the first few days of the federal response from 10 March onwards – for example, restrictions on travel and events, the closure of schools and universities, and the ending of the skiing season – were still based on the Epidemic Diseases Act, 15 March witnessed a rather extraordinary episode in Austrian parliamentarism.

On this Sunday, a set of bills, among them the Covid-19 Measures Act, was adopted by both chambers of Parliament within less than 24 hours, authenticated by the President and published in the law gazette. The Covid-19 Measures Act, which contains a sunset clause providing for its termination at the end of 2020, was since then at the core of efforts to combat the pandemic. It was this Act which allowed for the closure of businesses except for shops providing basic services, imposed limitations on entering public places, and made it obligatory to wear face masks. Some restrictions, especially those regarding access to public places, expired on 30 April 2020, after which a new ordinance came into force, the so-called easing ordinance (*Lockerungsverordnung*) (BGBl. II Nr. 197/2020).

In terms of institutions that shaped federal action, a key body was a newly established 'coronavirus taskforce'. It was curious that this taskforce, nominated and chaired by the Minister of Health, included national authorities and experts such as health professionals and mathematicians but had no representatives of the *Länder*.

Among the first federal measures were business closures affecting in particular hotels and cable-car businesses in Tyrol. These measures, as noted, were based on the 1950 Epidemic Diseases Act, which promised full compensation for losses in the amount of 'comparable extrapolated earnings'. To avoid such costly compensation, the Covid-19 Measures Act of 15 March not only enabled the Minister of Health to prohibit, through an ordinance, customers, and economic operators from entering business premises, but also simply excluded, once this ordinance was in force, the applicability of the compensation rules under the old law of 1950.

In a seminal judgment, the Constitutional Court held that this provision is no violation of the right to equality but is proportionate, given that the Covid-19 Measures Act established a substantial crisis management fund for the compensation of businesses closed after the ordinance (VfGH 14.07.2020, G 202/2020). This was not the only aspect of business closure that raised legal concerns. Shops with a sales area of less than 400 m² were allowed to reopen on 14 April 2020 and others only on 1 May. The Constitutional Court ruled that the relevant ordinance of the Minister of Health was against the law, as it had failed to justify this differentiation (VfGH 14.07.2020, V 411/2020).

The Covid-19 Measures Act did not allow for bans on entering business premises but enabled more far-reaching restrictions of freedom of movement. By means of an ordinance, entering public places may be prohibited by the Minister of Health throughout the country, by a governor for the territory of the respective *Land*, and by a district administrative authority for its district or parts thereof. The crux of the matter was that the relevant section 2 of the law explicitly referred to banning access to 'specific public places'. However, section 1 of the 'entry ordinance' (*Betretungsverordnung*) of the Minister of Health (BGBl. II Nr. 98/2020), which like the Covid-19 Measures Act came into force on 16 March, decreed a *general* curfew with only few exceptions, such as movement for covering the basic needs of daily life or for professional purposes. The Constitutional Court did not agree with the argument that the Act was unconstitutional due to a violation of article 18(1), which stipulates that '[t]he entire public administration shall be based on law'. It did hold, however, that the 'entry ordinance' was partly unlawful because its *general* prohibition was indeed too extensive to be covered by the Covid-19 Measures Act (VfGH 14.07.2020, V 363/2020).

A third controversial area of the federal response to the pandemic was the obligation to wear face masks. With effect from 15 June, masks were required only for public transport and in health-care facilities such as pharmacies, and no longer in shops, schools and restaurants. However, this easing of measures would not last for long. The fact that the duty to wear masks was broadened on 24 July to include postal offices, banks, and grocery stores – but not, for example, clothes shops and restaurants – again ignited public debate. A point of controversy was whether this differentiation was objectively justifiable and if the ordinance provided a credible explanation – all of which was exactly the same as what the Constitutional Court had demanded a little more than a week before then in its ruling (mentioned above) on the privileged reopening of smaller businesses.

The federal actions described above illustrate a double centralisation of decision-making, that is, an accumulation of power vertically at the national government level and horizontally in the hands of the executive branch. Indeed, conventional wisdom has it that emergency situations lead to a predominance of the (national) executive because the latter can respond speedily and decisively to a sudden crisis. This 'Schmittian' or 'post-Madisonian' view of emergency governance has been opposed by a study based on data on Covid-19 responses from more than a hundred countries (Ginsburg and Versteeg 2020). The authors claim that the conventional wisdom applies only to a specific kind of emergency, namely a national security crisis. Other kinds of emergencies, such as the Covid-19 pandemic, which are characterised by a dispersal of information with effective implementation depending to a much greater extent on local governments, the (national) executive would be structurally bound rather than unbound.

In Austria, the mostly unbound national executive was only occasionally challenged by the *Länder*, with the pushback again coming from the executive, only in this instance the subnational executive. The finding that Germany's Covid-19 governance entailed a 'self-disempowerment of parliament' (*Selbstentmächtigung des Parlaments*) (Möllers 2020) applies in Austria to both the national and subnational levels of government. While the speaker of the first chamber from day one explicitly emphasised the continuity of parliamentary activities, Parliament had few high moments in resisting the executive, one of them being the opposition's success in introducing a sunset clause to the Covid-19 Measures Act. However, the hasty enactment of complex omnibus bills and the, at best, ambivalent role of the second chamber, supposedly representing *Länder* interests, testify to the diminished role of parliamentarism.

Only in few instances did the Federal Council (*Bundesrat*) apply its tool of a suspensive veto (Constitution, article 42(1–4)). However, to see this as an expression of *Länder* influence would be a misrepresentation of the real circumstances. First, there was a strong partisan element, as two opposition parties, the social democratic SPÖ and the right-wing FPÖ, held a majority in the Federal Council (Palermo 2020). Secondly, the stated reasons for the veto were feared infringements of fundamental rights and a reduction of parliamentary scrutiny due to the hasty legislative process (Gamper 2020). Instead of federalism grounds, the vetoes were prompted by the traditional rationale of bicameralism as an opportunity to give bills a second thought, a line of argument key to the thinking of George Washington and other framers of the US Constitution. The broader problem of the concentration of power in the (national) executive (Lachmayer 2020) is best illustrated by the federal government's use of *internal* administrative orders to public officials (*Erlässe*) to regulate matters with *external* effects (which ought to be regulated through ordinances). Such a practice deprives people of legal remedies because internal orders are not subject to judicial review.

In response to mounting criticism, the Minister of Health promised to avoid legal missteps in the future, while the Chancellor's reaction was rather nonchalant. He called on lawyers not to engage in 'legal sophistry' (*juristische Spitzfindigkeiten*) and pointed to the fact that, at the next session of the Constitutional Court in June 2020, the legal measures would no longer be in force anyway, which was not necessarily true.[4] This prompted observers to ask sarcastically whether constitutional law is 'for the Court only' (Somek 2020) and emphasise that a 'good legislator' would be obliged *ex ante* to weigh up the proportionality of measures in an effort to avoid unconstitutionality. Compared to earlier legal measures, the 'easing ordinance' (*Lockerungsverordnung*), entering into force on 1 May, was indeed viewed positively by legal experts as 'more differentiated and precise' (Bernd-Christian Funk, quoted in Kroisleitner and Scherndl 2020).

Besides horizontal concentration of power in the hands of the executive, double centralisation also entails – in its vertical dimension – the predominance of the national government. This is exemplified, in particular, by national Covid-19 legislation regulating, on the basis of the competence for public health under article 10(1)(12) of the Constitution, a number of issues that normally fall within the responsibilities of the *Länder*. This continues to be the case even though some *Länder* demanded, in the run-up to the 'easing ordinance' of 1 May, more decentralisation and differentiation regarding the roll-back of restrictions. However, this ordinance regulates, for example, the entry to sports facilities and the organisation of events, matters usually falling within *Länder* responsibilities. As the federal competence for public health allows it in times of emergency to take measures otherwise reserved to the *Länder*, the competences of the latter are pushed into the background. When they would come to the fore again thus depends on the return to 'normality'.

In this light, the comprehensive reform of both the 2020 Covid-19 Measures Act and the 1950 Epidemic Diseases Act, which the Austrian parliament passed on 25 September (BGBl. I Nr. 104/2020), had the declared aim of partially reducing centralisation (see section 4.4.4). In contrast to earlier, hasty legislation during the pandemic, a comprehensive evaluation procedure took place, with some of the several thousand comments on the bill by private individuals and organisations leading to genuine improvement. Yet it was correctly observed, in a critical vein, that a thorough amendment of the two acts took as long as seven months since the start of the pandemic (Bußjäger, quoted in Marchart and Weißensteiner 2020).

Overall, the reform provided a legal basis for pandemic governance which is firmer, more precise, and in line with the proportionality principle. Importantly, sections 3–5 of the Covid-19 Measures Act now determine the modalities for restrictions on freedom of movement by ordinance more extensively and precisely and thus seek to remedy the problem of the 'entry ordinance' being declared unlawful. Another welcome change in regard to the rule of law is procedural, as an ordinance decreeing a future lockdown would have to be discussed with the Main Committee of the first parliamentary chamber and thus with all parties represented there. However, as the aim is to avoid countrywide lockdowns, more autonomy is henceforth granted to the *Länder*.

4.4.3 Länder action

The *Länder* adopted several measures, partly through ordinary legislation but above all through ordinances, to combat the pandemic. However, this did not materially alter the predominance of the centralist approach. At the outset, Tyrol had lockdown rules that deviated for several weeks from those of the rest of the country, in addition to which it prohibited entry to other *Länder*. But as Covid-19 spread more evenly across the country, subnational governments tended to align themselves with the national government. When restrictions began to be eased in a staggered way in mid-April and early May 2020, greater differentiation was demanded by some *Länder* and academic observers in the interests of economic recovery and greater acceptance of the restrictions by the population. Still, Austria's Covid-19 response largely remained uniform, even though infection clusters in some areas prompted certain subnational governments to take special measures, with school closures and stricter face mask regulations in early July in Upper Austria being a case in point.

The debate about greater *Länder* autonomy regained momentum as infection numbers grew in early September and coincided with the introduction of the abovementioned 'coronavirus traffic light system' (*Corona-Ampel*). Based on weekly risk assessments by a commission that assigned one of four colours – green, yellow, orange, or red – to each district, it was up to federal, *Länder*, and district authorities to adopt recommendations or legally binding measures. Local differentiation between districts was thus key to this plan.

However, the plan was derailed by two problems. First, the mixed composition of the commission – that is, five experts nominated by the national government, five civil servants from national ministries, and one representative from each of the nine *Länder* – resulted inevitably in tensions between scientific and political rationales for the risk assessments. While it was mostly the representatives of the federal and *Länder* governments within the commission that attempted to wield influence, one member suggested at the start of one of the first crucial meetings that the chief of staff of the Chancellor, without being part of the commission, briefly join in order to read out a declaration. This was rejected by the commission, on the argument that, to preserve its air of technocratic probity, political interventions should be avoided (even though political representatives outnumbered experts 14 to 5!). However, the *Länder* and local governments also tried to exert pressure on the commission. Whereas Vienna initially demanded a stricter risk assessment, the Mayor of Linz was outraged that his city was in the yellow and not green column and lambasted the 'coronavirus traffic light system' as arbitrary and a failure.

The second problem was that a sharp increase in infection numbers precisely at the time of the new system's introduction prompted the federal government to throw regional differentiation overboard. On 12 September 2020, it resorted to countrywide measures by issuing another amendment, already the 10th, of the 'easing ordinance' (BGBl. II Nr. 398/2020). Thus, the assignment of colours to the single districts became rather symbolic and at most useful for risk-awareness raising because the new uniform rules, which were lying – depending on the issue – between those districts initially categorised as yellow or orange, also entered into force in the many green districts. For example, the maximum number of persons for indoor events was reduced to 50, as opposed to the 200 initially foreseen for green and 100 for yellow, and a few days later was lowered further to 10.

Issues of autonomy and differentiation also emerged on another occasion, namely in late September 2020 during the reform mentioned above of federal Covid-19 legislation. The Minister of Health himself underlined that the reform was aimed at increasing *Länder* competences to enable them to co-define locally the measures that would best contain the pandemic (APA 2020). The new section 7 of the Covid-19 Measures Act clarifies the power to issue ordinances based on this law at the federal, *Land*, and district levels and envisages regional differentiation. A *Land* Governor may act, if there is no federal ordinance or decree, to provide additional measures, and a district administrative authority may act, if there is neither a federal nor a *Land* ordinance, to introduce additional measures.

Such autonomous decision-making runs into certain limits. First, *Land* and district ordinances that prevent people (with exceptions) from leaving their private living spaces need the approval of, respectively, the Minister of Health and the *Land* governor. Secondly, the minister must be informed about both the *Länder* and district ordinances before they enter into force. Thirdly, legal hierarchy is reflected in the provision that *Länder* ordinances may repeal district ordinances and that both can be repealed by ordinances from the Minister of Health. In practice, these hard instruments for restraining autonomy were not used during the period under review. Instead, the federal government merely expressed its misgivings when, for example, Vienna in September 2020 decided to go its own way by introducing guest registration in pubs and restaurants rather than following other *Länder* in setting closing hours at 22:00.

4.4.4 Local government action

Under the Constitution, district administrative authorities do not have the scope of autonomy comparable to that of the *Länder*, as they are merely subordinate units. Nevertheless, as instructions from the *Land* or federal governments cannot and/or do not determine, even more so in a complex emergency situation, all district actions, the leeway they give to local governments is significant in practice. In fact, it is the health departments of the districts that decide in concrete cases whom to quarantine or which businesses to close. Inasmuch as the implementation of numerous competences, both federal and from the *Länder*, is concentrated in the district authorities, the role they play in the state machinery is undramatic and often even unacknowledged, yet for all that, crucial (Bußjäger et al. 2018).

In the context of Covid-19, the extent to which they made a difference depended critically on the staff capacities each *Land* assigned to them and their approach to tackling the pandemic. For example, Innsbruck's authorities – which were in charge of dealing with the couple from Lombardy who were Austria's first identified Covid-19 cases – were far more efficient in testing and quarantining contact persons than the district commission of Landeck was in regard to the cases in Ischgl. Indeed, this comparison contributed to accusations that business interests hindered interventions by the authorities in Landeck. Precisely because they were so pivotal in implementing Covid-19 measures on the ground, district commissioners complained to the Minister of Health about ever-changing, unrealistic rules that were difficult to put into practice and criticised a lack of communication by the federal government (Wiener Zeitung 2020). The minister reacted by inviting them to a direct exchange but also pointed to his intensive talks with the health boards of the *Länder* and their duty – within indirect federal administration – to keep the districts informed.

While the Constitution generally accords municipalities a lesser role in health care than it does the districts, they were of course still critical in the fight against Covid-19, for instance in their efforts to provide information and coordinate the activities of local stakeholders, including volunteers. With local governments at the forefront of providing basic services, they were key to keeping crucial public sector activities running during the lockdown. There were urgent needs, for example, to switch to digitalised services and to reorganise child care and public transportation to suit the conditions dictated by the pandemic. Quite often municipalities came to the rescue of crisis-ridden local companies by deferring the payment of fees or even availing direct financial assistance. The role of municipalities was thus less concerned with the health emergency itself than with its impact, not least of all its economic impact.

4.4.5 Intergovernmental relations

Relations between governments were marked on the whole, especially in the early stages of the pandemic, by a high level of cooperation. However, this was not collaboration on an equal footing, as the *Länder* long felt comfortable with letting the federal government take the lead. Given the lack of significant pre-existing institutions of emergency management (see section 4.3), cooperative governance took place by means of general mechanisms of intergovernmental relations. Informal contacts as well as the Conference of the *Länder* Governors (*Landeshauptleutekonferenz*) played a role. At a gathering on 15 May 2020 of this conference, which is much more powerful in representing subnational interests than the second chamber (Kössler 2016: 363f), the governors expressly referred to 'successful federalism' as the recipe for making Austria 'healthy and strong again'.

This relatively harmonious picture does not mean, of course, that relations were devoid of failures of cooperation or outright conflict; indeed, intergovernmental tension increased over time. Early examples concerning restrictions of free movement included an internal order (*Erlass*) issued by the Minister of Health shortly before Easter to the *Länder* governors that they prohibit 'all meetings in a closed room attended by more than five persons not living in the same household'. Even though the federal government retracted the order, explaining that it had meant only to ban 'corona parties' and not families' Easter celebrations, there was a time lag during which district administrative authorities upheld the ordinances based on this order. The resultant confusion could have been avoided by more efficient intergovernmental communication.

Another controversy revolved around an ordinance in which Burgenland's governor stipulated that this *Land*'s most popular lake could be visited only by people who resided within 15 km of it. This was to avoid large crowds and thus a higher risk of infection. While section 2 of the Covid-19 Measures Act certainly allowed the governor to regulate access to a specific public place such as a lake, the federal government demanded uniform rules regarding swimming lakes. This episode is emblematic of how relations between single *Länder* and the national government differed because they showed different levels of subnational activism. For example, whereas Burgenland pushed to have its own solution, the *Land* Carinthia called for the national government to act and establish countrywide rules.

Subsequent conflicts related to measures imposed at Austria's borders when fears that holiday returnees would 'import' the virus led to the introduction of health checks. While the health departments of the districts carried out fever measurements and, where necessary, a coronavirus test, they were, from an organisational perspective, subject to their *Land* government and assisted by military troops sent by the federal government.[5] With traffic jams of several hours occurring at certain border crossings, the intergovernmental blame game would soon start. The Minister of Health stated that this *Land* had misinterpreted the relevant ordinance by performing more than just random checks, but Carinthia complained about a lack of clear communication.

When infection numbers increased rapidly in early September 2020 (despite the border checks), another field of intergovernmental friction came to the fore. The federal government accused certain *Länder* and the health departments of their districts of being too slow regarding so-called TTI ('testing, tracing, and isolating'). In turn, Vienna not only blamed everything on the allegedly premature lifting of the federal lockdown but also frantically started to increase staff capacity dedicated to these tasks. The *Länder* had been free to find different solutions. Indeed, some supported understaffed district health departments with civil servants from other departments or other districts, or with military troops provided by the federal government, while others relied primarily on hiring (medical) students on a short-term basis.

4.4.6 Intergovernmental fiscal relations

In Austria, most of the revenue at all levels of government is generated as part of a shared taxation system, and fiscal resources depend, in the absence of extensive constitutional regulations,[6] on an ordinary federal law, that is, the Financial Equalisation Law, which is adopted every four years and determines for each single tax the revenue portions of the various government levels. Even if the legislative process involves tripartite talks, negotiators are in fact not on an equal footing, and *Länder* and municipalities 'really have no legal alternative but to accept the determination of fiscal relations by the federal government' (Bußjäger 2005: 61). Eighty-four per cent of the total revenue raised in Austria falls within this shared taxation system, and from these funds 68 per cent have gone since 2018 to the federal government, 20 per cent to the *Länder*, and 12 per cent to the municipalities (Federal Ministry of Finance n.d.). The fact that virtually all lucrative sources are shared taxes entails that the economic downturn in the wake of Covid-19 would have an equal impact on all three government levels, especially due to diminishing receipts from corporate and personal income taxes.

However, revenue shortages from joint taxes are, in relative terms, particularly damaging for the *Länder* because they do not enjoy much fiscal autonomy. Admittedly, they are allowed to 'invent' taxes not mentioned in the Financial Equalisation Law. But the latter is so comprehensive that it does not leave much space for this. Despite perennial discussions (or sham fights), increased tax autonomy has never been realised due to a certain reluctance on the part of the *Länder* and to the fact that the federal government offers them only marginal taxes with limited revenue.

As for Austria's municipalities, they faced significant income losses in shared taxes, which in 2018 accounted for 39 per cent of their revenues,[7] as well as in certain exclusive local taxes. Receipts from a municipal tax (*Kommunalsteuer*) that employers have to pay based on the gross income of their employees were expected to shrink by 20–40 per cent. Reduced payments due to rising unemployment and a widely used partial furlough scheme (*Kurzarbeit*) account for that. Tight municipal budgets were also the result of reduced income from tourist taxes or fees for public services, such as child care. At the same time, municipalities are responsible for many basic services, such as water supply, so their room for manoeuvre in cutting costs was limited. Clearly, the financial impact of the pandemic on municipalities was highly differentiated, with those reliant on tourism or other businesses hard-hit by Covid-19 bearing the brunt.

As early as 15 March 2020, when the Austrian parliament passed the first pandemic-related bills, a support package was announced, including direct emergency help, credit guarantees, and tax deferments. For municipalities, EUR 1 billion was to be provided to cover local investments under a 50 per cent co-financing scheme. However, it was likely that some municipalities would fail to reach the co-financing quota. Moreover, the aid received was forecast to be in effect equalised by EUR 1.1 billion that municipalities would lose in revenue due to tax cuts envisaged in Austria's recovery package to stimulate the economy (Mitterer 2020). In view of shrinking resources, it was certain that intergovernmental fiscal relations would remain tense.

4.5 Findings and policy implications

When it comes to health care and federalism, it has been a mantra of critics, especially health economists (Trukeschitz et al. 2013: 174) but so too the Austrian Court of Auditors (Rechnungshof 2010), that far-reaching *Länder* competences have resulted in fragmentation and an inefficient proliferation of hospitals with more beds than are actually needed. The irony is that the high numbers of hospital beds, not least of all in ICU units, turned out to be a major asset in Austria's Covid-19 response. There is a good chance that decentralised service provision will come to be appreciated again and that the creed of efficiency, often idolised as an undisputed guiding principle within mindsets strongly inclined towards centralisation, will be re-assessed. A question, then, is whether this will be limited to the era of Covid-19 or lead to lasting long-term change.

This same question of permanent or merely temporary change is also key when it comes to considering the centralisation that the Covid-19 emergency brought about. There can be little doubt that a double centralisation of decision-making occurred in the early stages through an accumulation of power horizontally in the hands of the executive branch and vertically at the national government level. In May 2020, it was claimed, for good reason, that Covid-19 turned Austria into a 'decentralized de facto unitary state' (Bußjäger 2020b). Nevertheless, these tendencies – set in motion without using constitutional emergency powers – do not reflect a profound change but rather re-emphasise trends towards centralisation that were already in existence in 'normal times'. To be sure, there were certain cautious efforts to reduce centralisation for the sake of more autonomy and differentiation in autumn 2020, namely the 'coronavirus traffic light system' and the new rules for ordinances under the reformed federal Covid-19 legislation. But the sustainability of these efforts is in doubt and they are unlikely to alter the underlying centralist tendencies.

It is therefore nearly impossible to assess whether Austria's federal dispensation has been a boon or bane in managing the pandemic. The truth is that federalism has hardly been noticeable in the making of key decisions at the time of this writing. It is thus somewhat misleading to argue that the country 'fared surprisingly well in the current crisis' despite its 'strong federalism' (Czypionka 2020). First, the largely centralised management of the pandemic follows from the fact that the public health competence of the national government under article 10(1)(12) of the Constitution overshadows for the duration of the emergency the *Länder* competences and enables it to intervene in what are otherwise subnational prerogatives. Second, this key provision envisages public health as a matter for indirect federal administration. On the one hand, this form of mixed administration compels all authorities to cooperate; on the other, the federal government has legal instruments to enforce its will vis-à-vis the state governors, even if their power of instruction meets factual limits, for example in the staff capacities of the subordinated authorities (Bußjäger 2020a). While district administrative authorities have considerable functions in practice, even more so in a complex emergency like Covid-19, and the *Land* Governor is central because of his or her instructions to the districts and other members of the *Land* government, one person remains at the top of the legal hierarchy: the Minister of Health. Politically, of course, he is also dependent on these subordinate authorities for implementation and is thus to some extent forced to compromise.

It is true that the Minister of Health came to be challenged more and more and that intergovernmental relations suffered increasingly from disputes as the pandemic dragged on. However, these conflicts were not as numerous and fundamental as they were in many other countries. To some extent, this is linked to the well-known argument that Austria, due to its societal homogeneity, has a higher tolerance for centralism than other countries because there is, compared to multinational federations with territorially based distinctiveness, clearly less pressure towards decentralisation (Erk 2004). On closer inspection, many of what appear to be intergovernmental conflicts are skirmishes following the logic of party politics. Several of the disputes in autumn 2020 concerned Vienna and have to be seen in the context of tensions between the conservatives leading the national government and the Social Democrats ruling the capital which were further amplified in the run-up to elections in Vienna on 11 October. True intergovernmental conflicts based on ambitions of the *Länder* to go their own way remained relatively limited compared to other countries. Nonetheless, the onset of a second wave of infection saw increasing tension, with subnational governments being more proactive in some instances and the national government explicitly urging them to be more active and adopt stricter measures in other instances. Austria therefore still oscillates between, on the one hand, cautious attempts towards greater autonomy and differentiation and, on the other, the move from national unity to a de facto unitary state, one which has characterised the country's particular brand of 'pandemic federalism'.

Notes

1 From a legal point of view, these are, at one and the same time, municipalities and district administrative authorities. On their role, see Kössler and Kress (2021).
2 Several countries made use of this right in spring 2020, among them, for instance, Estonia, Romania and Serbia.
3 The constitutional lawyer Bernd-Christian Funk quoted in Brickner (2020).
4 The Constitutional Court could also have decided to hold an extra session until 30 April 2020 when the legal measures were still in force. Moreover, even legal acts not in force anymore in June could still have had legal effects and thus have been far from irrelevant. For instance, the ordinance regulating entry to public places was the basis for fines challenged in ongoing administrative penalty proceedings; the fact that the Court invalidated parts of this ordinance meant that these fines were not payable anymore.
5 The involvement of the army might seem odd to an external observer. But beyond military defence (Constitution, article 79(1)), the civilian administration may assign to the Austrian army several additional tasks, among them 'to render assistance in the case of natural catastrophes and disasters of exceptional magnitude' (article 79(2)(2)).
6 Article 13 of the Constitution merely refers to the Financial Constitutional Law of 1948, which provides only general principles for tax allocation and abstract types of taxes and itself authorises the federal legislator to assign taxes concretely through the Financial Equalisation Law.
7 For an examination of the shares of various municipal income components and how they are affected by Covid-19, see Biwald and Mitterer (2020).

References

APA. 2020. '*Anschober: Corona-Ampel soll nicht mehr jede Woche umgeschaltet werden*', *Der Standard*, 15 September, https://www.derstandard.at/story/2000120036372/anschober-will-kommunikation-wieder-einfacher-machen (accessed on 10 November 2020).

Biwald, Peter and Karoline Mitterer. 2020. '*Städte und Gemeinden in der Corona-Krise: Ist ein Rettungspaket notwendig?*', *KDZ*, http://kdz.eu/de/aktuelles/blog/staedte-und-gemeinden-der-corona-krise-ist-ein-rettungspaket-notwendig (accessed on 14 November 2020).

Brickner, Irene. 2020. '*Anschober und Co stolpern über ein veraltetes Gesetz und Fehler von früher*', *Der Standard*, 2 August, https://www.derstandard.at/story/2000119117395/anschober-und-co-stolpern-ueber-ein-veraltetes-gesetz-und-fehler (accessed on 10 November 2020).

Bußjäger, Peter. 2005. 'Reforms on Fiscal Federalism in Austria', in Gerhard Robbers (ed.), *Reforming Federalism: Foreign Experiences for a Reform in Germany*. Bern: Peter Lang.

Bußjäger, Peter. 2020a. 'COVID-19 Crisis Challenging Austria's Cooperative Federalism', *Föderalismus-Blog*. 28 April, https://www.foederalismus.at/blog/covid-19-crisis-challenging-austria%E2%80%99s-cooperative-federalism_235.php (accessed on 14 November 2020).

Bußjäger, Peter. 2020b. '*Das B-VG im exekutiven, dezentralisierten de-facto Einheitsstaat, oder: Souverän ist, wer das Ende des Ausnahmezustands definiert?*', *100 Jahre B-VG*, 20 May, https://www.uibk.ac.at/oeffentliches-recht/100-jahre-b-vg/das-b-vg-im-exekutiven-dezentralisierten-de-facto-einheitsstaat.html (accessed on 14 November 2020).

Bußjäger, Peter, et al. 2018. *Kontinuität und Wandel: Von 'guter Polizey' zum Bürgerservice: Festschrift 150 Jahre Bezirkshauptmannschaften.* Vienna: New Academic Press.

Consumer Protection Association. 2020. 'Class Action: Coronavirus-Tyrol', https://www.verbraucherschutzverein.at/Corona-Virus-Tirol/ (accessed on 9 December 2020).

Czypionka, Thomas 2020. 'Austria's Response to the Coronavirus Pandemic: A Second Perspective', *Cambridge Core Blog*, 12 April, https://www.cambridge.org/core/blog/2020/04/12/austrias-response-to-the-coronavirus-pandemic-a-second-perspective/ (accessed on 14 November 2020).

Erk, Jan. 2004. 'Austria: A Federation without Federalism', *Publius*, 34(1): 1–20.

Federal Ministry of Finance. n.d. '*Besteuerungsrechte und Abgabenerträge*', https://www.bmf.gv.at/themen/budget/finanzbeziehungen-laender-gemeinden/besteuerungsrechte-abgabenertraege.html (accessed on 9 December 2020).

Gamper, Anna. 2020. 'Austrian Federalism and the Corona Pandemic', *Föderalismus-Blog*, 5 June, https://www.foederalismus.at/blog/austrian-federalism-and-the-corona-pandemic_237.php (accessed on 14 November 2020).

Ginsburg, Tom and Mila Versteeg. 2020. 'The Bound Executive: Emergency Powers during the Pandemic', Virginia Public Law and Legal Theory Research Paper No. 2020-52. Public Law Working Paper No. 747. University of Chicago.

Kössler, Karl. 2016. 'Reform of the Second Chamber or Its Perpetuation? The Austrian Dilemma and Its Implications for the Italian Senate', *Istituzioni del Federalismo*, 37(2): 339–70.

Kössler, Karl and Annika Kress. 2021. 'European Cities between Self-Government and Subordination: Their Role as Policy-Takers and Policy-Makers', in Ernst Hirsch Ballin et al. (eds.), *European Yearbook of Constitutional Law 2020: The City in Constitutional Law.* T.M.C. Asser Press, 273–302.

Kostera, Thomas. 2013. 'Subnational Responsibilities for Healthcare and Austria's Rejection of the EU's Patients' Rights Directive', *Health Policy* 111: 149–56.

Kroisleitner, Oona and Gabriele Scherndl. 2020. '*Lockerungsverordnung im Detail:Was darf ich mit wem machen?*', *Der Standard*, 1 May, https://www.derstandard.at/story/2000117230404/lockerungsverordnung-im-detail-was-darf-ich-mit-wem-machen?ref=article (accessed on 10 November 2020).

Lachmayer, Konrad. 2020. 'Austria: Rule of Law Lacking in Times of Crisis', *VerfBlog*, 28 April, https://verfassungsblog.de/rule-of-law-lacking-in-times-of-crisis/ (accessed on 14 November 2020).

Marchart, Jan M. and Nina Weißensteiner. 2020. '*Mit fünf fragwürdigen Gesetzespassagen gegen die Pandemie*', *Der Standard*, 16 September, https://www.derstandard.at/story/2000120029100/mit-fuenf-fragwuerdigen-gesetzespassagen-gegen-die-pandemie (accessed on 14 November 2020).

Mitterer, Karoline. 2020. '*Corona-Krise trifft Gemeinden auch 2021 stark: Weitere Unterstützungsmaßnahmen sind erforderlich*', *KDZ*, http://kdz.eu/de/presse/corona-krise-trifft-gemeinden-auch-2021-stark (accessed on 10 November 2020).

Möllers, Christoph. 2020. '*Parlamentarische Selbstentmächtigung im Zeichen des Virus*', *VerfBlog*, 26 March, https://verfassungsblog.de/parlamentarische-selbstentmaechtigung-im-zeichen-des-virus/ (accessed on 10 November 2020).

OECD. 2020. 'Health at a Glance 2017: OECD Indicators. How Does Austria Compare?', https://www.oecd.org/austria/Health-at-a-Glance-2017-Key-Findings-AUSTRIA.pdf (access 9 December 2020) (accessed on 9 December 2020).

Palermo, Francesco. 2020. '*La gestione della crisi pandemica in Austria: regolarità costituzionale e qualche distonia politica*', *DPCE Online*, 43(2), http://www.dpceonline.it/index.php/dpceonline/article/view/979 (accessed on 10 November 2020).

Palermo, Francesco and Karl Kössler. 2017. *Comparative Federalism: Constitutional Arrangements and Case Law*. Oxford: Hart Publishing.

Rechnungshof. 2010. '*Verwaltungsreform Problemanalyse Gesundheit und Pflege*', https://www.rechnungshof.gv.at/rh/home/home_1/home_6/Verwaltungsreform_2011.pdf (accessed on 10 November 2020).

Somek, Alexander. 2020. 'Is the Constitution Law for the Court Only? A Reply to Sebastian Kurz', *VerfBlog*, 16 April, https://verfassungsblog.de/is-the-constitution-law-for-the-court-only/ (accessed on 10 November 2020).

Trukeschitz, Birgit, Ulrike Schneider and Thomas Czypionka. 2013. 'Federalism in Health and Social Care in Austria', in Joan Costa-Font and Scott L. Greer (eds.), *Federalism and Decentralization in European Health and Social Care*. Palgrave Macmillan.

Wiener Zeitung. 2020. 'Lokale Macht und Ohnmacht', *Wiener Zeitung*, 29 August, https://www.wienerzeitung.at/nachrichten/politik/oesterreich/2073177-Lokale-Macht-und-Ohnmacht.html (accessed on 9 December 2020).

5

MANAGING THE COVID-19 CRISIS IN A DIVIDED BELGIAN FEDERATION

Cooperation against all odds

Patricia Popelier and Peter Bursens

5.1 Introduction

When it recorded its first case of Covid-19 on 3 February 2020, Belgium was in the midst of a political crisis. Since the fall of its government in December 2018 and elections in May 2019, political parties had still not succeeded in forming a new federal government. The antagonism between the two major parties, the Flemish nationalist *Nieuw-Vlaamse Alliantie* and the francophone social democratic *Parti Socialiste*, was intensified by the elections, which resulted in deepened division between Flemish and Walloon voters and an unprecedented rise of extremist parties on either side of the spectrum. Meanwhile, a caretaker minority government stayed on, backed by temporary parliamentary support, until a new government was formed eventually on 1 October 2020, now backed by a parliamentary majority of seven parties – a transition that took place at a moment when infections were on the rise again.

This chapter examines how a divided Belgian federation responded to the Covid-19 pandemic, with the period of analysis extending from February to October 2020 and thus covering the full cycle of the first wave – including the outbreak in February, the peak in spring, and the low point in summer – and the beginning of a second outbreak at the end of summer. The shift from the first to the second wave coincided with the start of a new federal government, a turn of affairs that was accompanied by some changes of response, among them to the approach taken to intergovernmental relations (IGR).

With a population of 11.5 million, Belgium is a relatively small country, but it is deeply divided along converging cleavages between the north (Dutch-speaking, prosperous, and voting predominantly centre-right) and the south (French-speaking, less prosperous, and voting predominantly left). To accommodate these tensions, the country transformed itself over three decades from a

DOI: 10.4324/9781003166771-7

unitary, decentralised state into a dyadic federation with confederal traits; subsequent reforms decentralised it further.

Belgium thus consists of six overlapping federated entities: three communities with language- and culture-related competences (Flemish, French, and German) and three regions (Flemish, Walloon, and Brussels) with economic- and territory-based competences. However, politics revolves around the two major (French-speaking and Dutch-speaking) linguistic communities. When the Covid-19 crisis hit Belgium, even the French-speaking press, hitherto centralist in spirit, agreed that the country was split into two separate democracies.[1]

Public concern in Belgium about the coronavirus mounted during the spring break at the end of February when Covid-19 case numbers began to rise dramatically, especially in the north of Italy, where many Belgians go skiing; as they returned from their travels, so the number of domestic infections increased. It was nevertheless only on 13 March 2020, two days after Covid-19 claimed its first fatality in Belgium, that the federal government initiated health measures, following which a more drastic lockdown was imposed on 18 March.

By mid-April, at the height of the crisis, Belgium was at the top of the list of Covid-19 deaths per capita worldwide, with a fatality rate of 359 per million residents.[2] Unlike those of other countries, its statistics included fatalities – mostly in elderly homes – that were probably caused by Covid-19 but not officially confirmed as such (Wilmès 2020: 5). Still, the coronavirus undoubtedly hit hard in Belgium. The country's high population density, its open economy at Europe's crossroads, and the return of tourists from heavily infected areas in the Italian, Austrian and French Alps, help to explain this fact.

In April, reports emerged that the economy was beginning to stagnate due to the pandemic, and in May, Belgium announced its first exit measures from the nationwide lockdown. Others followed in quick succession, until the signs of a second outbreak came to notice at the end of July. Further relaxation measures were put on hold, and new restrictions were introduced, or older ones reinstated. However, in September, schools were able to reopen for the new school year, albeit under tight conditions. At that point in the year, the government decided, in spite of a rising number of infections, not to impose stricter measures but to relax contact arrangements again in order to keep citizens motivated.

As Belgium has a high-performing health-care system, the maximum capacity of its hospitals was never exhausted. The main problem lay in the area of prevention: it had no strategic supply of face masks and lacked testing capacity. Consequently, and despite a travel ban, the virus spread quickly in elderly homes and residential care centres. Many of the subject-matter domains relevant to the crisis were competences of the federated communities, but there was immediate and widespread consensus that, for the country to fight Covid-19, the federal government had to take the lead.

At first, no distinction was made between regions, in that public data did not specify the location of infections and hospitalisations. This changed at the start of the second wave of the pandemic, when a ministerial decree ordered local authorities to determine in which shopping streets it would be mandatory to wear face masks, and also empowered them to take additional preventative measures (Ministerial Decree of 24 July 2020, article 13). Local governments, until then subordinate implementers of central policy, now came to the fore.

In the sections that follow, this chapter explains the Belgian system of power allocation and IGR and provides an overview of government action at the federal, federated, and local levels of authority. This will reveal three important findings. First, Covid-19 – perhaps temporarily – turned dual federalism into cooperative federalism, with the federal government occupying a prominent position in inter-governmental decision-making. Secondly, the local level of authority popped up as a relevant actor that should be factored into the design of future systems of pandemic crisis management. Thirdly, calls in Belgium for institutional reform should keep in mind that, whatever the result of such reform, it is crucial to provide clarity in the allocation of competences and to develop a scheme for more efficient inter-governmental coordination and cooperation, especially in the case of pandemics.

5.2 The federal constitutional and legislative framework

5.2.1 The allocation of competences

Belgium follows a model of dual federalism, with an allocation system based on exclusivity. This means that, as a rule, matters lie within the legislative and administrative competence of the federal authorities, the communities, or the regions, to the exclusion of the other entities. A side effect of exclusivity is fragmentation: if the federal government loses control over transferred matters and is not able to intervene in the general interest or secure inter-regional solidarity, it is inclined to transfer only parts of the matter and set restrictions on its use (Popelier 2021a). This entails that parts of a policy field are attributed to the federated entities, whereas others remain within the ambit of central powers, making it difficult to develop coherent and encompassing policies without cooperation among entities (Happaerts et al. 2012: 444). It also means that competences are formulated in a detailed way, with specific conditions and exceptions.[3]

Several of the matters related to preventing and containing Covid-19 were transferred to the communities, albeit with many exceptions. Together, there are four categories of community competences: person-related competences and competences in education, culture, and languages. Each is discussed below.

In terms of the Special Majority Law on the Reform of Institutions, health care, including residential-care institutions, is a community matter that falls under the category of person-related competences (article 5, section 1, I). However, in the development of this law, only specific aspects of health care were transferred to the communities, and even those aspects contained several exceptions that remained federal. For example, organic laws and financial laws on hospitals remain federal, as do basic and financial rules pertaining to medical institutions as well as to health and disability insurance. Also, only the federal government can impose an obligation to vaccinate. By contrast, promoting and providing vaccinations and taking quarantining and contact tracing measures are (mostly) community matters, whereas the federal government has the power to issue basic rules, for example with regard to the right to privacy.[4] In addition, the communities have the power to issue preventative regulations only for specific matters and institutions, while general rules remained a federal competence. A number of social-welfare community competences are closely associated with health care, including child care, family care, and elderly care.

Education is the sole competence that was transferred in its entirety by the Constitution itself, barring only three exceptions: determining the beginning and end of compulsory schooling, setting minimum standards for granting diplomas, and administering the teachers' pension scheme; the latter all remained federal competences (Constitution, article 127, sections 1, 2). Finally, cultural competences – applying to areas such as youth policy, libraries, museums, fine arts, and sports and leisure activities (Special Majority Law on the Reform of Institutions, article 4) – were transferred to the communities, mostly without specific exceptions.

Preventative measures that impact on business operations and labour conditions, such as the closure of shops and promotion of telework, are federal matters. In turn, measures to mitigate the economic consequences of pandemic response fall under both federal and regional competences. Economic affairs such as tourism and commercial rentals are a regional competence, but many of their aspects remain federal, such as financial policy, commercial law, labour law, and social security (Special Majority Law on the Reform of Institutions, article 6, section 1, VI). As a result, during the 2020 pandemic, different subsidy mechanisms were developed at the federal and regional level. Preventative measures in response to Covid-19 also affected other regional competences, such as public transport.

Finally, at supranational level, the European Union (EU) limited Belgian authorities' discretion in combating the Covid-19 pandemic. For example, the regulation of medicines remains a residual federal competence but is controlled mostly at the EU level. Also, the principles of free movement prohibit border control and closure, except in the case of serious threat and for a limited period of time. On that basis, the federal government, by ministerial decree, closed the country's borders on 20 March 2020 (Vanheule 2020: 1448). Further restrictions arose from coordinated action by the European Council; the European Commission also engaged in coordination efforts, in its case ones that were directed, for instance, at public procurement of protective gear and at repatriating EU citizens from countries throughout the world.

5.2.2 The absence of an emergency clause

Belgium is a dual federation, which means that the federal and federated jurisdictions are conceived as separate entities with exclusive powers and on an equal footing; by implication, the federal government has no overriding powers.

Fittingly, the Constitution does not even mention a state of emergency, conventionally the occasion for centralisation of power in the national executive branch – an emergency situation is only implied where it provides that it is the King who declares the existence of a state of war (article 167, section 1). The federal government does have residual powers, but these must respect the constitutional allocation of powers.

This raises the question of whether the federal government may invoke police powers to encroach upon federated policy domains, for example when closing schools and museums, prohibiting cultural and sports events, or deciding under which conditions such organisations and activities can resume. One could argue that crisis management in the case of a pandemic is inherently part of the government's residual emergency powers, given that the risk of infection threatens the entire country, which though small is densely populated.

However, the Council of State, the supreme administrative court in Belgium, warned on various occasions that the federal government does not have the exclusive residual competence to take all urgent matters but that each government is instead responsible within its own field of competences.[5] Its suggestion that a cooperation agreement or explicit legal solution be adopted was not acted upon, though. Indeed, one could argue equally that because sources of infection are concentrated in specific regions, a differentiated approach is what is called for, and that police powers are inherent to the executive office at all tiers of government.

5.3 Preparedness for a national disaster: The institutional framework

Following an EU Decision, member states are under a duty to communicate information to the EU network operated by the European Centre for Disease Prevention and Control (ECDC) (EU Decision 2013). To this end,[6] a Protocol was concluded between the federal government and the communities to establish a National Focal Point.[7]

The same Protocol also established a Risk Management Group (RMG) and a Risk Assessment Group (RAG). The first is composed of representatives from the federal and subnational ministries of health and decides on notification and control measures. The second is an advisory body composed of experts from the health authorities and epidemiologists of the Belgian Institute for Health (Sciensano), along with medical scientists from universities on both sides of the language divide, who are invited ad hoc to the body. The RAG takes care of the daily surveillance of potential health threats and prepares risk assessments. The politically responsible body is the Inter-ministerial Conference on Public Health, composed of the ministers responsible for public health at the federal and community levels; the coordinating crisis manager is appointed by the federal government. It is, however, up to each entity to implement the decisions within its respective range of competences (Protocol 2018, article 6, section 1).

5.4 Rolling out measures to contain the pandemic

5.4.1 Taking the initiative

As mentioned, the Covid-19 health crisis struck Belgium in the middle of a political crisis. Given the dual nature of Belgian federalism and the extensive powers communities have in health policy, one would have expected them to take the initiative in response to the pandemic. Nonetheless, there seemed to be wide consensus that – in consultation with the communities and regions – it was the federal government that had to take the lead.

The most visible body during the first wave of infection was the National Security Council (NSC), the composition of which reflects that it was established with terrorism threats in mind. It consists of the Prime Minister, the ministers of justice, defence, home affairs and foreign affairs, the vice-ministers, and other ministers in matters under their competence (Royal Decree of 28 January 2015), in this case the Minister of Health. To deal with the Covid-19 pandemic, the NSC was extended to the regional minister-presidents. It was supported by the National Crisis Centre, which has three monitoring and advisory bodies: the RAG, the RMG, and the Scientific Committee Coronavirus. These bodies report to an Evaluation Cell (CELEVAL) consisting of representatives of health administrations and advisory bodies at national and subnational levels; in turn, CELEVAL reports to the different governments.

The NSC convened for the first time on 10 and 12 March 2020. On 13 March, the federal phase of the coordination of Belgium's pandemic response was announced and the first measures taken: cultural, social, festive, sports, and youth activities as well as religious services were prohibited; cultural, festive, recreation, and sports establishments as well as bars and restaurants were closed; and non-food stores were closed on weekends (Ministerial Decrees of 13 March 2020). Only four days later, several political parties, still unable to form a government, agreed to give the minority government of Sophie Wilmès full powers, with the promise to request a new vote of confidence after six months (Royal Decree of 17 March 2020).

Then, on 27 March, the government received special powers to take measures to address the crisis and mitigate its consequences, if need be by passing Acts of Parliament (Laws I and II of 27 March 2020 authorising the King to take measures to combat the spread of the coronavirus (Covid-19)), albeit with several formal and informal guarantees. For example, special power decrees have to be ratified by Parliament within one year, in addition to which 10 political parties acted as watchdogs in weekly meetings to discuss the Covid-19 decrees.

In the end, these special powers have not been used for preventative measures. They were taken by ministerial decree, even though their constitutionality was doubtful (Popelier 2020a, 2020b). On 18 March, the Minister of Internal Affairs decreed a more severe lockdown, one that included the closure of schools, further restrictions on shops, and a ban on travelling abroad other than for essential purposes (Ministerial Decree of 18 March 2020).

CELEVAL was replaced on 6 April by a multidisciplinary expert group, the Group of Experts in Charge of the Exit Strategy (GEES), consisting of medical, economic, statistical, legal, and financial experts and tasked with developing an exit strategy from Belgium's initial lockdown. At the start of a second wave of infections, GEES was replaced by CELEVAL, the membership of which was broadened and included representatives of scientific research institutes, business, and the event sector, as well as medical, psychology, and health economics experts.

Political parties in power at both the regional and federal level, aware of the need for urgency, seemed to agree that the federal government has a residual power in regard to health crisis management; it was less clear, though, on how far this power extends. For example, the federal government started a programme for contact tracing but had to leave it to the communities once the Council of State made it clear that this competence (mostly) remained with the communities.[8] In another example, protective masks and equipment were simultaneously procured at several levels of government, with major issues arising in mid-April 2020 about quality requirements for materials and the use of testing kits. The responsible federal minister himself complained about 'absurd' situations regarding competences and coordination (Andries 2020).

Either way, the proportionality (or loyalty) principle demands that measures cannot make it impossible or arduous for other entities to pursue their policies unless these entities are involved in the decision-making. This means that regardless of who has the final say in which matter, governments are forced to cooperate. In practice, political actors in 2020 chose to allow the federal government to take the lead, but communities and regions could implement the measures according to their competences. This sometimes led to awkward results as when, for example, a federal ministerial decree stated that communities should plan for a resumption of teaching activities on the basis of expert advice (Ministerial Decree of 15 May 2020, article 4): even though it was undisputed that emergency measures should rely on expert advice, it was not for the federal minister to impose procedural requirements.

In a third phase of pandemic governance, a differentiated approach was taken after all, one that hence brought local entities to the fore. Mayors and provincial governors have police powers of their own, but in March 2020 a ministerial decree announced the federal phase of the coordination of the coronavirus crisis (Ministerial Decree of 13 March 2020a), a regime in terms of which local entities were to be merely implementers of federal and federated decisions.

In July, however, more detailed information was made available as to where exactly new outbreaks were situated. A ministerial decree that ordered face masks to be worn in specific places, including in shopping streets, required that mayors delineate those streets; it also allowed mayors and provincial governors to take 'complementing' and, where necessary, 'additional' measures.

On this basis, the provincial governor of severely hit Antwerp province made it compulsory to wear face masks in public and imposed a (controversial) nightly curfew (Ordinance of 29 July of the Governor of the Province of Antwerp). In addition, the Flemish government, when its own system proved inadequate, reluctantly permitted local entities to develop their own system of contact tracing.

The discussion above presented the chronology of the measures taken. In the following sections, we dig deeper into the type of measures taken by the different government levels and then turn to IGR. Federal actions were taken mostly by the government – the federal parliament remained largely absent. Also, whenever a ministerial decree touched upon the powers of the federated entities, the executives of the regions and communities took care of the implementation without much involvement from the respective parliaments. This was the trend particularly in the French Community and the Walloon and Brussels regions.

5.4.2 Federal action

At the federal level, five types of measures were taken: (1) preventative, (2) health care, (3) exit, (4) socio-economic, and (5) measures to mitigate other measures. Several measures were challenged in the Council of State.

5.4.2.1 Preventative measures

Preventative measures to contain the spread of the virus in 2020 came in two waves. In the first wave, shops were closed, with some exceptions for essential services such as food shops and pharmacies; firms were ordered to close or switch to teleworking; bars and restaurants were closed (except for takeaways); school, cultural, sports, recreation, and social establishments were closed and (almost) all activities forbidden; people were ordered to stay at home except for essential activities (including walks); and travel abroad was forbidden.

These decisions were taken after long negotiations, with Flemish politicians preferring the Dutch approach that gave more consideration to economic activities, and French-speaking politicians leaning more towards the French approach which prioritised public health. In the end, all parties agreed on a drastic lockdown, even if this intruded in subnational domains. For example, although Flemish political parties preferred to keep schools open and it is the case that education is a community competence, they agreed that teaching activities should be suspended by a federal ministerial decree.

When a second wave was looming in mid-July, measures were less drastic (Ministerial Decree of 10 July 2020). Shops, bars, and restaurants stayed open conditional on certain preventative measures; the wearing of face masks was obligatory in specific public places and shopping streets; dance halls, discotheques, wellness centres, and hammams were forbidden; people could gather only in groups of a maximum of 10 persons, with some exceptions; non-essential travel was allowed within the EU with the exception of 'red zones'; and close contact was limited to five persons per household. Some local authorities, at the municipal level as well as at provincial level used the opportunity provided by the ministerial decree to take additional measures to counter local surges of infections.

5.4.2.2 Health-care measures

Steps were taken to give health-care providers full capacity in terms of staff, infrastructure, and equipment. These included regulations on the sale, distribution, commissioning, and use of rapid self-tests, medical devices, personal protective equipment and biocides, and on the triage of potentially infected persons.

5.4.2.3 Exit measures

Exit measures enabled the relaxation of initial controls and reopening of business and other services. On 24 March 2020, the NSC announced a phased exit strategy that would begin in early May and gradually allow greater social and economic activity, including the phased reopening of schools (a community competence). In its decision-making, the NSC relied on the advice of the multidisciplinary expert group GEES. The measures followed one after the other at a surprisingly fast pace until, at the end of July, signs of a new outbreak forced the government to put further relaxations on hold and take a new set of preventative measures.

5.4.2.4 Socio-economic measures

Steps were also taken to mitigate the pandemic's socio-economic consequences. Among these were measures to support ('viable') firms by means of government guarantees for credit granted by credit institution, lower value-added tax (VAT) rates for restaurants, or subsidies for self-employed persons who were temporarily unable to pursue their activities. Employees could fall back on temporary unemployment relief, a system already in existence but now amended with simplified procedures and increased wages.

5.4.2.5 Measures to mitigate other measures

Measures were adopted to deal with the repercussions that preventative measures had for ongoing activities, obligations, and requirements. For instance, the functioning of essential services such as federal administrations and the national rail network had to be ensured, and measures put in place to discontinue or extend terms, for example in litigation procedures.

5.4.2.6 Challenges in the council of state

The special powers above were used mainly for type 5 measures and only occasionally for type 3 or 4 measures. Most type 4 measures were based on Acts of Parliaments, whereas all type 1 and 2 measures were issued by a ministerial decree. The ministerial decrees were challenged before the Council of State on several occasions. Within the period under review, the Council ruled on suspension requests only in urgent procedures and dismissed them all.

In these cases, it showed great reluctance to interfere with the government's crisis management. At first, it held that the Minister of Health has 'the widest discretion to fight an unprecedented and most serious international health crisis' (Council of State, No. 247.452 Stihl and Fedagrim, 27 April 2020, para. 30). This was not repeated when it came to the exit measures. Here, the government was given merely 'wide' discretion, but a duty of care was imposed on it which required that crisis measures do not depart from relevant facts, be established with care, and be weighed against all the interests at stake (Council of State No. 248.151 Vandonghen, 17 August 2020).

However, the Council referred to expert advice and consultation only as an aid to support the crisis measures – it accepted that the government took an even stricter position than what was recommended by experts (Council of State Nos. 248.131 BV The Masters, 10 August 2020; 248.132 BV Harman, 10 August 2020). In addition, when fairground stallholders criticised measures for being disconnected from the realities of their sector, the Council reiterated that the government was advised by expert committees but it did not examine whether in this instance the fairground sector had been consulted (Council of State No. 248.151 Vandonghen, 17 August 2020). The Council thus missed an opportunity to give the government guidance on how to balance safety concerns and fundamental rights.

5.4.3 State action

Actions by the communities and regions fell into the same five categories as did federal action.

- All three communities implemented the ministerial decrees by closing down primary and secondary schools within their respective jurisdictions and prohibiting visits in retirement homes.
- Regions simplified procedures for the construction and utilisation of infrastructure for medicines or medical equipment and activated emergency plans for hospitals. All levels of government (including some municipalities) simultaneously engaged in the procurement of medical supplies such as face masks and protective gowns.
- The communities implemented federal exit measures for those establishments within their sphere of competences, such as schools, museums, and residential care centres.
- The regions put in place a series of financial compensations and guarantee schemes for businesses that were closed or limited in operation, in addition to administering the federal temporary unemployment scheme for employees

of these businesses. They also provided for rental price adjustments, subsidies for day-care, and the like.

- The regions guaranteed minimal public transport services by bus and tram and facilitated the extension of rental agreements. Regions and communities extended terms for ongoing administrative procedures and made arrangements for the functioning of administrations and other public services.

The Flemish and German-speaking communities took action mostly on the basis of specific legal authorisations. By contrast, the Walloon Region, the French Community, and the Brussels Region quickly adopted a Special Powers Act on the basis of which the governments made arrangements without prior parliamentary involvement and with the possibility to amend or bypass parliamentary acts. The scope of these special powers was unheard of; moreover, the parliaments of regions and communities that granted special powers had either adjourned or substantially reduced their activities (Bouhon et al. 2020).

We can conclude that the communities and regions were, to a large extent, the implementers of federal type 1 and 2 measures. At the same time, they were closely involved in the federal decision-making that led to these measures. Also, they had wide discretion to take measures in the other categories, within their sphere of competence. Interestingly, communities chose to coordinate their actions even where they had some policy discretion, for example in the reopening of schools. This was welcomed especially in Brussels, where both the French and Flemish communities have jurisdiction – indeed, it would have been difficult to explain why measures were more stringent in one (Francophone) school or cultural establishment than in a similar (Flemish) establishment around the corner.

Overall, the communities did not always give evidence of better crisis management than the central government. They were criticised in particular for slow progress in contact tracing, to the point that municipalities were eager to take over.

5.4.4 Local government action

The regions are responsible for local authorities; accordingly, regional governments inform and support local authorities. The 'federal phase' of crisis management implied the coordination of measures at the federal level and implementation and enforcement at the local level (municipalities and provinces). As a result, local entities predominantly played a role in the enforcement of type 1 measures; in regard to type 4 measures, they pledged to support local businesses.

In addition, the ministerial decree of 24 July 2020 allowed mayors and provincial governors to take measures in case of a local surge in infections. They had to notify the competent regional administration, as well as the provincial governor, who has a coordinating function. Mayors could, for instance, make it compulsory to wear face masks in crowded environments over and above the places already indicated in the ministerial decree. The latter stipulated that local measures were enforceable through criminal sanctions.

In one instance, the NSC called on the governor of the Province of Antwerp to take additional measures to address the deteriorating epidemiological situation in the province in the final weeks of July 2020. This resulted in the governor issuing an ordinance on 29 July that, among other things, made face masks mandatory in all public and publicly accessible places, changed the closing hours of bars and restaurants from 01:00 to 23:00, and imposed a curfew from 23:30. The latter was the most contested of these measures and was challenged before the Council of State. However, the petitions were rejected without a decision on their merits.

Several mayors of municipalities also took additional measures (for instance, in regard to closing hours of cafés and obligatory facemasks in public), depending on the epidemiological situation. They had police powers to act in urgent circumstances, but the measures had to be subsequently ratified by the city council. By stepping in in this way, local government showed its usefulness in addressing health crises, an observation which may inform future state reform.

5.4.5 Intergovernmental relations: A virus-driven push for cooperation

In Belgium, IGR usually take place in the Concertation Committee and inter-ministerial conferences and through cooperation agreements (Popelier 2021b). The central body is the Concertation Committee, which consists of the prime ministers and ministers from the federal and federated levels of authority. It is characterised both by linguistic parity (French–Dutch) and parity in federal and federated government representatives. The committee organises sectoral inter-ministerial conferences for the discussion of high-level policy issues such as state reform, the environment, or foreign policy, with these conferences often leading to cooperation agreements (Poirier 2002: 34).

Formal IGR is accompanied by informal IGR, which plays out mainly in interaction between the party elites of majority parties at different levels of government. Informal IGR functions as a mechanism for reducing conflict – before matters reach the Concertation Committee, they are usually addressed out of sight of the public eye and resolved among the governing party leaders or among ministerial cabinets (Poirier 2002: 34).

Belgium is designed as a fragmented, multinational, dyadic, and dual type of federalism where legislative as well as administrative powers are allocated on the basis of exclusivity. Transfers of powers to the communities and regions are the usual outcome of deadlock at the federal level, where antagonistic Flemish and French-speaking partners govern in a pseudo-confederal manner (Pas 2004: 160). Belgian dual federalism was therefore designed to prevent IGR as much as possible (Adam 2019: 591; Swenden and Jans Maarten 2006: 886).

At the same time, as mentioned, exclusivity entails fragmentation: policy fields are broken down into detailed dimensions and scattered over different levels of authority. As shown in a previous section, social and health policy, of crucial importance in the Covid-19 crisis, is one of these fragmented policy fields. Paradoxically, this fragmentation in turn forces the entities to cooperate and thus to engage in IGR.

Dual and dyadic federalism also explains the particular form that Belgian IGR takes, given that it is based on a multipolar playing field of federal and federated levels of authority but is also influenced by bipolar politics (Poirier 2002: 26). IGR in Belgium, as elsewhere (Swenden 2006: 190; Trench 2006: 227), is confined mainly to the executive level, where it takes place through negotiations in informal inter-ministerial consultations, inter-ministerial conferences, or formally in the Concertation Committee and through cooperation agreements concluded by the executives. IGR is thus easier when the ruling parties at the regional level are also coalition partners in the federal government.

Incongruent government formations, however, have become more common. During the Covid-19 pandemic, the federal minority emergency government in no way reflected the regional governments. In particular, the major political parties – the socialist party *Parti Socialiste* in the Walloon Region and French Community, and the nationalist party *Nieuw-Vlaamse Alliantie* in the Flemish Community – were not part of the federal coalition.

Intergovernmental relations, generally speaking, are dominated by federal governments (Trench 2006: 229), but this is not so in Belgium: even in regard to EU policies, where the federal level plays a coordinating and gatekeeping role, the regions and communities have become dominant role-players (Beyers and Bursens 2006: 1062). This poses a risk in that the absence of a dominant federal actor creates a bias towards the joint-decision trap, which can limit the effectiveness of governance (Trench 2006: 229); however, such IGR in the context of dual federalism may also engender a more integrated federalism.

In Belgium, this is particularly the case in matters that involve international decision-making. The intensity of intergovernmental cooperation and coordination has led scholars to argue that Belgium, in this arena, has moved towards cooperative federalism (Beyers and Bursens 2013: 277; Van den Brande 2012: 429).

Nonetheless, securing cooperation and compromise during the 2020 pandemic was an arduous task. This became clear when Belgium was the only EU member state that had to abstain when the Union responded to Covid-19 by mobilising funds from the European Structural and Investment Funds and making them available under cohesion rules. The reason was that the Flemish political party *Nieuw-Vlaamse Alliantie* argued that, under the logic of European cohesion policy, most of the funding to Belgium would go to the Walloon part, whereas the Flemish part was the most affected by the virus.

Initially, though, intergovernmental cooperation went surprisingly smoothly. As mentioned, there was consensus that the federal government should take the lead, with the NSC opening to involve the minister-presidents of the Communities and Regions. At press conferences, minister-presidents were seated prominently next to the Prime Minister to demonstrate intergovernmental accord. In addition, the governments could fall back on the protocol and institutions mentioned in section 3. This activated, inter alia, the RMG, with representatives from the federal and federated entities as well as the Interministerial Conference of Health.

The press conferences, however, followed long and difficult meetings that were held to reach compromise on thorny issues such as the shutdown of schools. Experts who participated in the decision-making complained about the innumerable committees and officials who were involved and the absence of leadership to take charge in the event of disagreement. Also, there was some competition in the purchasing of face masks and protective gear, with both the federal and community governments having placed orders. When contact tracing at the community level got off to a difficult start, the Flemish Minister of Welfare pointed a finger at deficient data inflow from the federal platform and unadjusted protocols for information-sharing, arguing that the Flemish system of contact tracing had been hampered by insufficient test capacity and appealing for the establishment of an intergovernmental committee and taskforce to solve the problem (Flemish Parliament 2019–2020). Likewise, local authorities complained about regional government failures in implementing track-and-trace policies, to the point that they threatened to install local systems.

As a result, prominent political actors put new state reforms on the agenda, albeit that they had differing views. Some advocated for the centralisation of crucial domains in order to combat future pandemics more effectively; others demanded even further decentralisation to avoid complex and slow decision-making. Experts and health-care workers, having dealt on the ground with the consequences of Belgium's complex system of governance, pleaded above all for unity of command, regardless of the direction future state reform takes.

5.4.6 Intergovernmental fiscal relations

Needless to say, the impact of the coronavirus crisis weighed heavily on the budgets of the federal, federated, and local entities. The National Bank predicted that the Belgian economy would suffer permanent damage and public finances be hit hard. The outlook for 2020 showed a decrease in gross domestic product (GDP) of 10 per cent per resident and sovereign debt – already burdensome before the crisis – rising to 120 per cent of the GDP, that is, twice as high as it would have been without the crisis (National Bank 2020). In addition, it was forecast that the budget deficit of the Belgian federation would rise to 6 per cent of GDP, the bulk of which would be shouldered by the federal level.

The financial capacity to carry the costs differed among the regions, with the Walloon Region being the poorest entity in terms of GDP and the Flemish Community the most prosperous.[9] A fiscal equalisation programme was in place, with fees for the communities (with social and cultural competences) on the basis of need, and for the regions (with economy and territory-based competences) on the basis of performance. Still, the variation in wealth inevitably resulted in differing room for manoeuvre for regional subsidy mechanisms.

At the time of this writing, no changes to fiscal federalism principles were on the agenda. The new federal government agreement of 1 October 2020 entrusted only two federal ministers with the task of preparing a new state reform and gave little detail. Ultimately, however, a deal on future fiscal federalism mechanisms will have to be concluded. The differential impact of Covid-19 economic costs would undoubtedly complicate the operation of the new federal government with seven political parties on board.

5.5 Findings and policy implications

The core features of the Belgian federal system determine which actors and government levels come to the fore, how they respond, and how they interact. Among these features are an intricate division of powers, dual federalism with exclusive competences, vertical IGR, and a split party system. Moreover, incongruent government coalitions resulting from split electoral constituencies probably hindered cooperation and information exchange, although their precise impact is difficult to assess.

The most crucial finding is that, similar to what happened in the policy domain of EU and foreign affairs, the Covid-19 pandemic in Belgium was an external factor that reshaped *de jure* dual federalism into de facto cooperative federalism. The legal scheme of competence allocation was interpreted creatively. As a rule, matters are allocated on the basis of exclusivity, with the federal and federated entities situated as equal partners. By contrast, crisis management in 2020 was considered a federal competence cutting across exclusive community and region competences, contrary to previous Council of State opinions, and reducing the federated entities to implementers of federal policy. Only in a later phase, advising on a parliamentary Pandemic Act, did the Council of State (2021) develop a new theory to legitimize this situation, thereby fixing this behaviour for the future.

This occurred with the full agreement of the federal and federated authorities. While the federal level was put in charge, federal policies and decisions were made on the basis of intergovernmental cooperation and implemented by the federated entities whenever the policies and decisions applied to their competences. At the same time, intergovernmental cooperation and coordination lacked unity of command, resulting in slow, complex decision-making. Moreover, the absence of an adequate pre-existing legal framework for crisis management caused confusion and, particularly at the outset of the crisis, made decision-making onerous in a situation requiring speed of response.

Another finding is the rise of local authorities as relevant actors in the Belgian multi-tiered system. Initially mere enforcers of federal measures, they gained a more prominent position at the start of the second wave of infections when granted the power to enact additional measures in a system of differentiated crisis management; they also established partnerships when the Flemish contact tracing system proved deficient. In a later phase, they would also contribute to a successful vaccination campaign. The appearance on the scene of local authorities is quite remarkable. The successive state reforms of the last 50 years were designed to mitigate adversarial relations between regional entities and resulted in decentralisation to the regional level. The Covid-19 health crisis revealed, however, that the designers of Belgian federalism neglected the potential contribution of a level further down – local government – not only in the implementation but the design of public policies.

The pandemic triggered calls for institutional reform, especially regarding the division of competences in public health policies. The new government agreement envisaged a new state reform in 2024. In all likelihood, the reforms will be based less on an evaluation of how the Covid-19 crisis was managed than on the interests and demands of the parties that formed the new federal government. Despite the uncontested centralist approach to crisis management, the crisis did not appear to have enhanced Belgium's federal 'esprit'. The Flemish-nationalist *Nieuw-Vlaamse Alliantie* put on the table proposals for a further decentralising state reform. The party was not a member of the new government, but as the major Flemish political party it was very likely to influence the position of the coalition partners. Also, its support would be crucial for the next state reform, considering the special majority requirements.

Demands for further decentralisation, especially in the domain of health policy, were also voiced by the coalition partner, the CD&V (*Christen-Democratisch en Vlaams*). The precarious financial position of the French-speaking entities stood to facilitate such a development, as a deal would imply federal financing yet regional policy autonomy, the latter being favoured as well by the *Parti Socialiste*, the dominant French-speaking player.

Whether such an outcome would be sustainable in the light of an already ailing federal level seems doubtful. Moreover, decentralisation will not obviate the crucially important need for cooperation should Belgium be hit by another pandemic. One reason is that a pandemic cuts across a wide range of policy domains; another is that, considering the density of the Belgian population, crisis management in one region inevitably impacts on that in another – all the more so in the case of Brussels, where communities have overlapping competences.

The architects of a seventh state reform thus have the responsibility to provide clarity on the allocation of competences and to develop clear and efficient schemes for coordination, cooperation, and lines of command in crisis management policies. Preferably, the local level should be factored in too. Belgium's experience in 2020 shows that crisis management should combine, on the one hand, a centralist approach with unity of command and, on the other, a differentiated approach respecting and utilising the autonomy of the regional and community level as well as local authorities.

Notes

1 The headline in *La Libre Belgique* read, 'La Fracture'; in *L'Echo*, 'La Belgique coupée en deux'; in *La Capitale*, 'La fin de la Belgique'; and in *Le Soir*, 'Deux Belgiques'.
2 For epidemiological data, see Sciensano (2020).
3 For an overview of the allocation of competences relevant to the Covid-19 pandemic, see Van Nieuwenhove and Popelier (2021).
4 See Council of State, Legislative Branch Opinion No. 67.423/3 of 26 May 2020; Opinion No. 67.425–427 of 26 May 2020.
5 See Council of State, Legislative Branch Opinion 47.062/1/V of 18 August 2009; Opinion 53.018/VR of 13 May 2013; Opinion 53.932/AV of 27 August 2013.
6 The mandate of these three bodies also applies in case of health threats of national concern.
7 Protocol to establish the generic structures for sectorial health management of crises for public health and their method for the implementation of the International Health Regulation (2005) and Decision No. 1082/2013/EU on serious cross-border threats to health of 5 November 2018', *Official Gazette* 14 December 2018 (Protocol 2018).
8 Council of State. 2020. Opinion No. 67.423/3 of 26 May 2020.
9 See https://www.statistiekvlaanderen.be/nl/bruto-binnenlands-product-per-inwoner-0 (after factoring in the commuting component to Brussels Capital).

References

Adam, Ilke. 2019. 'Defying the Traditional Theses: Intergovernmental Relations on Immigrant Integration in Belgium', *Regional & Federal Studies*, 29(5): 591–612.
Andries, Simon. 2020. 'Ik heb te veel absurditeiten gezien. Ons systeem werkt niet', *De Standaard* 30 May.
Beyers, Jan and Peter Bursens. 2006. 'The European Rescue of the Federal State: How Europeanisation Shapes the Belgian State', *West European Politics*, 29(5): 1057–78.
Beyers, Jan and Peter Bursens. 2013. 'How Europe Shapes the Nature of the Belgian Federation: Differentiated EU Impact Triggers Both Co-operation and Decentralization', *Regional & Federal Studies*, 23(3): 271–91.
Bouhon, Frédéric et al. 2020. 'L'Etat belge face à la pandémie de Covid-19: esquisse d'un régime d'exception', *Courier Hebdomadaire Crisp No. 2446*.
Council of State. 2021. Advice 68.936/AV of 7 April 2021.
EU Decision 2013. Decision No. 1082/2013/EU of the European Parliament and the Council of 22 October 2013 on Serious Cross-Border Threats to Health, *Official Journal* 5 November 2013, L293/1.
Flemish Parliament (2019–2020). Commission Report. No. 289/5, 23, 24.
Happaert, Sander, Simon Schunz and Hans Bruyninckx. 2012. 'Federalism and Intergovernmental Relations: The Multi-Level Politics of Climate Change Policy in Belgium', *Journal of Contemporary European Studies*, 20: 441–58.
National Bank. 2020. 'The Belgian Economy's Recovery from the Coronavirus Crisis will be Difficult', https://www.nbb.be/en/articles/belgian-economys-recovery-coronavirus-crisis-will-be-difficult-and-budget-deficit-2022-will (accessed on 1 December 2020).
Pas, Wouter. 2004. 'A Dynamic Federalism Built on Static Principles: The Case of Belgium', in G. Alan Tarr, Robert F. Williams and Joseph Marko (eds), *Federalism, Subnational Constitutions, and Minority Rights*. Westport: Praeger.
Poirier, Johanne. 2002. 'Formal Mechanisms of Intergovernmental Relations in Belgium', *Regional & Federal Studies*, 12(3): 24–54.

Popelier, Patricia 2020a. 'COVID-19 Legislation in Belgium at the Crossroads of a Political and a Health Crisis', *TPLeg*, 8(1–2): 131–53.

Popelier, Patricia. 2020b. 'Crisisbeheer bij Ministerieel Besluit', *Tijdschrift voor Wetgeving*, 23(4): 282–291.

Popelier, Patricia. 2021a. 'Exclusive Powers and Self-Governed Entities: A Tool for Defensive federalism?', in Ferran Requejo and Marc Sanjaune (eds), *Defensive Federalism*. Routledge (forthcoming).

Popelier, Patricia. 2021b. 'Intergovernmental Relations in Belgium: Obstacles for Effective Cooperation in Dyadic Federalism', in Yonatan Fessha, Francesco Palermo and Karl Kössler (eds), *Intergovernmental Relations* (forthcoming).

Sciensano. 2020. https://datastudio.google.com/embed/u/0/reporting/c14a5cfc-cab7-4812-848c-0369173148ab/page/QTSKB (accessed on 1 December 2020).

Swenden, Wilfried. 2006. *Federalism and Regionalism in Western Europe: A Comparative and Thematic Analysis*. Basingstoke and New York: Palgrave Macmillan.

Swenden, Wilfried and T. Jans Maarten. 2006. 'Will It Stay or Will It Go? Federalism and the Sustainability of Belgium', *West European Politics*, 29(5): 877–94.

Trench, Alan. 2006. 'Intergovernmental Relations: In Search of a Theory', in Scott L. Greer (ed.), *Territory, Democracy and Justice: Regionalism and Federalism in Western Democracies*. Basingstoke and New York: Palgrave Macmillan.

Van den Brande, Karoline. 2012. 'Intergovernmental Co-operation for International Decision-making in Federal States: The Case of Sustainable Development in Belgium', *Regional & Federal Studies*, 22(4): 407–433.

Van Nieuwenhove, Jeroen and Patricia Popelier. 2021. *De bevoegdheidsverdeling en de coördinatie tussen de bevoegde overheden in de strijd tegen de Covid-19 pandemie*, Tijdschrift voor Wetgeving (forthcoming).

Vanheule, Dirk. 2020. '*Reizen in tijden van corona. Een lockdown van en aan de grenzen?*', *Rechtskundig Weekblad* 1448.

Wilmès, Sophie. 2020. Prime Minister Wilmès, Questions Plenary Session, Question 9, Integral Report, House of Representatives 9 April, afternoon session, CRIV 55 PLEN 035.

6

WEAK INSTITUTIONS, POSITIVE RESULTS

The European Union's response to Covid-19

Beniamino Caravita, Simone Barbareschi, Francesco Severa, Sergio Spatola and Adriano Dirri[1]

6.1 Introduction

The European Union (EU) experienced two waves of infection during the Covid-19 pandemic in 2020. The first wave, extending from March to May, came to notice when infections began to be detected in northern Italy on 21 February, after which the coronavirus spread across all 27 EU member states, with Italy and Spain initially the hardest hit countries. At the end of summer in Europe, this was followed by a second wave of the pandemic, in which contagion again affected the entirety of the EU but was characterised by faster rates of infection and had a heavy impact even on states, such as Germany, which fared relatively well in the first wave.

As at 31 October 2020, the EU had recorded a total of 10,020,313 cases and 273,734 deaths; economically, the effects of the first wave were keenly felt by the most fragile states, such as Italy and Spain, but during the second wave, it became clear that the pandemic was posing a serious economic threat to both the EU as a whole and each and every member state. The outbreak of Covid-19 put a major squeeze on the EU's institutional and economic framework, and the crisis it brought about shook the foundations of European integration.

This was all the more so because the pandemic found the EU already divided from within, on the one hand facing contestation by numerous member states (notably Poland, the Czech Republic, Slovenia, and Hungary) and, on the other, deeply concerned by Britain's exit, which came to pass on 31 January 2020, only a few weeks before the start of the pandemic. As a result, many reforms to the European Treaties were on the table, especially in regard to the empowerment of the European Parliament. In this context, the economic crisis underlined the division between the richer (the Netherlands, Belgium, and Germany) and poorer (Italy, Spain, and Greece) EU countries.

DOI: 10.4324/9781003166771-8

This chapter aims to highlight the impact of Covid-19 on the federalising process of the EU. The main issues at stake are the dialectical relationship between the intergovernmental and supranational perspectives. The chapter describes the EU's response to the pandemic by analysing the EU's competence in disaster management and public health as well as the financial tools that exist for addressing economic crisis. Moreover, it assesses the role of the principle of solidarity and cooperation during the 2020 pandemic, with the focus on the European Commission and the financial measures that were adopted.

6.2 The EU institutional and legislative framework

6.2.1 The EU system

In this brief overview of the European institutional system, what is important to highlight is the constitutional nature of the EU: that is, it is not simply an international organisation, as it can enact legislation that is immediately applicable in its member states (Schütze 2020). The EU, in view of the economic scope of its federalising process, may be compared to a federal state. It is strikingly different, however, in its lack of two other typically federal areas: defence and foreign policy. Moreover, its notorious lack of strong democratic legitimacy prevents it from being traced back to the traditional liberal-democratic systems of government. Indeed, a true supranational dynamic fails to form in Europe, as EU institutions are forced to confront elected governments in member states.

As Fabbrini (2008) has argued, the EU may be defined as a 'compound democracy', a term referring to an institutional model characterised by a multiplicity of separations of power. The idea behind such a model is that neither member states nor individual institutions can gain a monopoly of decision-making. This function is thus entrusted to a subtle equilibrium and balancing between the different influences of the various institutional and political actors. Therefore, the functioning of the EU system is based on a partnership between the various institutions and on a mixture of functions, bound by the principle of loyal collaboration (Treaty on European Union, article 13, para. 2). The legislative and budgetary functions, for instance, are entrusted to the concurrent participation of Parliament and the Council (Fabbrini 2008).

A key role is played by the European Council, composed of heads of state or government of the member states, which stems from its political function. Although the Council does not exercise legislative power, it is the engine of the EU in that, for instance, it is empowered to define its general political direction, examine any subject of common interest, and, above all, decide on the revision of the treaties.

The European Parliament is the representative unit of the citizens of the Union and is elected, in its current composition of 751 members, every five years on a proportional basis, in consultation with all member states. In turn, the Council of the EU (the Council) is composed of government ministers from each EU country according to the policy area to be discussed. In regard to the approval of community acts, Parliament and the Council play an equal role in the ordinary legislative procedure; in regard to budgetary procedure, the two institutions have a co-decision role, both in the formulation and in the decision phase.

Next, the role of the European Commission is crucial because it retains the power of legislative initiative in the EU. According to article 17 of the Treaty on European Union, the Commission acts as the Union's 'government'. Its president is nominated by the European Council and elected by the European Parliament. Subsequently, the Council, in conjunction with the President-elect, adopts the list of commissioners. In addition to the role of proposal, which can be requested by Parliament and the Council, the Commission has other powers: (1) control over compliance with the obligations deriving from the treaties by the member states (infringement procedure); (2) administrative execution; and (3) inspection and supervision with respect to the division of responsibilities between the EU and the member states.

As for the European Court of Justice, it is a real judicial body. On the one hand, it exercises control over the lawfulness of the acts and conduct of EU institutions; on the other, it seeks to ensure correct and unambiguous interpretation of EU law.

The institutions above are supported by two financial institutions: the European Central Bank (ECB) and European System of Central Banks (ESCB). The first, based in Frankfurt am Main, has the task of directing EU monetary policy and authorising the issuance of the euro. The second – directed by the central banks of each member state – has the task of controlling price stability and contributing to the EU's general economic policies (Raffiotta 2020).

The complexity of the European institutional model makes it difficult for the EU to respond promptly and effectively in cases of extraordinary need and urgency. It is known that the supranational dynamic, flanked by and often opposed to the intergovernmental one, is not equipped with its own tools for immediate intervention. In fact, urgent measures must be agreed upon in the Council, even in the face of situations of grave risk and danger that involve the entire continent.

6.2.2 European health law and disaster management

The framework of EU health law derives from article 168 of the Treaty on the Functioning of the European Union (TFEU). The implications of the framework are numerous (Hervey and Bishop 2017), but what is significant here is that it lays down the competences of the member states and that of the EU, which are exclusive, shared, and supporting competences (Azoulai 2014).

Article 168 states that health protection shall be ensured in all EU policies and activities, which makes health a transversal policy. Nevertheless, the primary role is played by the member states, with national governments retaining this responsibility in managing the pandemic. In fact, paragraph 1 of article 168 affirms that 'Union action, which shall complement national policies, shall be directed towards improving public health' and that, among other things, '[s]uch action shall cover the fight against the major health scourges'. The EU encourages cooperation among member states by supporting their actions and seeking to strengthen and coordinate dialogue between them (article 168, para. 2). It has rightly been observed that the EU 'mainly acts as a hub for rapid information exchange and coordination of national crisis' (Pacces and Weimer 2020: 286).

The complementary nature of the power of the EU in health law and policy is also understood on the basis of article 2, paragraph 5 of the TFEU. In certain matters, including the protection and improvement of human health, the Union may carry out actions to support, coordinate, or supplement the actions of member states without superseding their competences as listed in article 6 of the TFEU. This balance of power between the EU and member states is exemplified by article 168, even though paragraph 4 of that article lays down two derogations to the general principle.

In fact, on one hand, the TFEU allows the EU to overcome the limited power of the EU in health policies, by stating that the EU, in order to achieve the objectives in article 168, may adopt, through ordinary legislative procedure,

a.   measures setting high standards of quality and safety of organs and substances of human origin;
b.   measures in the veterinary and phytosanitary fields which have as their direct objective the protection of public health; and
c.   measures setting high standards of quality and safety for medicinal products and devices for medical use.

In the second derogation, the EU is empowered to 'adopt incentive measures designed to protect and improve human health and in particular to combat the major cross-border health scourges, measures concerning monitoring, early warning of and combating serious cross-border threats to health …' (TFEU, article 168, para. 5).

On the other hand, the same paragraph excludes any harmonisation of the laws and regulations of member states. In this regard, paragraph 7 further specifies that 'Union action shall respect the responsibilities of the Member States for the definition of their health policy and for the organisation and delivery of health services and medical care', including 'the management of health services and medical care and the allocation of the resources assigned to them'.

This short appraisal highlights the complementary nature of EU health law and policy and the constraints upon it, albeit that the power of the EU has been considered broader than what can be ascertained from the core provisions. It has been argued that the holistic approach may lead to a wider range of legal options for the EU through the interplay of the provisions of the treaties, such as the precautionary and proportionality principles and the right to health care in article 35 of the European Charter of Fundamental Rights (Purnhagen et al. 2020).

Similarly, the scope of article 168, paragraph 7 may be broader, given the emphasis placed on cooperation between the Union and its member states and between the member states themselves. As the experience of Covid-19 has shown, it is better to speak in terms of interconnections and symbiotic relationships between the levels of the Union and the states (Guy 2020: 3).

During the 2020 pandemic, lack of cooperation and coordination between the Union and the member states emerged specifically in relation to one of the pillars of the EU: the free movement of persons. The Schengen Borders Code (Regulation EU 2016/399) allows the suspension of controls on external borders in case of a threat to public policy (article 2, para. 21; article 6, subpara. 6) and internal borders (article 25) in case of serious threat to public policy or internal security. The EU response in this regard was compromised in that internal borders were gradually closed by the member states.

The EU has no power to declare a state of emergency since this is not included among its exclusive competences. The coordinator of the European Emergency Response is the European Commissioner for Crisis Management, under which administration falls the EU Civil Protection Mechanism. In the context of Covid-19 and the economic crisis to which it led, the EU had to discuss and adopt new and broader economic mechanisms than it had in the past.

6.3 Preparedness for disaster: The institutional framework

As noted, the EU does not have competence in health matters and disaster management: it thus plays the role of coordinator for the member states. This is the operative logic of the EU Civil Protection Mechanism, the legal basis of which lies in article 196 of the TFEU. The Mechanism was established in 2001 and reformed in 2013 with the adoption of Decision No. 1313/2013/EU (Widmalm et al. 2019: 11–12). Its purpose is

> to strengthen the cooperation between the Union and the member states and to facilitate coordination in the field of civil protection in order to improve the effectiveness of systems for preventing, preparing for and responding to natural and man-made disasters. (article 1, para. 1)

The Mechanism is clearly designed for a 'classical' disaster along the lines of a natural disaster (Bouckaert et al. 2020: 769), but it was strengthened in March 2019 by RescEU, an ad hoc tool that uses EU internal funds, pre-committed national funds and Union co-financing to enhance the EU's capabilities to face a major emergency (Purnhagen et al. 2020: 299; Widmalm et al. 2019: 177). RescEU was created particularly for providing assistance when member states are affected by unexpected disasters and collective capacity is insufficient.

The EU's framework for crisis preparedness and responding to cross-border health threats was adapted after previous viral outbreaks such as severe acute respiratory syndrome (SARS) and bird flu (H1N1). The reform of 2013 was aimed at providing rules on epidemiological surveillance, early warnings, and combating serious cross-border threats to health. At its core, once again, are cooperation and complementation of national policies in regard to managing epidemiological threats.

The main operative tools are the Early Warning and Response System (EWRS) and Health Security Committee (HSC), composed of representatives of member states (generally health ministers) and tasked with exchanging information about disease outbreaks within and outside the EU. In addition, the European Centre for Disease Prevention and Control (ECDC) monitors outbreaks and provides guidance on risk management. The ECDC, together with the HSC, plays an important role in managing pandemics, as it did during the Zika and Ebola outbreaks; nevertheless, the agency is hampered by, among other things, a lack of financial resources and cooperation among member states (Renda and Castro 2020: 276–7).

Last but not least, the operative tool for providing medical equipment such as masks, gloves, and ventilators is the Joint Procurement Agreement (JPA), introduced in 2014. The JPA has the task of boosting the EU's capacity to buy medication and vaccines before and during health crises. It is thus a further instrument aimed at fostering greater cooperation in matters of public health (Azzopardi-Muscat et al. 2017).

Regarding economic aid, what tools did the EU have at its disposal when the pandemic began? We refer to the measures adopted in the aftermath of the 2008–2012 financial crisis (Tuori and Tuori 2014; Morrone 2015) and their implementation until December 2019. There are two areas of intervention: the measures taken to overcome the financial crisis and those adopted to overcome the sovereign debt crisis. Both can be summarised by grouping, on the one side, the institutional and regulatory responses and, on the other, those at the policy level.

At the institutional level, the EU established the European System of Financial Supervision (ESFS) and the Banking Union (BU) for member states which desire to participate. At the policy level, it enhanced micro-prudential and macro-prudential rules for banks; established a banking crisis management system; and strengthened the regulatory framework for the non-banking system, which includes insurance and occupational pensions, non-bank financial intermediaries, and market infrastructure sectors (Hinarejos 2015: 15).

As for measures taken to face the sovereign debt crisis, in terms of policies the EU established the European Financial Stability Mechanism (EFSM), the European Financial Stability Facility (EFSF), the European Stability Mechanism (ESM), and the European Fiscal Board (EFB). Economic governance undoubtedly changed due to the global financial crisis of 2007/2008 (Fabbrini 2015). Thus, the EU was more than ready to face a further economic crisis, both in terms of coordination between member states and in terms of financial measures, thanks in particular to the policies of the ECB, with its injection of liquidity buffers and bail-in options, during the mandate of Mario Draghi, president of the ECB between 2011 and 2019 (Waibel 2020; Bofinger 2020).

These were the main response mechanisms available to the EU for facing pandemic threats and economic crises. It has to be acknowledged that, in matters of health policy, the EU's network of agencies was not designed for engaging directly with a full-scale pandemic like Covid-19; moreover, the economic crisis of 2020 is regarded as the worst Europe has faced since the end of the Second World War.

6.4 Rolling out measures to contain the pandemic

6.4.1 Taking the initiative

Although it has been said that the EU lives off crises (Cassese 2016; Matthijs 2020), the Covid-19 pandemic was an unprecedented situation for the EU. Therefore, it should not be a surprise that, at the outset, its response was inadequate, coordination was missing, and EU institutions hesitated to act. Indeed, the measures taken were not decisive in preventing the outbreak.

In January 2020, an alert was issued on the EWRS by the Directorate General for Health and Safety, after which the HSC met on 17 January. Subsequently, on 28 January the Council of the European Union decided to activate the Integrated Political Crisis Response (IPCR) mechanism. The mechanism is, in particular, the EU framework for the coordination of cross-sectoral crises. The role of this body was later enforced when the Council, on 2 March, escalated the IPCR mechanism to full activation mode for coordinating EU response measures at presidency-led roundtables with the participation of the Commission, the European External Action Service, the office of the President of the European Council, affected member states, and relevant EU agencies and experts.

This was the first stage of coordination of the EU but, when the outbreak in Italy took place and the first red zones were declared, the main issue at stake was the closure of internal borders. In late February, within the EU, internal border control was under the spotlight. On 24 February 2020, with the outbreak in Italy already underway, the European Commissioner for crisis management was confident in the capacity of Italy and the EU to respond to the outbreak. Likewise, the Commissioner for Health and Food Safety stressed that the key points would have been cooperation, coordination, and keeping the borders open, with the closure considered as a disproportionate measure.

Of the same view was the Council of the European Union, which on 20 February 2020 highlighted the need for coordination between member states in the field of monitoring and surveillance, diagnosis and treatment and communications, research, and development. Furthermore, the Council, on the basis of Decision No. 1082/2013/UE, called upon the Commission to promote cross-sectoral information-sharing and cooperation on surveillance, risk management, and assessment, with the support of the HSC and UCPM, and to activate existing funding mechanisms to support member states in facing the outbreak; and to examine all available possibilities, such as joint procurement, to facilitate access to personal protective equipment (PPE) needed by member states.

Hence, the EU's initial action was to provide expertise and foster coordination. To this end, on 17 March 2020, the Commission appointed a new EU advisory panel on Covid-19. It was tasked to advise the Commission president, Ursula von der Leyen, on the measures to be taken, and to help the Commission in the development of guidance for member states in order to ensure science-based and coordinated national risk management. In addition, the HSC added a further forum for coordinating measures against the Covid-19 outbreak, with this body composed of national health ministers and chaired by the Commission. This structure thus entails the Commission and the HSC supported by the ECDC, scientific and technical bodies, and the newly established advisory panel (Pacces and Weimer 2020: 291).

A more concrete instrument for providing medical supplies was the JPA, which emerged, with RescEU, as the main vehicle at the EU level for purchasing medical equipment such as PPE, ventilators, and devices for testing. At the end of February 2020, the Commission launched the first of four joint procurement competitions; these were concluded in March, even though the first went defunct (McEvoy and Ferri 2020: 8; Sdanganelli 2020: 2339). In the interim, the Commission created a strategic RescEU stockpile of medical equipment, the budget for which amounted to EUR 50 million, with 90 per cent of it financed by the Commission and the balance by member states; the stockpile was managed by the Emergency Response Coordination Centre. The Commission's other initial measure was allocating EUR 232 million for boosting preparedness, prevention, and containment.

The more critical issue remained border control. The first member state to unilaterally close its border was Austria, which did so on 11 March 2020 when the World Health Organization declared the pandemic. Many others decided to follow suit. On 16 March, the Commission eventually introduced border controls in terms of article 25 of the Borders Code and established guidelines for an integrated approach. The closure of internal borders was a milestone in the management of the crisis, one that marked the moment when EU institutions became aware of the unique health and economic crisis they were facing (Brehon 2020: 5; Maurice et al. 2020: 1–2).

6.4.2 EU action

The border closures in the EU may be considered the red line for awareness of the magnitude of the crisis; as such, the need for significant and coordinated action became the main concern. The first step was the meeting of the Council on 10 March 2020, at which the EU's priorities were set out: limiting the spread of the virus, ensuring the provision of medical equipment, promoting research, and tackling the pandemic's socio-economic consequences. The second conference, held on 17 March, focused on the provision of medical equipment, particularly masks and respirators, and helping EU citizens stranded in third-party countries.

From this moment on, intergovernmental relations became the engine of the EU institutions. For instance, on 18 March 2020, EU transport ministers, together with the European Commission, joined forces to keep priority traffic moving in order to maintain economic continuity, protect the health and safety of transport workers, and ensure their free movement across borders (the situation was discussed further at a meeting of foreign affairs ministers on 23 March and 6 April). On the same date, the Council went on to give the go-ahead to support member states from the EU budget through the approval of legislative proposals that would free up funds to support small- and medium-sized enterprises (SMEs) and strengthen investment in products and services necessary to bolster health services in response to the crisis.

On 19 March 2020, EU ministers relevant to the Commission's proposal on the Coronavirus Response Investment Initiative (CRII) presented their positions and plans for a possible reallocation of EU funds for new initiatives to address the social and employment consequences of Covid-19. Soon afterwards, finance ministers agreed to ease EU fiscal rules and apply maximum flexibility so as to allow member states to take all necessary measures to support health, the civil protection system, and the economy.

On 26 March 2020, after the extraordinary G20 leaders' video conference, European Council members held a third video conference on Covid-19. Upon the assessment of the EU's response to the pandemic, the member states invited the Eurogroup (the informal body for informal meetings of the ministers of the euro area member states) (Craig 2017) to present proposals within two weeks. Once a slot waiver[2] was adopted to help airlines, the EU amended legislation on structural and investment funds to accommodate greater flexibility and release EUR 37 billion, which was allocated to the CRII and EU Solidarity Fund.

In April 2020, the contagion escalated, as did its socio-economic impact. On 8 April, the Council approved a further use of so-called cohesion resources, offering a second package of measures, the Coronavirus Response Investment Initiative Plus (CRII+), to free up other money from EU structural funds for crisis-related operations. The development ministers, for their part, gave the green light to a package with overall financial support amounting to more than EUR 20 billion drawn from existing external action resources. This aid was followed by two financial decisions. First, Eurogroup contemplated three immediate safety-nets for workers, businesses, and member states and prepared the ground for a recovery fund; secondly, the Council adopted two amendments to the EU 2020 budget that made an additional EUR 3.1 billion available in funds to purchase and distribute medical supplies, boost the production of testing kits, build field hospitals, and transfer patients for treatment in other member states.

In May 2020, concrete action was taken. On 8 May, for instance, Eurogroup agreed on standardised terms for Euro-area countries to access the ESM Pandemic Crisis Support. Member states were allowed access to 2 per cent of their gross domestic product (GDP) to finance direct and indirect health care as well as preventative measures related to Covid-19. On 19 May, the EU adopted a temporary scheme to help workers keep their jobs during the crisis. Under the scheme, the European Commission would raise funds on international capital markets on behalf of the EU, while the member states would be able to request up to EUR 100 billion in loans under favourable terms to help finance sudden and severe increases of national public expenditure in response to the crisis in specific areas. Support to the audio-visual, cultural, and creative sector; aid to help transport companies and authorities, a EUR 3 billion assistance package for neighbouring partners; and recovery measures for the EU tourism, aviation, and railway sectors all followed from those actions.

May 2020 closed with two important events. In the first, the Board of Directors of the European Investments Bank (EIB) reached an agreement on the new pan-European guarantee fund to support businesses. This was the second of the three safety-nets, worth EUR 540 billion, for jobs and workers, businesses, and member states, after the Support to mitigate Unemployment Risks in an Emergency (SURE) was adopted by the Council on 19 May. In the second event, the European Commission issued its proposal for a recovery fund and the EU's long-term budget, the multiannual financial framework (MFF) for 2021–2027. Consequently, the President of the European Council called for a meeting for this purpose in mid-July.

In addition, ministers dealt with the future of the EU in this recovery programme. Specifically, they addressed research and innovation, space, safe sport activities, digital priorities, internal border controls and free movement of persons, trade policy implications, and resilient labour markets. Last but not least, they considered how to shape Europe's digital future and reinforce the EU4Health programme and its objectives for 2021–2027, with the focus on strengthening the resilience of health systems and promoting innovation in the health sector.

After the adoption of a recommendation on the gradual lifting of the temporary restrictions on non-essential travel into the EU for residents of some third-party countries, the Council provided a temporary derogation from certain provisions of EU legislation in order to facilitate swift development of a vaccine against Covid-19.

The month of July 2020 was notable for a new proposal for the EU's long-term budget and recovery package ahead of the European Council session on 17–18 July, in which, after bitter negotiations between two very distant positions, EU leaders agreed on an extraordinary EUR 750 billion recovery package in the context of the European budget for 2021–2027. That aside, a more decisive effort was prompted on the implementation of testing and tracing, as well as on research on a vaccine for the coronavirus.

6.4.3 Evaluating solidarity and cooperation

The issues of solidarity and cooperation flow like subterranean rivers in the EU, underlying every political and legal debate on its future (Battaglia 2020; Borger 2020), be it in areas such as migration, tax policy, economic integration, or even Brexit. Solidarity, federal loyalty, and cooperation are at stake in federal systems and federalising processes generally. This is true as well of the EU, where these principles were developed during the European integration, mostly by the European Court of Justice (Lanceiro 2018: 74 ff).

The Lisbon Treaty introduced the principle of solidarity in article 3, paragraph 4, of the Treaty on European Union and of 'sincere cooperation' in article 4, paragraph 3, of the same, which imposes the duty that 'the Union and the Member States shall, in full mutual respect, assist each other'. These provisions are inter-linked with each other as well as with article 13, which enshrines the duty of loyalty and fairness between EU Institutions.

It is worth recalling that solidarity is often under the spotlight due to its link to the issue of migration, in regard to which solidarity is specifically enforced by articles 78, paragraph 3, and 80 of the TFEU; nonetheless, migration has been a key point of contention since 2015. Similarly, the principle of solidarity has been challenged in the field of political economy, in the context of the inadequacy, or 'austerity' of approach which the EU, here largely influenced by its richer member states, has adopted.

Consequently, tests of solidarity and cooperation in the EU have become routine (Casolari 2014). The Covid-19 pandemic in 2020 was a further occasion for stress-testing the EU framework – in this instance, however, a framework under an extraordinary burden. On one hand, there were calls for solidarity among member states; on the other, differing economic interests, as well as the North-South divide, overshadowed the development of inter-state trust and solidarity. Although solidarity is a yardstick for measuring the success or failure of the EU, it remains undefined in the Union's policies. Hence, what shall be considered here is the institutional performance, the praxis, both of the EU institutions (in particular the Commission) and of member states (Beaucillon 2020a: 688).

Initially, the Commission's response to the coronavirus was hesitant, but as the pandemic worsened, it acted on the basis of the principle of solidarity. That was evident in the case of the Civil Protection Mechanism and RescEU, described above, which aimed at coordinating member states and the collective response by the Commission. Denmark, Greece, Hungary, and Sweden joined Germany and Romania as host states of the RescEU medical equipment reserve which is available for distribution across Europe in medical emergencies (Beaucillon 2020b: 395–98). In a similar vein, European public procurement is an additional soft-law tool for fostering solidarity in concrete ways, in this instance by supporting member states in purchasing medical equipment. The Commission highlighted the relevance of the tool by publishing a guide on using the public procurement framework in the context of Covid-19. The purpose of the guide was to foreground the advantages of the European procurement process, such as its flexibility and transparency.

The Commission demonstrated involvement and solidarity with member states by underlining their common interests in combating the pandemic (Baratta 2020: 370–373). Another example is the Guidelines on EU Emergency

Assistance in Cross-Border Cooperation in Healthcare related to the Covid-19 crisis, funded by the Solidarity Fund and developed to help national health-care systems under pressure. Among other things, the document provided for emergency transfers of patients in intensive care and the coordination of requested and offered intensive care places for patients (Capuano 2020: 28). The Commission also took action by proposing the provision of emergency aid on the basis of article 122 of the TFEU in the matter of economic policy (financial assistance in case of exceptional occurrences) and by adjusting the general budget of the Union (Beaucillon 2020b: 398).

The Commission initiated these measures, but ultimately decisions in regard to them lay with the European Council, the forum of EU leaders (the Master of the Treaties). These remarks lead us to the more problematic intergovernmental relations that obtained between member states. From the outset of the crisis, the response to the most affected country, Italy, was uncoordinated and bilateral. Only Austria provided assistance to it on the basis of the Civil Protection Mechanism (Beaucillon 2020b: 388–91). Shortly afterwards, the bone of contention between member states was the EU budget. The North-South division between member states was pronounced, especially because the so-called frugal four (the Netherlands, Austria, Denmark, and Sweden) advocated a meagre recovery fund based on loans instead of grants. Hence, evaluating the EU's solidarity in the face of the Covid-19 crisis entails examining the financial measures that were taken.

6.4.4 Intergovernmental fiscal relations

This section considers the main policies the EU adopted to support employment, businesses, and the economy in response to the Covid-19 pandemic. These may be summarised in terms of three themes: introducing flexibility into tax rules and the EU budget, the mobilisation of the EU budget, and the expansion of monetary policies.

6.4.4.1 Flexibilisation of EU fiscal and budgetary rules

The first assessment on the pandemic's socio-economic effects dates back to European Council conclusions on 'Competitiveness'. In the document of 27 February 2020, the Council, based on a note shared by the Commission, stated that the pandemic would have the effect of reducing the economic growth of the EU.

Upon the request of member states already affected at the time, the Commission, first of all, proposed to the Council that it deviate from the normal budgetary obligations of the Stability and Growth Pact (SGP) (Keppenne 2019) through the use of article 173, paragraph 3(b) of the TFEU (Domenicali 2020: 459–60). The latter, known as the 'general escape clause', allows for deviation from (1) the process of approaching the medium-term objective, (2) the stability and convergence programmes, and (3) correction in the event of an excessive deficit.

The choice to use this clause, rather than the so-called unusual event clause, is to be traced back to the involvement of the entire euro area in the pandemic crisis. This does not indicate that the EU has used a rule designed for this type of event. As we will see regarding other financial measures, the EU has interpreted the rules, taking advantage of the experience of the last decade. Indeed, it is certain that the clause was not designed to encourage an economic recovery of the euro area, but for the sole purpose of system stability.

Furthermore, the Commission accompanied the deviations above with derogatory measures from the European regulatory framework. A derogation was envisaged from the rules on state aid not because of individual programmes proposed by each member state but for cumulative and simultaneous adoption by all member states. This method of application freed the member states as regards the choice of ways to support their economies. The only constraints, in fact, were the temporary nature of the measures, the connection to the assumptions set by the Commission, and to the verifiability of the measures taken (Domenicali 2020: 460).

It is precisely this last requirement that made it possible to affirm an expansion of the political orientation of each member state in this matter. The consequence is that the clause is transformed from an exceptional to a general instrument to safeguard the economic and financial stability of the euro area.

6.4.4.2 Mobilisation of the EU budget

The Commission, having realised that the crisis would be Europe-wide, complained that the EU budget was too small for addressing its socio-economic dimensions. It thus reallocated part of the European funds to deal with the crisis, creating a package of EUR 37 billion of structural funds (CRII) and implementing it via the CRII+. The three measures considered strategic were supporting health care, protecting short-term employment positions, and assisting SMEs.

The approval of the funding package made it necessary to amend the regulations governing the Common Provisions Regulation, European Regional Development Fund, and European Maritime and Fisheries Fund. The amending regulation grants flexibility to the states both in relation to the transfer of the sums allocated between the three cohesion funds (European Regional Development Fund, European Social Fund, and Cohesion Fund) and between different categories of regions, both in relation to the methods of expenditure and the criterion of thematic cohesion.

The same system of flexibility and modification of the destination of allocations was used for the EU Solidarity Fund. Finally, about EUR 3 billion in funds were used to directly support the health systems of the member states, through the EU emergency support instrument for the health-care sector. With regard to the mobilisation of the EU budget, this was the instrument for the extraordinary measure of the Next Generation EU recovery fund (discussed below).

6.4.4.3 Expansion of monetary policies

The ECB confirmed, with the Pandemic Emergency Purchase Programme (PEPP), the use of unusual monetary policies previously developed in the aftermath of the global financial crisis of 2008. The PEPP, which had a total budget of EU 750 billion, was limited in duration to 2020 and it was flexible in the forms of debt it made available through the central banks that include the ESCB. In addition, the ECB provided for the extension of eligible assets for the purposes of the Corporate Sector Purchase Programme and interventions on interest rates and financing transactions as well as support measures for the disbursement of bank loans with the simultaneous relaxation of disbursement criteria.

6.4.4.4 Next Generation EU

The adoption of the Next Generation EU recovery fund was a major step forward because its purpose was to increase the European budget by 0.6 per cent. The increase was to obtain liquidity in the financial markets through debt operations. Furthermore, a reform of the Union's own resources was envisaged.

The debt of the Union must have a maximum threshold of EUR 750 billion. The sums obtained from the operation were to be diverted to the member states, in part through loans and partly through direct funding, for the achievement of the EU's strategic objectives. One of the key features is the role of the European Commission: the latter's role was strengthened in that the Commission sets the agenda and verifies the recovery plan of each member state.

The device for recovery and resilience, according to article 175, paragraph 3, of the TFEU, is a structural fund aimed at reinforcing cohesion. It should enable member states to recover more quickly and increase their future resilience. As for the timing of disbursement to the member states and the terms of commitment of the sums, 70 per cent had to be committed by the beneficiary countries in 2021 and 2022 and the remaining 30 per cent by the end of 2023. However, all funds had to be spent by 31 December 2026.

Finally, as regards distribution criteria, for the two-year period 2021–2022 funds were to be based on population, per capita GDP, and average unemployment rate in the last five years (2015–2019) compared to the EU average. For 2023, on the other hand, the loss of real GDP observed over 2020 and the cumulative loss of real GDP observed in the 2020–2021 period would replace the average unemployment rate in equal percentages. That being noted, own resources constitute the real innovative core of the 'extraordinary' instrument; in fact, resources from carbon tax, financial transactions, and business income were often extolled as the beginning of this path.

In conclusion, Europe managed to capitalise on the decade spent consolidating its regulatory framework after the 2008 financial crisis by harnessing these gains in order to offset the socio-economic impact of the pandemic more quickly. It is clear that the extraordinary increase of the EU budget represents an opportunity to revive the process of European integration, pursue the unification of the political economy, and build a fiscal union that transcends the differences among member states (Fasone 2020). In fact, several studies now consider the separation between economic and monetary policy to be irreconcilable (Howarth and Verdun 2020; Demertzis and Wolff 2019). The latter is no longer considered relevant to the economic development of the member states. An all-too-recent and vivid example is provided by the repercussions that the monetary policies of the ECB have had on the economic policies of each member state.

6.5 Findings and policy implications

The Covid-19 pandemic was an important test for the EU and a turning-point in European history. It forced a rethinking of the EU's fiscal and budgetary rules, as well as its instruments for providing financial assistance to ailing states. After an initial phase of weak coordination in managing the emergency, especially within the health-care sector, European institutions decided to implement more effective measures when it came to economic governance.

It can be argued that during 2020 a new political reasoning began to prevail, one focused no longer on the intergovernmental dynamic but on a new centrality of European institutions and therefore on the more properly supranational dynamic. The European conundrum and its federalising process have been shaped by moments of integration and moments where the division between member states seemed to give way to disintegration (Vollaard 2018). Currently, the EU is fractured not only by economic differences between the North and the South but by diverse geopolitical interests (Atlantic, Continental, and Mediterranean). In juxtaposition to this, supranational institutions were created to mediate between member states, among them the Commission, the ECJ, and, more recently, the ECB.

This dialectical relationship may be measured by European policy, especially in times of crisis. In this perspective, then, the outcome of the European Council session of July 2020 may be considered a step forward more for the integration dynamic than for the intergovernmental dynamic. The latter has led, even perhaps in a despotic manner, European processes in the last decade; by the same token, enforcing the supranational dimension raises the issue of democratic legitimacy which has so weakened EU supranational institutions. Consequently, the risk is that the interests of the member states will prevail, along with their respective nationalisms. Indeed, even the European Parliament, the sole legislative body directly elected by European citizens, plays only a marginal role in determining EU policies. In this regard, before the pandemic took the limelight, a Conference on the Future of Europe was planned and the call was for, among other things, the empowerment of the European Parliament.

The European Council decisions of July 2020 did not propose a definitive solution to the European integration process, but they did open a new perspective. This led member states of the Union to accept the guarantees and negotiations of the European institutions in the management of economic tools for supporting the economy of the member states. Moreover, the pandemic showed that, despite the huge allocation of funds, the EU is not able to face emergencies as such. The issue on the table is, hence, to rethink the distribution of the EU competences in order to bolster the Union's response in the future to emergencies such as pandemics. To sum up, the lesson that can be learnt from Covid-19 is that there is a need for concrete solidarity, and in this regard, the actions of the Commission have revealed that it is crucial in the management of crisis situations.

Notes

1 This chapter is part of the research undertaken by 'Osservatorio sui processi di governo e sul federalismo' and also a product of the Project of Research of National Interest (PRIN 2017): 'Where is Europe going? Paths and perspectives of the European federalising process' (Principal Investigator: Prof. Beniamino Caravita).
2 To control congestion at airports, airlines are assigned fixed periods, or slots, during which their planes may land or take off. The rule is that if an airline fails to use a certain proportion of its slots, it loses them to its competitors. Slot waivers were intended to allow airlines to reduce flights to only necessary ones, without the risk of forfeiting their commercially valuable slots.

References

Azoulai, L. 2014. *The Question of Competence in the European Union.* Oxford: Oxford University Press.

Azzopardi-Muscat, N. et al. 2017. 'The European Union Joint Procurement Agreement for Cross-border Health Threats: What Is the Potential for This New Mechanism of Health System Collaboration?', *Health Economics, Policy and Law*, 12(1): 43–59.

Baratta, Roberto. 2020. 'EU Soft Law Instruments as a Tool to Tackle the COVID-19 Crisis: Looking at the "Guidance" on Public Procurement through the Prism of Solidarity', *European Papers*, 5(1): 365–73.

Battaglia, Francesco. 2020. 'Il principio di leale cooperazione nel Trattato di Lisbona. Una riflessione sulle vicende legate al recesso del Regno Unito dall'Unione europea', *Federalismi. it*, 19: 23–53.

Beaucillon, Charlotte. 2020a. 'European Solidarity in Times of Emergency: An Introduction to the Special Focus on COVID-19 and the EU', *European Papers*, 5(1): 687–9.

Beaucillon, Charlotte. 2020b. 'International and European Emergency Assistance to EU Member States in the COVID-19 Crisis: Why European Solidarity Is Not Dead and What We Need to Make It Both Happen and Last', *European Papers*, 5(1): 387–401.

Bofinger, Peter. 2020. 'The ECB's Policy under the Presidency of Mario Draghi: A Curse or a Blessing for Europe?', *European Journal of Economics and Economic Policies: Intervention*, 17(2): 171–82.

Borger, Vestert. 2020. *The Currency of Solidarity.* Cambridge: Cambridge University Press.

Bouckaert, G. et al. 2020. 'European Coronationalism? A Hot Spot Governing a Pandemic Crisis', *Public Administration Review*, 80(5): 765–73.

Brehon, N-J. 2020. 'The European Union and the Coronavirus', Policy Paper No. 553, European Issues – Foundation Robert Schumann Foundation, pp. 1–10.

Capuano, Valeria. 2020. 'Covid-19 e libera circolazione dei servizi sanitari: un esempio di solidarietà europea?', *AISDUE, Sezione 'Coronavirus e diritto dell'Unione'*, 3: 21–31.

Casolari, Federico. 2014. 'EU Loyalty after Lisbon: An Expectation Gap to Be Filled?', in Lucia Serena Rossi and Federico Casolari (eds), *The EU after Lisbon: Amending or Coping with the Existing Treaties?* Basel: Springer.

Cassese, Sabino. 2016. 'L'Europa vive di crisi', *Rivista trimestrale di diritto pubblico*, 3: 779–90.

Craig, Paul. 2017. 'The Eurogroup, Power and Accountability', *European Law Journal*, 23: 234–49.

Demertzis, Maria, and Guntram B. Wolff. 2019. 'What Are the Prerequisites for a Euro Area Fiscal Capacity?', *Journal of Economic Policy Reform*, 23(3): 267–72.

Domenicali, Caterina. 2020. 'La Commissione europea e la flessibilità "temporale" nell'applicazione del Patto di Stabilità e Crescita', *Federalismi.it*, 19: 453–62.

Fabbrini, S. 2008. *Compound Democracies: Why the United States and Europe Are Becoming Similar*. Oxford: Oxford University Press.

Fabbrini, S. 2015. *Which European Union? Europe after the Euro Crisis*. Cambridge: Cambridge University Press.

Fasone, Cristina. 2020. 'Le conclusioni del Consiglio europeo straordinario del 21 luglio 2020: una svolta con diverse zone d'ombra', *Diritti comparati*, 21 July.

Guy, Mary. 2020. 'Towards a European Health Union: What Role for Member States?', *European Journal of Risk Regulation*, 11: 307–316.

Hervey, Young and Louise E. Bishop (eds). 2017. *Research Handbook on EU Health Law and Policy*. Cheltenham: Edward Elgar.

Hinarejos, A. 2015. *The Euro Area Crisis in Constitutional Perspective*. Oxford: Oxford University Press.

Howarth, David and Verdun, Amy. 2020. 'Economic and Monetary Union at Twenty: A Stocktaking of a Tumultuous Second Decade: Introduction', *Journal of European Integration*, 42(3): 287–93.

Keppenne, Jean-Paul. 2019. 'Fiscal Rules', in Federico Fabbrini and Marco Venturozzo (eds), *Research Handbook on EU Economic Law*. Cheltenham: Edward Elgar.

Lanceiro, Rui Tavares. 2018. 'The Implementation of EU Law by National Administrations: Executive Federalism and the Principle of Sincere Cooperation', *Perspectives on Federalism*, 10(1): 71–102.

Matthijs, Matthias. 2020. 'Lessons and Learnings from a Decade of EU Crises', *Journal of European Public Policy*, 27(8): 1127–1136.

Maurice, Eric, Thibault Besnier and Marianne Lazarovici. 2020. 'Restoring Free Movement in the Union', *Policy Paper No. 562, European Issues – Foundation Robert Schumann Foundation*, pp. 1–9.

McEvoy, E. and Delia Ferri. 2020. 'The Role of the Joint Procurement Agreement during the COVID-19 Pandemic: Assessing its Usefulness and Discussing Its Potential to Support a European Health Union', *European Journal of Risk Regulation*, 11: 1–13.

Morrone, A. (eds). 2015. *La Costituzione finanziaria. La decisione di bilancio dello Stato costituzionale europeo*. Torino: Giappichelli.

Pacces, Alessio M. and Maria Weimer. 2020. 'From Diversity to Coordination: A European Approach to COVID-19', *European Journal of Risk Regulation*, 11(2): 283–96.

Purnhagen, Kai P. et al. 2020. 'More Competences than You Knew? The Web of Health Competence for European Union Action in Response to the COVID-19 Outbreak', *European Journal of Risk Regulation*, 11(2): 297–306.

Raffiotta, Edoardo Carlo. 2020. 'La Banca centrale europea a dieci anni dal Trattato di Lisbona tra emergenze e la ricerca di un'identità', *Federalismi.it*, 19: 345–60.

Renda, Andrea and Rosa Castro. 2020. 'Towards Stronger EU Governance of Health Threats after the COVID-19 Pandemic', *European Journal of Risk Regulation*, 11(2): 274–82.

Schütze, R. 2020. *An Introduction to European Law*. Cambridge: Cambridge University Press.

Sdanganelli, Gloria. 2020. 'Il modello europeo degli acquisti congiunti nella gestione degli eventi rischiosi per la salute pubblica', *DPCE Online*, 43(2): 2323–46.

Tuori, Kaarlo and Klaus Tuori. 2014. *The Eurozone Crisis: A Constitutional Analysis*. Cambridge: Cambridge University Press.

Vollaard, Hans. 2018. *European Disintegration: A Search for Explanations*. Cham: Palgrave Macmillan.

Waibel, Michael. 2020. 'The EU's Most Influential Economic Policy-maker: Mario Draghi at the European Central Bank', *European Journal of International Law*, 31(1): 345–52.

Widmalm, Sten, Charles Parker and Thomas Persson (eds). 2019. *Civil Protection Cooperation in the European Union How Trust and Administrative Culture Matter for Crisis Management*. Cham: Palgrave Macmillan.

7

MANAGING THE CORONAVIRUS PANDEMIC IN SWITZERLAND

How federalism went into emergency mode and struggled to get out of it

Eva Maria Belser[1]

7.1 Introduction

Switzerland was a federation calmly polishing its aged edifice of power-dividing and -sharing when it was hit by the coronavirus pandemic. What occurred next felt like a hurricane blowing through the country's institutional landscape. In mid-March 2020, three weeks after the first person tested positive for Covid-19, the venerable pillars of Swiss constitutional law – federalism, democracy, the rule of law and human rights – seemed to tremble. The Federal Council declared a state of emergency, and the country underwent a period of centralisation of power such as it had never witnessed before. Parliaments changed into speechless institutions, cantons into mere recipients of orders, and all simply waited for the next press conference by the national executive to find out what rules were to be obeyed and what rights and freedoms were still left. What had happened? Moreover, what are the consequences of a crisis in which federalism was regarded as too complicated, democracy too slow, the rule of law too flexible, and human rights too individualistic to protect public health effectively?

The Swiss coronavirus pandemic story starts at the end of February 2020. When Italy reported its first cases, Switzerland's federal authorities – under the leadership of the Federal Office of Public Health – established a taskforce to carry out an information campaign on health-protection measures. At the same time, cantons started to prepare for the pandemic, with some declaring an emergency situation, others banning large events, and others yet deciding to wait and see. When the first Swiss Covid-19 case was confirmed, the Federal Office of Public Health continued to assess the risk for the general public as moderate and recommended that the 8.6 million Swiss inhabitants regularly wash their hands and sneeze into their elbows. The Swiss population, benefiting from a

DOI: 10.4324/9781003166771-9

high-performing health system and mandatory social health insurance system, seemed well prepared to face a major health crisis.

However, the country's age demographics – with only 20 per cent of the population younger than 20 years, 61 per cent between 20 and 64 years, and 19 per cent over 65 – would soon prove to be one of the reasons for an increasing fatality rate (Federal Statistical Office n.d.). The high density of the population also posed a challenge to containing the spread of the virus. Only about 15 per cent of the population live in rural areas, while the rest are concentrated in urban areas, such as Zurich, Geneva, Basel, Bern, and Lausanne, or in agglomerations (Federal Statistical Office 2020). In addition, the population's high mobility affected the pandemic and its management: given the small size of the country and its division into 26 cantons, thousands of workers and consumers commute across cantonal borders daily, and even small and medium-sized enterprises operate across borders.

In examining the federal aspects of Switzerland's pandemic management, I argue that federalism did not fail during the pandemic – as numerous actors claimed – but was put in emergency mode as foreseen in the Constitution and the Epidemics Act. Federal structures thus did not hinder prompt and effective pandemic responses but were flexibly adapted to new circumstances: since cantons were unable individually or jointly to act quickly to control a virus indifferent to cantonal borders, concentrating power at the federal level was in line with the principle of subsidiarity. Although it felt like a mighty storm severely disrupting the institutional landscape, the pandemic response putting federalism in emergency mode at first worked to plan.

However, I will show that the country struggled to find its way into a new pandemic normalcy. One of the reasons for this is that since the end of the first wave in June 2020 when the epidemic regime was downgraded from being 'extraordinary' to being 'special', both tiers of government hoped for the other to introduce restrictive measures controlling the pandemic – and to pay for the ameliorative measures softening their effects. The principle of fiscal equivalence – namely that whoever decides, pays – thus seems to generate a negative struggle over competences ('someone else should do it'). Hence, it seems clear that Switzerland should revisit certain aspects of its institutional setup in order to deal better with the federal dynamics that arise during protracted emergencies.

7.2 The federal constitutional and legislative framework

As happens in most aggregative federations, the Swiss Federal Constitution enumerates the federal competences while residual powers are vested with the cantons. Cantonal autonomy is extensive and includes institutional, legislative, administrative, and fiscal matters. With the Covid-19 pandemic, the constitutional and legislative framework on epidemics and on emergency rules set the scene for the country's response measures.

7.2.1 Constitutional and legislative powers in health matters

Health, in general, is a cantonal matter. The Confederation, however, has a constitutionally limited mandate to issue legislation in enumerated fields, among them 'the combating of communicable, widespread or particularly dangerous human and animal diseases' (Federal Constitution, article 118, paragraph 2 lit. b). The Federal Act on Epidemics was adopted in 1970 but revised entirely in 2013 to improve the country's preparedness for fast-spreading diseases and to clarify emergency rules (Belser and Mazidi 2020). As the Act also provides a legal basis for introducing compulsory vaccination for specific groups, such as people at risk or particularly exposed in case of a health crisis, opponents of vaccines called for a popular referendum. However, the Swiss population, borne of its experiences with severe acute respiratory syndrome (SARS) and other recent epidemics, approved the law in a popular vote. All measures of the Federal Council preventing or combating the spread of Covid-19 are based on this law and thus cannot be said to lack democratic legitimacy.

The Epidemics Act applies a three-stage model. In 'normal' situations, the federal tier, in consultation with the cantons, determines aims and strategies, but it is up to the cantons to prevent and control diseases (Bergamin and Mazidi 2020: 15–16; Stöckli 2020: 18–19). There is some evidence that the normal situation was not managed appropriately in the recent past (Zeltner 2018: 15–16). Apparently, numerous cantons have not complied with national aims (in particular regarding the stocking of protective materials), preferring to invest financial resources for the health sector in seemingly more urgent matters (such as cancer and dementia); in turn, the federal authorities have failed to use their surveillance powers to insist on observance of the national strategy. The Covid-19 pandemic thus hit a country that was not as prepared as it should have been.

In 'special' situations – in which the country found itself from 28 February to 16 March 2020 and again since 20 June up to the time of writing – the Federal Epidemics Act entrusts the Federal Council with a clearly defined extra set of competences that otherwise would be cantonal matters. The council may ban or limit events, close schools and other public institutions or private enterprises, or restrict their way of operating, prohibit people from accessing or leaving a building or an area, and ban or restrict certain activities within defined zones. However, it may use these special competences only after consulting with the cantons – a rule ensuring, first, that the loss of cantonal autonomy is compensated for by institutional cooperation and, secondly, that the cantonal governments, which are in charge of the health sector and aware of the situation on the ground in the areas under their jurisdiction, contribute appropriately to the making of special rules (Bergamin and Mazidi 2020: N17–20; Kley 2020: 272; Stöckli 2020: 19). During the crisis in 2020, it became clear that the special situation was not sufficiently regulated and that the concurrent competencies, combined with the absence of joint bodies monitoring the disease and coordinating actions, raised the risk of conflicts in competence.

Finally, when the situation is declared 'extraordinary', the Federal Council may take any necessary measure for the entire country or some parts of it; in such a case, prior consultation with the cantons is no longer mandatory according to the Epidemics Act, albeit still mandated by the Constitution to the extent possible. This situation – in which the country found itself between 17 March and 19 June 2020 – is foreseen but not regulated by law and leaves numerous questions open (Bergamin and Mazidi 2020: N21–22; Stöckli 2020: 19–21). In particular, it is unclear how far the federal competences reach, whether the Federal Council is bound by federal law or may amend it and whether the cantons are allowed to go beyond the federal rules.

7.2.2 Constitutional and legislative emergency powers

The Federal Constitution provides the Federal Assembly and Federal Council with emergency powers. 'If extraordinary circumstances require', the parliament may issue ordinances or decrees to safeguard the external and internal security of Switzerland, with these ordinances or decrees exempted from the usual optional referendum that would otherwise delay parliamentary laws from entering into force (Federal Constitution, article 165). In the past and during the Covid-19 crisis, parliamentary emergency powers have not been relevant.

In contrast, the slightly more restrictive executive emergency powers are deployed regularly. The Federal Council can use emergency power in international relations and in case of serious threats to external and internal security (Federal Constitution, articles 184 and 185) and may, in direct application of the Constitution, 'issue ordinances and rulings in order to counter existing or imminent threats of serious disruption to public order or internal or external security' (article 185, paragraph 3). The emergency ordinances must be limited in duration and necessary to protect fundamental legal values such as peace, life, and public health.

In recent times, the Federal Council has used its emergency powers on several occasions. For instance, in 2001 it issued an ordinance prohibiting Al-Qaeda. The ordinance was limited in duration – to two years – but was extended three times before it was finally transposed into an ordinance of Parliament in 2011 and emergency legislation of Parliament in 2014, which itself was later extended. Numerous constitutional scholars claimed that such perpetuation of emergencies violated the Constitution (Biaggini 2017b: N10b; Künzli 2015: N43; Saxer 2014: N108). The Federal Council also used its emergency powers in 2007 and 2008 to order the destruction of plans containing information about atomic bombs. Here, its use of emergency powers was criticised for interfering in the sphere of the judiciary (Biaggini 2017a: N17; Brunner et al. 2020: 688; Saxer 2014: N109–111).

Most famously, the Federal Council made extensive use of its emergency powers during the financial crisis of 2008. The executive adopted a comprehensive programme to support the Swiss finance system and bailed out the private bank UBS, arguing that the bank was 'too big to fail'. This case was particularly controversial, as the claimed emergency was of an economic – and private – nature and views were deeply divided on whether the bankruptcy of a bank constituted a serious threat to national security (Kley 2011: 133–4). In the notorious UBS case, the Federal Supreme Court supported the view that emergency situations were not limited to serious threats to peace, life, and public health but could result from an economic and social crisis (Federal Court Decision, BGE 137 II 431, paragraph 4.1). Various scholars criticised the judgment, arguing that it opens the doors too widely to emergency powers.

The contentious use of emergency powers led to a number of legislative amendments. In 2011, a Federal Act on the Safeguard of Democracy, Rule of Law and Capacity to Act in Extraordinary Situations entered into force. It obliges the Federal Council to inform parliamentary commissions immediately when it uses emergency powers and states that executive ordinances cease to be effective if they are not submitted to Parliament within six months (Government and Administration Organisation Act, article 7(d), paragraph 2). There is, however, still no agreement on the limits of emergency powers. While most agree that emergency powers do not allow the Federal Council to violate the Constitution, there is an ongoing dispute as to whether they permit the council to break or amend parliamentary laws (Saxer 2014 N101–104; Stöckli 2020: 24–5). The Federal Council based all economic aid and Covid-19 recovery measures on its constitutional emergency powers. It informed parliamentary commissions and, after a few months, submitted the Federal Covid-19 Act to Parliament in compliance with the six-month' deadline.

In sum, two parallel emergency regimes unleashed unprecedented executive powers at the federal level. The Federal Council implemented the Federal Epidemics Act, on which it based all health-related measures and also used the general emergency clause of the Constitution for all economic-support measures.

7.3 Preparedness for a national disaster: The institutional framework

As the cantons are competent to deal with health issues, they all have a ministry of health headed by one the members of the collegial cantonal government. The 26 ministers of health are represented in the inter-cantonal conference of cantonal health ministers, a crucial body of horizontal and vertical cooperation. All cantons have cantonal doctors in charge of the test-trace-quarantine-isolate approach and empowered to issue binding orders for individuals. Cantonal health laws provide for emergency rules, mostly by establishing taskforces, as do most security and police laws. When the Covid-19 pandemic struck the country, most cantons thus established special health, security, and coordinating taskforces. Some of them were foreseen by law, others were formed ad hoc. The composition, tasks, and procedures were not always transparent, with the mushrooming of bodies having led to some confusion about who was doing what.

On the federal level, the Epidemics Act provides for a special taskforce operating under the leadership of the Federal Office of Public Health. It was headed by its director, but a senior official called Daniel Koch, omnipresent at press conferences, soon became 'Mr Corona' and the public face of the federal pandemic strategy. In addition, an ad hoc taskforce was established with the mandate to coordinate action and support the Federal Council in its decision-making. In this body, all federal ministries and the army were represented to ensure horizontal policy coordination. The general secretary of the inter-cantonal conference of cantonal governments was also a member of this federal taskforce. The latter was supported by three affiliated ad hoc bodies, one representing the economy, one civil society, and a third, named the Swiss Covid-19 Science Task Force, academia. All of these bodies were rapidly set up to counter criticism that the Federal Council was neglecting the interests of private economic actors, failing to involve non-governmental organisations, and not being guided sufficiently by scientific evidence.

The burgeoning of emergency bodies can be taken as a sign that Switzerland's institutions were not ideally prepared to face a major crisis. The institutions provided for by law were centred on health issues and not up to the task of coordinating a comprehensive pandemic response. The cantonal and federal ad hoc taskforces suffered from other shortcomings. As they were not regulated by law, or regulated only by internal directives, their composition, competences, and procedures had to be contrived in a hurry. As for the supporting bodies that shot up out of the ground, it was unclear who had nominated whom and according to what criteria. Like the federal taskforce itself, they were composed predominantly of men, a reminder that, in the absence of rules, the old gentlemen's club inexorably takes over. On 8 March, women activists were demonstrating with placards that read, 'Not My Taskforce'.

7.4 Rolling out measures to contain the pandemic

Switzerland's pandemic response can be divided into three phases. The cantons were the first to act, but when the Federal Council declared an extraordinary situation, most powers shifted to the central level. Once the situation was downgraded to being special, the Confederation and cantons struggled to sort out their respective competences and coordinate their actions.

7.4.1 Taking the initiative

At the end of January 2020, the federal authorities established a special taskforce closely cooperating with the cantonal health authorities and immediately launching an information campaign about sanitary measures. Ticino and other southern cantons were soon expressing fears that the pandemic, then raging in Northern Italy, would cross the border and that federal measures were insufficient to contain it. However, their request that borders be closed was not taken up by the federal authorities. On 25 February, the Federal Office of Public Health confirmed the first Swiss Covid-19 case, in Ticino. The patient was put in an isolation unit, and all contact persons were notified and placed in quarantine by the cantonal health authorities.

As the coronavirus spread, the cantons started to prepare for an epidemic by establishing special task forces (Uri and Glarus), or setting up quarantine apartments (Bern). They traced infections and put hundreds of people in quarantine. Ticino was the first canton to issue preventative measures: it prohibited major events, such as popular carnival festivities, and banned spectators from hockey matches. At the outset, Ticino was hardest hit by the pandemic, with its health facilities conveying horrifying messages to the rest of the country. Later, the Lake Geneva region (Geneva, Vaud, and Valais) reached the highest numbers of cases and began to take measures. Other cantons, however, had not yet reported any cases.

After an extraordinary meeting on 28 February 2020, the Federal Council declared a 'special situation' under the federal Epidemics Act and immediately used its new powers to ban large-scale events involving more than a thousand people. The cantons enforced the federal ban and were allowed to issue stricter rules. Basel Stadt, Basel Landschaft, and Zug opted for a maximum of 200 persons at events and Aargau, for 150; other cantons obliged event organisers to give notifications of events or carry out risk assessments; and others yet adopted a wait-and-see approach. However, as the infection rate increased exponentially, the test-trace-contact-isolate strategy broke down in some cantons and health care systems began to reach capacity. By mid-March, it was clear that, left to their own devices, the cantons were unable to cope with the pandemic.

7.4.2 Federal action

On 13 March 2020, the Federal Council decided to issue stricter national rules. It imposed border controls on persons entering from Italy and closed all schools throughout Switzerland. It also banned events with more than a hundred participants, a rule which – after some hesitancy – also applied to ski resorts, thus abruptly ending the Swiss ski holiday season. In restaurants, bars, and discos, a maximum of 50 people was allowed. At the same time, the Federal Council made up to CHF 10 billion in emergency aid available to cushion the economic impact of the pandemic response. This aid was immediately available to enterprises, which could get government-backed loans from their banks within hours – the Federal Council insisted on prompt aid without bureaucratic hassles.

Only three days later, the Federal Council declared an 'extraordinary situation'. The next day, lockdown rules were issued. All public and private events were prohibited, and all but essential shops were closed, as were markets, restaurants, bars, and entertainment and leisure facilities. Only pharmacies, petrol and railway stations, banks, post offices, hotels, public administrations and social institutions, food stores, takeaway outlets, canteens, and food-delivery services stayed open. Hospitals, clinics, and medical practices had to forego non-urgent medical treatments. The Federal Council also authorised the deployment of up to 8,000 members of the armed forces to assist the cantons; introduced checks at the borders with Germany, Austria, and France; and imposed entry bans. Two days later, these rules were extended to Spain and all non-Schengen states, and visa processes were suspended. Again, two days later, on 20 March, the Federal Council issued a new series of measures. It banned gatherings of more than five people, prohibited the collection of signatures for popular initiatives and referenda, and issued a standstill on deadlines on the collection of signatures. It also approved an impressive additional aid package of CHF 32 billion, bringing the total economic relief measures up to CHF 40 billion.

At the peak of the first wave of Covid-19 infections, the concentration of power in the hands of the Federal Council was extraordinary. The federal executive issued and amended one emergency ordinance after the other, with no obligation to consult Parliament or cantons. Only a few of these ordinances, such as the ones relating to border control or the deployment of the army, concerned matters that were typically federal competences – most of them, such as those to do with health, education, the economy, and cultural activity interfered in spheres normally governed by the cantons. The federal government actions reduced cantons to mere implementation agencies that were no longer allowed to decide on their own how to run their hospitals, schools, or other institutions.

Although this upscaling of competences is provided for by the Constitution and the Epidemics Act, its effect took many by surprise. The concentration of power occurred not only vertically but also horizontally; as a result, it was not the Confederation which was in charge, only its executive. In mid-March, when the Federal Assembly decided to suspend its sessions, the chambers of Parliament were deserted. The members of both chambers returned home to their domiciles and left the scene to the executive and its councillors (Caroni and Schmid 2020: 211–12). It became clear that Parliament was ill-prepared to operate during a health emergency. There were few rules on the involvement of parliamentary commissions in decision-making, and no preparedness for the legislature to function as an e-parliament.

In the cantons, the situation was equally concerning. With direct democratic mechanisms having been suspended, direct democracy in Switzerland was on hold as well. When some cantonal parliamentarians attempted to open their session, they were told by the federal authorities that their meeting fell under the prohibition of gatherings of more than five people (Bergamin and Mazidi 2020: N51–4; Uhlmann 2020: N5–16). Local assemblies, crucial actors in local self-administration, were similarly prevented from operating. Everyone, except the Federal Council and its administration, seemed to obey the stay-at-home recommendation.

Most actors, including the media, seemed to approve of this dominance by the Federal Council. However, as time went by, and as people recovered from the shock and learnt how to work effectively from home, the executive's extensive use of emergency powers became a subject of controversy. The effects of the lockdown measures on fundamental rights and freedoms, on the one hand, and the autonomy and participation rights of cantons, on the other hand, were enormous – and not all of the measures respected the principle of proportionality and subsidiarity (Belser et al. 2020: 5–7; Märkli 2020: 62–4). Some of the executive ordinances, for instance, were in conflict with federal parliamentary laws, while others, especially those relating to direct democratic rights, conflicted with the Federal Constitution (Biaggini 2020a: 254–6). The rule that signatures for a popular initiative must be collected within 18 months and for an optional referendum within 100 days are provided for by the Constitution itself. If the Federal Council could simply override these constitutional rights, what else could it do?

Given that direct democracy constitutes the main instrument of government accountability, its suspension raised fundamental questions about the control of power (Biaggini 2020b: 281–2). Aggrieved Swiss citizens typically collect signatures for referenda rather than applying to the courts. Notoriously, judicial review is limited: it applies fully to cantonal acts only and is limited when federal norms are at stake. As a rule, acts of the Federal Council may not be challenged in the Federal Supreme Court (Federal Constitution, article 189, paragraph 4). Thus, the judiciary has no mandate to review the declaration of special or extraordinary situations or emergency ordinances (Gerber 2020: N6–13; Märkli 2020: 62). When local, cantonal, and national populations and their representatives were silenced, scheduled referenda votes postponed, and the collection of signatures suspended, there was no one left to counterbalance the emergency powers of the Federal Council – and in such a situation, the limited powers of the federal judiciary seemed especially problematic.

The media customarily took it upon themselves to function as public watchdogs and urged federal civil servants to exercise their individual judgment rather than blindly follow orders from above. Nevertheless, the country was governed by central executive rule for three months in an unprecedented and largely uncontrolled way (Belser et al. 2020: 2–4). While it lasted, few actors seemed overly troubled, holding to the view instead that the exigencies of the pandemic necessitated fast and uniform action. The fact that there were few concerns about abuse of power was probably due to the generally high level of trust in institutions as well as the unique structure of the Federal Council.

In Switzerland, the concentration of power at the federal level does not mean that one strong individual takes over – it means seven take over. Uncompromising and polarising personalities are typically not elected members of the Federal Council, as they cannot succeed in a collegial body. In addition, all the linguistic groups of the country and all four major parties are represented, given that the government is elected by a 'magic formula' guaranteeing the inclusion of all relevant groups. During the emergency, the president of the Federal Council remained a *prima inter pares* member of a collegial body that continued to base its decisions on consensus. The composition of the Federal Council and its way of functioning thus served as an inbuilt check on power. The fact that the left-wing

Social Democratic Party, the centrist Christian Democratic People's Party, the Liberals, and the right-wing Swiss People's Party all had one or two federal councillors represented contributed to making the executive orders acceptable to most.

Indeed, at press conferences, the Federal Council took care to speak in several languages and always be represented by more than one member. Attentive observers could tell that the Minister of Home Affairs and the President, both Social Democrats, would often have liked to issue stricter rules but that the Minister of Finance, a member of the People's Party, prevented this from happening (*Neue Zürcher Zeitung* 2020). The Federal Council hence seemed able to balance different interests, views, and priorities even in the absence of the usual checks and balances.

In April 2020, parliamentary commissions and chamber presidents resumed work, were consulted by the Federal Council, and made extensive use of parliamentary mechanisms to get involved in the decision-making processes (Caroni and Schmid 2020: 712). While the Federal Council continued to issue or amend dozens of emergency ordinances, the Federal Assembly reconvened in May for an extraordinary session dedicated to Covid-19, one it used mostly to endorse and widen the Federal Council's economic support programmes. During the regular session in June, Parliament approved the Federal Covid-19 Act, thereby creating a parliamentary basis for further economic support actions to be decided upon by the Federal Council. By delegating far-reaching spending powers to the executive, Parliament made it clear that it considered the Federal Council the most appropriate actor to manage the crisis.

Beginning in mid-April 2020, the Federal Council decided to ease its lockdown measures. At this point it started to dawn on observers that although the Swiss constitutional and statutory framework was rather well prepared for leading the country through a carefully managed emergency situation, it gave no clue about how to get out of it (Belser and Mazidi 2020). Who was to decide on the transition to a more normal situation, or to design, plan, and finance it? As there were no clear answers and pressures were mounting to get cantons back in control, the Federal Council decided on 19 June, when infection and hospitalisation rates had stabilised at a low level, that the situation was no longer extraordinary but special. Parliament was back in session, and cantons back in charge.

However, the rules applying to the special situation were unclear. While the Federal Council now insisted that cantons should act proactively, the same cantons asked the centre to take back control as soon as the weather cooled and case numbers rose. Precious time was lost in the summer months during which no one really seemed in control and official communication was scarce. While some cantons used the time in between the waves of infection to scale up their testing-and-tracing capacity, others hoped there simply would be no second wave – or that the Federal Council would again take over if they were wrong about this. When infection rates duly started to increase once more at the end of summer, the Federal Council agreed to issue an order for masks to be worn on public transport, as it seemed exceedingly impractical to expect train passengers to adjust their behaviour to the dictates of a new jurisdiction every time they crossed another cantonal border. For the rest, the Federal Council leaned back and bade the cantons to go forth and craft tailor-made responses of their own. While some did so, others did not.

By the end of October 2020, Switzerland was about to become Europe's latest Covid-19 hotspot. The second wave of infection hit it badly, yet both the national and cantonal tiers were hoping for the other to intervene and issue more restrictive measures. Mandatory masks seemed to be the only thing they could agree on – mostly because masks do not harm business and consequently provoke no demands for economic aid. On 28 October, the Federal Council decided on light and flexible lockdown rules, and – after much hesitation – provided CHF 30 million to cushion their economic effects. The cantons were asked to design their own rules and chip into the economic relief programmes. At the time of this writing, they were still pondering how far they should go.

7.4.3 Cantonal action

When the federal authorities took control of the pandemic response, the role of cantons was unclear. It was undisputed, even during the extraordinary situation, that it was up to them to implement the pandemic response. But could they issue their own emergency regulations? Could they be stricter, as the Canton of Ticino and most French-speaking cantons would have liked to be, or only more generous when it came to cushioning the economic shock? While this matter was being debated in scholarly commentary, the federal authorities expressed the view that the national-level pandemic response was exhaustive and did not allow cantons to go beyond it. The official argument was that diverse rules would lead to confusion, but the hidden concern was that cantons with stricter rules would ask for more financial support from the national emergency relief pot than others. Scholars argued in vain that cantons more adversely affected by the pandemic should be allowed to issue stricter rules – at least if they agreed to take responsibility for the economic effects of these rules (Belser et al. 2020: 4–7).

In order to resolve a serious conflict between the Federal Council and the Canton of Ticino, the Covid-19 ordinances opened so-called crisis windows allowing cantons to go beyond the national lockdown measures under defined circumstances, thereby retroactively legalising a cantonal ban on construction work (Bergamin and Mazidi 2020: N49–50; Bernard 2020: 63–4). The Lex Ticino, designed to accommodate an upset cantonal government, was removed as soon as the situation in the canton's hospitals improved. Disputes about the respective competences and financial responsibilities persisted, however, getting worse even as the curve flattened.

The non-application of the usual institutional mechanisms produced other hiccups. The insufficient involvement of cantons in the making of rules shaped some norms which the cantons found difficult to implement. After all, the federal health authorities were used to strategic planning and coordination only and lacked practical experience on the ground. When the Federal Council decided to ease measures and return from the extraordinary to the special situation, the country experienced an unprecedented, and disconcerting, struggle over competences and roles. The cantons had been asking for greater involvement, but the sudden retreat of the Federal Council caught them by surprise. 'Mr Corona' took his retirement and so, seemingly, did the federal government.

As it turned out, the cantons were not overly eager to take measures. It was politically unattractive to ban events or close institutions – and there was heavy economic pressure not to do so. Given the small size of most cantons, expected free-rider effects also severely reduced cantonal willingness to act. Why should Basel, Zurich, or Vaud ban events – and contend with requests for economic relief by the organisers – when their sports and cultural offerings attracted visitors from a large region? Why should national football games be allowed at some places and not in others? The federal authorities, however, did not share this interpretation of the principle of subsidiarity and continued to encourage the cantons to act – and to do so rapidly. Overall, the country seemed lost and its institutions incapable of taking timeous, appropriate action. It was then that journalists coined a new term for federalising, '*föderalen*', meaning to shift responsibility to the cantons when it is inexpedient to act (Karpiczenko 2020).

It was only in October 2020, when the country was already badly hit by the second wave of Covid-19 that cantons started to issue stricter rules, to limit the operation of institutions, and to impose cantonal lockdown measures. While the Federal Council still urged the cantons to do more, it announced new national measures at the end of October. On 28 October, it amended the Covid-19 ordinance to prohibit discos and clubs, to require bars and restaurants to close at 11 pm, to ban sporting and cultural events with more than 50 people, to expand the mandatory wearing of masks, and to oblige universities to suspend face-to-face teaching. With the exception of the increasingly active corona sceptics, most actors approved of the new national involvement, though while criticising the Federal Council for not simultaneously announcing an economic support programme.

7.4.4 Local government action

The role of local government in implementing pandemic control measures was crucial. Cities and villages were at the forefront of enforcing such measures. They adapted public buildings, in particular schools and health centres, to suit the new hygiene requirements, closed parks, removed benches, controlled events and enterprises, and enforced mask-wearing. At the same time, local governments did not issue their own pandemic responses, for instance by banning events or closing institutions on their own. The fact that this did not happen can probably be explained by the small size of most communes – Swiss territory is divided into 2,200 local governments, many of which have less than a thousand inhabitants. As for the large cities, they were able to voice their concerns within their respective cantons.

To look beyond pandemic regulations, local governments were often highly innovative when challenged by the health crisis. They set up health and support teams, operated emergency lines, called households, offered help, and encouraged and coordinated neighbourhood support. Numerous municipalities also sought to complement federal and cantonal economic relief measures, including by supporting local enterprises with direct aid, such as encouraging consumers to buy locally and by issuing and subsidising coupons. Undoubtedly, local governments were in the best position to provide rapid aid to individuals and enterprises in difficult situations. As most of the municipalities are in charge of social assistance and thus of supporting those not aided by the federal social security system, they also had the greatest interest in timeously offering help and encouraging private support networks.

7.4.5 Intergovernmental relations

The participation of Swiss cantons in federal decision-making is generally strong. Cantons are represented in the second chamber of the Federal Assembly, and – more importantly – have the right to participate in the federal decision-making process, in particular in the legislative process (Federal Constitution, article 45). In 2020, consultation and information-exchange between the Confederation and the cantons always took place, even during the extraordinary situation. However, in the early phase, cooperation was patchy. The representation of cantons in the Federal Council's ad hoc taskforce was clearly insufficient and a real coordination body lacking. The general secretary of the conference of cantonal governments had no mandate to speak on behalf of the cantons, which were affected differently by the pandemic and had differing views about the best way forward. He could play the role only of a transmission channel for information.

Over time, vertical cooperation improved. The return to the special situation made it clear that no federal measures were allowed to be taken without the involvement of the cantons. The experiences showed that this was not only a constitutional duty but a practical need. The federal administration was not well positioned to design effective measures in cantonal spheres of competences. It lacked data – a tremendous concern throughout the pandemic – and hands-on knowledge about testing capacities, information channels, and health and education structures. Strong cooperation also proved to be necessary in the field of federal competences. The decision of the Federal Council to close the border to Northern Italy threatened the health system in Ticino relying on thousands of health workers commuting daily, while controlling the border to France severely affected all economic sectors of Geneva and the functioning of the international organisations based in the canton.

As most cantons are unreasonably small in the context of an increasingly mobile population, horizontal cooperation is a crucial feature of Swiss federalism. Conferences of cantonal governments and conferences of ministers of police, health, and education coordinate and harmonise cantonal policies and laws and seek to ensure that the concerns of the cantons are heard in Bern (Belser 2020: 285 ff.). However, in February and March 2020, horizontal cooperation was largely dysfunctional. The members of cantonal governments were overwhelmed by the task of dealing with the health crisis and its effects in their cantons. Although informal talks were never suspended, it was only after a few months that the inter-cantonal conferences resumed operating in their usual manner and that the conference of health ministers and the affiliated association of cantonal officers of health raised their voices and coordinated their actions.

7.4.6 Intergovernmental fiscal relations

Switzerland's federalism is characterised by a high level of fiscal decentralisation. Cantons issue and implement their own norms – and pay for it – and are in charge of implementing federal laws – and pay for it as well. Local governments adopt their own rules and fulfil federal and cantonal tasks delegated to them. The delivery and financing of most public services is thus heavily devolved to the cantons and local governments. The important role of the cantons and communes is also reflected on the revenue side, as each tier of government raises taxes and fees and none is over-dependent on transfers and grants.

Intergovernmental fiscal relations are guided by the constitutional principle of fiscal equivalence, composed of two elements: on the one hand, the collective body that benefits from a public service bears the costs thereof; on the other hand, the collective body that bears the costs of a public service may decide on the nature of that service (Federal Constitution, article 43(a), paragraphs 3 and 4). Hence, fiscal equivalence ensures that those benefiting from, financing and deciding on the provision of public goods are the same. The system is complemented by a scheme of vertical as well as horizontal financial equalisation designed to reduce the differences in financial capacity among the cantons, guarantee all cantons a minimum level of financial resources, and compensate for excessive financial burdens due to geographical or socio-demographic factors (Federal Constitution, article 135, paragraph 2).

The pandemic deeply challenged these intergovernmental fiscal relations. All of a sudden, federal authorities took costly decisions for which the cantons and communes were not prepared. National hygiene and sanitary norms made the running of all institutions significantly more expensive. More importantly, there were controversies about the sharing of the costs of economic recovery. What also upset the cantons was the fact that the Federal Council obliged hospitals and other health services to abstain from all non-urgent treatments, even in cantons which at that time hardly had any Covid-19 cases. At a high cost, all cantonal health services thus prepared for Covid patients and, while waiting for the wave to hit the hospitals, ran out of work and income.

Intergovernmental fiscal relations probably explain most of the hiccups in the Swiss reaction to the pandemic. For several months, for instance, the testing strategy was debated. The cantons used very different strategies to test people and thus were more or less effective in applying the test-trace-quarantine-isolate strategies. Their point of view was that the federal tier would have to pay for extra costs when issuing a binding national test strategy. Worse, the transmission of data was disastrously dysfunctional. For a long time, no actor seemed able to come up with reliable information on tests, test results, the use of hospital beds and intensive care units, and fatalities. It was obvious that preparation and cooperation in this field were sorely needed and that the numerous taskforces were navigating in the dark. Improving the data situation was hindered by financial disputes: Who should be in charge of a reliable health data system and finance its speedy establishment? Although many actors expressed concern about data protection (Vokinger 2020: 420–2), the hidden concerns were of a financial nature.

When the Federal Council downgraded the situation from extraordinary to special and urged the cantons to take over, financial matters were crucial in preventing prompt pandemic responses. In fact, the Federal Council, which had adopted large financial-support packages and increased social payments, was eager to step back. The cantons, however, were not keen to ban events or issue lockdown rules, as those suffering from the effects would turn to them for relief. Even when infection rates started to increase rapidly in September 2020, cantons hesitated to act and hoped for the Federal Council to keep control. It was at this moment that federalism seemed to fail the country, by hindering timely and adequate responses to the health crisis. Both the federal and cantonal tiers were eyeing each other, hoping for the other to act – and take financial responsibility for these actions.

7.5 Findings and policy implications

In normal times, the limited role of the Confederation and the far-reaching autonomy of the cantons and the communes raise little interest. During the pandemic, though, federalism seemed to matter and hoary debates about the right balance between unity and diversity resurfaced. Should there be cantonal or national lockdowns? Should cantons be allowed to decide on their testing strategies and tracing approach? Should they be allowed to control their borders, or at least discourage their populations from travelling? Such debates had not been witnessed in the country for a very long time.

The Swiss system of power-dividing and power-sharing impacted strongly on the management of the coronavirus pandemic. While the federal system had been put in emergency mode with ease, the real issue seemed to have been about how to adapt the system to an ongoing and dynamic emergency. The first reaction, that of concentrating power at the centre, fortunately gave way to more nuanced views. After all, nationwide measures are rarely proportionate, and certainly not in pandemics – during 2020, they were not far-reaching enough for those regions severely hit by Covid-19, while going beyond the necessary in regions not yet or no longer experiencing peaks in case numbers. As far as they limit human rights, the constitutionality of national restrictive measures must be questioned. Limitations of the right to education and health, to family and private life, and to economic activity and free movement must be kept to what is strictly needed at a particular time and place. The full implementation of human rights thus mandates tailor-made pandemic responses, which can be orchestrated top-down, as they are in some unitary states, or designed bottom-up. The latter has the advantage of being more legitimate and effective than the former. Regional and local actors, familiar with governing their region and resourced to do so, are in a better position than others to judge the necessity of restrictive measures and to lift them as soon as possible.

Although democracy had been suspended for months, it was back in operation by October 2020. The Federal Assembly operated behind Perspex panes, and its commissions reclaimed their right to be informed and consulted by the government. Direct democracy was also back, and the new Covid-19 ordinance made it clear that event bans did not apply to cantonal parliaments and other political assemblies, including demonstrations, which could take place provided that protection plans were in place. The profound challenges to the institutional architecture of the country, however, are very likely to leave traces.

At the federal level, it seems crucial to establish emergency-proof checks and balances. Among the options under discussion is that the Federal Council should no longer be allowed to empower itself by declaring a situation extraordinary, or to disempower itself during an emergency; instead, a parliamentary commission should be involved (Stöckli 2020: 49; Stöckli et al. 2020). During a crisis, parliament should be involved permanently and prepared for such involvement, in particular by getting ready to operate as an e-parliament (Caroni and Schmid 2020: 719–20; Stöckli et al. 2020). It has also been debated whether the mandate of the Federal Supreme Court should be expanded to allow for the abstract review of federal emergency ordinances (Stöckli 2020: 46; Stöckli et al. 2020).

At the cantonal level, it is mostly inter-cantonal collaboration that raises questions. How crisis-resistant can a federal system be which relies so strongly on the horizontal cooperation of 26 autonomous actors? Is it possible to inform and consult all of them or to allow all of them to sit in a joint emergency body? While the current practice of including only one cantonal representative on the national taskforce seems clearly insufficient, opening up the body to 26 actors appears to be inappropriate. An improvement of the situation thus seems to require profound changes in the field of intergovernmental relations and, eventually, the transformation of inter-cantonal conferences into supra-cantonal bodies. If such a change were successful, a representative delegation of the cantons could sit in a joint body with federal delegates and share responsibility for the planning, design, and implementation of the management of pandemics. Such stronger coordination seems essential to ensure a prompt and coherent response, to prevent spillover effects and, just as importantly, jointly sort out financial matters. As the latter will have long-term effects on all tiers of government and affect their room for manoeuvre in the future, the current hide-and-seek under way at the time of this writing must give way to negotiated solutions. After all, 'let's talk' has always been the motto of Swiss federalism – the country's political actors should walk that talk, even if they are wearing masks and visors.

Note

1 The author wishes to express her gratitude to MLaw Simon Mazidi, research assistant and PhD student at the University of Fribourg, for his invaluable support in the preparation of this chapter.

References

Belser, Eva Maria. 2020. 'Heading Together: Intergovernmental Relations and Horizontal Law-Making by Swiss Cantons', in Alain-G. Gagnon and Johanne Poirier (eds), *Canadian Federalism and Its Future: Actors and Institutions*. Montreal and Kingston: McGill-Queen's University Press.

Belser, Eva Maria and Simon Mazidi. 2020. 'Does Swiss Federalism Need Oxygen Treatment after Being Hit by the Covid-19 Crisis?' *UACES Territorial Politics Blog*, 2 June, https://uacesterrpol.wordpress.com/2020/06/02/does-swiss-federalism-need-oxygen-treatment-after-been-hit-by-the-covid-19-crisis/ (accessed on 11 October 2020).

Belser, Eva Maria, Bernhard Waldmann and Andreas Stöckli. 2020. 'Der schweizerische Föderalismus funktioniert auch im Krisenmodus', *IFF Newsletter 2/2020 COVID-19*, 7 April, https://www3.unifr.ch/federalism/de/assets/public/files/Newsletter/IFF/Newsletter_COVID-19_Beitrag_Belser_Stoeckli_Waldmann.pdf (accessed on 11 November 2020).

Bergamin, Florian and Simon Mazidi. 2020. 'Kompetenzabgrenzung zwischen Bund und Kantonen bei der Bekämpfung von Epidemien: Erste Einschätzungen unter besonderer Berücksichtigung der COVID-19-Verordnungen', *IFF Newsletter 2/2020 COVID-19*, 7 April, https://www3.unifr.ch/federalism/de/assets/public/files/Newsletter/IFF/Bergamin.Mazidi_Kompetenzabgrenzung%20zwischen%20Bund%20und%20Kantonen_COVID-19.pdf (accessed on 11 October 2020).

Bernard, Frédéric. 2020. 'La répartition des compétences entre la Confédération et les cantons en situation de pandémie', *Zeitschrift für Schweizerisches Recht* Sondernummer 'Pandemie und Recht': 55–67.

Biaggini, Giovanni. 2017a. Kommentar zu Art. 184. *BV Kommentar, Bundesverfassung der Schweizerischen Eidgenossenschaft*, 2nd ed. Zurich: Orell Füssli Verlag AG.

Biaggini, Giovanni. 2017b. Kommentar zu Art. 185. *BV Kommentar, Bundesverfassung der Schweizerischen Eidgenossenschaft*, 2nd ed. Zurich: Orell Füssli Verlag AG.

Biaggini, Giovanni. 2020a. 'Notrecht in Zeiten des Coronavirus – Eine Kritik der jüngsten Praxis des Bundesrats zu Art', 185 Abs. 3 BV. *ZBl* 121: 239–67.

Biaggini, Giovanni. 2020b. 'Der coronavirusbedingte Fristenstillstand bei eidgenössischen Volksbegehren – eine Fallstudie zur Tragfähigkeit von Art,' 185 Abs. 3 BV. *ZBl* 121: 277–87.

Brunner, Florian, Martin Wilhelm and Felix Uhlmann. 2020. 'Das Coronavirus und die Grenzen des Notrechts, Überlegungen zu einer ausserordentlichen Lage', *AJP* (6): 685–701.

Caroni, Andreas and Stefan G. Schmid. 2020. 'Notstand im Bundeshaus, Die Rolle der Bundesversammlung in der (Corona-) Krise,' *AJP* (6): 710–21.

Federal Statistical Office. 2020. 'Bevölkerung: Panorama', https://www.bfs.admin.ch/bfs/en/home/statistics/catalogues-databases/publications.assetdetail.13695287.html (accessed on 11 November 2020).

Federal Statistical Office. n.d. 'Mortality, Causes of Death', https://www.bfs.admin.ch/bfs/en/home/statistics/health/state-health/mortality-causes-death.html (accessed on at 11 November 2020).

Gerber, Kaspar. 2020. 'Rechtsschutz bei Massnahmen des Bundesrats zur Bekämpfung der Covid-19-Pandemie, Am Beispiel der Schliessung von öffentlichen Einrichtungen für das Publikum und der Schutzkonzepte', *sui-generis*: 249–64.

Karpiczenko, Patrick. 2020. 'Föderalen', NZZ am Sonntag, 14 November, [third image], https://nzzas.nzz.ch/magazin/bildstrecke/karpipedia-ueber-bros-renitente-jasser-und-feigen-foederalismus-ld.1586933 (accessed on 27 November 2020).

Kley, Andreas. 2011. 'Die UBS Rettung im historischen Kontext des Notrechts', *ZBl* 130: 123–38.

Kley, Andreas. 2020. 'Ausserordentliche Situationen verlangen nach ausserordentlichen Lösungen. – Ein staatsrechtliches Lehrstück zu Art. 7 EpG und Art.' 185 Abs. 3 BV. *ZBl* 121: 268–76.

Künzli, Jörg. 2015. 'Kommentar zu Art. 185', in Bernhard Waldmann, Eva Maria Belser and Astrid Epiney (eds), *Bundesverfassung, Basler Kommentar*. Basel: Helbing Lichtenhahn Verlag.

Märkli, Benjamin. 2020. 'Notrecht in der Anwendungsprobe - Grundlegendes am Beispiel der COVID-19-Verordnungen', *Sicherheit & Recht* (2): 59–67.

Neue Zürcher Zeitung. 2020. 'Der Bundesrat im Krisenmodus: von General Berset bis zu Skeptiker Maurer – die Rollenverteilung im Kampf gegen das Virus', 1 April, https://www.nzz.ch/schweiz/bundesrat-im-krisenmodus-von-general-berset-bis-zu-skeptiker-maurer-die-rollenverteilung-in-der-coronakrise-ld.1549352 (accessed on 23 November 2020).

Saxer, Urs. 2014. 'Kommentar zu Art. 185', in Bernhard Ehrenzeller, Benjamin Schindler, Rainer J. Schweizer and Klaus A. Vallender (eds), *Die schweizerische Bundesverfassung, St. Galler Kommentar*, 3rd ed. Zurich, St. Gallen: Dike.

Stöckli, Andreas. 2020. 'Regierung und Parlament in Pandemiezeiten', *Zeitschrift für Schweizerisches Recht* Sondernummer 'Pandemie und Recht': 9–54.

Stöckli, Andreas, Eva Maria Belser and Bernhard Waldmann. 2020. 'Gewaltenteilung in Pandemiezeiten', *Neue Zürcher Zeitung*, 26. May 8.

Uhlmann, Felix. 2020. 'Kompetenzen des Kantonsrates unter dem Notverordnungsrecht (Coronavirus) und weitere Fragen. Kurzgutachten zuhanden Kantonsrat Zürich', 19 March, https://www.ius.uzh.ch/dam/jcr:cf4f83e9-4ef0-4e15-a1d6-ba6427184478/WP%20Kurzgutachten%20vom%2019.%20M%C3%A4rz%202020.pdf (accessed on 11 November 2020).

Vokinger, Kerstin Noëlle. 2020. 'Die digitale Bekämpfung von Covid-19 und die Rolle des Bundes (rates)', *Schweizerische Juristen-Zeitung* 116: 412–23.

Zeltner, Thomas. 2018. Zukünftiger Bedarf im Bereich Koordinierter Sanitätsdienst. Gutachten zuhanden des Vorstehers des Eidgenössischen Departementes für Verteidigung, Bevölkerungsschutz und Sport (VBS), 18 December, https://www.newsd.admin.ch/newsd/message/attachments/59943.pdf (accessed on 11 October 2020).

8

THE COVID-19 PANDEMIC IN THE UNITED KINGDOM

A tale of convergence and divergence

Paul Anderson

8.1 Introduction

The United Kingdom of Great Britain and Northern Ireland is a plurinational union state consisting of four parts: England, Wales, Scotland, and Northern Ireland. It has 66.8 million inhabitants, the vast majority of whom reside in England. As the largest nation, England accounts for approximately 85 per cent of the UK population (56.3 million), followed by Scotland (5.4 million), Wales (3.1 million), and Northern Ireland (1.9 million). The UK has an ageing population with circa 20 per cent of the population aged 65 years and over, many of whom live in rural and coastal areas. The urban population of the UK is about 56 million, while the rural population is approximately 11 million (ONS 2020a).

The plurinational nature of the UK state is manifest in the distinct and at times competing understandings of nation and statehood in the devolved territories (Scotland, Wales, and Northern Ireland), each of which has its own constitutional and political identity. In the late 1990s, a highly asymmetrical form of political devolution was implemented in Scotland, Wales, and Northern Ireland, while England, notwithstanding its status as the largest constituent nation, became a constitutional anomaly. Two decades after the implementation of devolution, 'the English question' continues to garner traction in territorial debates, but reforms to English governance remain limited; the UK government doubles up as both a UK-wide and English government.

The UK was one of the countries worst affected by the Covid-19 crisis in 2020. From the first case of infection on 31 January 2020 until 31 October of that year, it registered more than 46,000 deaths, the highest rate in Western Europe.[1] Despite the warnings of the World Health Organization (WHO), the UK government was rather slow to respond to the threat of the crisis and sought to delay the implementation of social distancing measures until absolutely necessary. This delay was

DOI: 10.4324/9781003166771-10

compounded by support among some officials for 'herd immunity', that is, the notion that allowing the virus to spread naturally would ultimately build up enough resistance in the population. After a public outcry and strong condemnation from medical experts, the UK government abandoned this approach in favour of social distancing measures and, ultimately, a state-wide lockdown.

The National Health Service (NHS) is the collective name for the four health systems of England, Scotland, Wales, and Northern Ireland. Health has been a devolved matter since 1999, but even prior to this, the health services in Northern Ireland and Scotland were managed by their respective territorial offices in the UK government. Safeguarding the NHS from being overwhelmed by the coronavirus pandemic was a primary reason advanced by the UK government in its moves to secure a state-wide lockdown on 23 March 2020. The government's slogan 'stay at home, protect the NHS, save lives' reflected this priority. In keeping with it, temporary hospitals were constructed, retired healthcare professionals returned to work, and thousands of non-emergency operations were cancelled to free up space in hospital wards.

Public support and appreciation for the NHS and its staff were shown through a weekly 'clap for carers' during the first wave of the pandemic. Likewise, Prime Minister Boris Johnson repeatedly praised the dedication of NHS staff, especially after he was admitted to hospital while suffering from the virus. Despite acknowledgment that the NHS weathered the first wave rather well, this success was overshadowed by a chronic shortage of personal protective equipment (PPE), a lack of testing capacity for NHS workers, and thousands of deaths in both hospitals and care homes.

This chapter examines the evolution of the UK response to the pandemic during the first wave from January to October 2020. At the time of writing, the UK was in the midst of a second wave of infections, but analysis of the first wave already reveals many of the dynamics and tensions within the devolved system that were continuing to gain traction in the second wave. The politics of the pandemic that played out during the first wave demonstrated the decentralised nature of the response in the UK, but while local capacity was harnessed at the national level (Scotland, Wales, and Northern Ireland), local capacity in English regions was generally stifled by ineffectual central government direction. The main findings show how the pandemic raised the profile of devolution more than any other event in the last two decades. It points, however, to a limp federal spirit, particularly in the context of collaboration, and underlines the urgency for new and more imaginative thinking to reform and rejuvenate the Westminster-centric model of intergovernmental relations (IGR).

8.2 The constitutional and legislative framework

The UK is neither a unitary nor federal state but a union of nations with autonomous executives and legislatures in Scotland, Wales, and Northern Ireland. The Scottish Parliament, Welsh Parliament, and Northern Irish Assembly follow the reserved-powers model of devolution, whereby legislative competence is granted in all areas not specifically 'reserved' in the respective statutes for each nation (Mitchell 2009).

In the two decades since the inception of devolution, the coronavirus pandemic is the biggest public health issue faced by all levels of government. In consonance with the devolution models in each territory, important jurisdictions affected by the pandemic – health care and education, to name just two – are the responsibility of the devolved governments in Scotland, Wales, and Northern Ireland. In England, the absence of a devolved institution means that the UK government is also the English government and thus the UK government's Department for Health and Social Care focuses largely on health policy in England, albeit some aspects of health policy (e.g., human fertilisation and surrogacy) remain 'reserved' to the UK government. Emergency powers dealing with public health infections are detailed in different legislative acts for the different nations: the Public Health (Control of Disease) Act of 1984 for England and Wales, the Public Health etc. (Scotland) Act of 2008, and the Public Health Act (Northern Ireland) of 1967. Other emergency legislation exists to deal with civil emergencies across the whole of the UK – the Civil Contingencies Act of 2004 – but this was developed to reflect the various devolution settlements, involving concordats of agreed frameworks for cooperation with each devolved nation.

In recent years, political devolution has been strengthened by the devolution of further competences as well as fiscal levers and has also involved processes of 'power transfer' in the shape of 'devolution city deals' in England (Sandford 2020: 26). Fiscal devolution remains fairly limited for all three devolved institutions, but each enjoys broad competence over important policy areas such as economic development, as well as responsibility in areas to contribute to economic growth, including transport and infrastructure. Nonetheless, the devolved governments have access to limited reserves, and the fiscal frameworks of the Scottish, Welsh, and Northern Irish governments place significant constraints on the borrowing powers of the devolved governments. Consequently, the devolved governments had and have limited capacity and resources to mitigate the economic impact of Covid-19.

8.3 Preparedness for a national disaster: The institutional framework

All four nations in the UK have existing legislation to manage the spread of infectious diseases. While legislation varies in the nations (except for England and Wales, which are covered by the same Act), the Acts share similar powers to prevent, protect, and control a significant risk to human health. Through a system of action and surveillance, these Acts endow government ministers, local authorities, and magistrates with powers to issue regulations to prevent onward transmission of infectious viruses.

The Civil Contingencies Act of 2004 is the main piece of legislation for responding to national emergencies in the UK. This legislation provides a framework enabling public authorities to respond to a range of emergencies: environmental disasters, health pandemics, protests, and terrorist attacks. In line with the Act, government ministers can use emergency regulations to introduce sweeping powers to deal with an emergency, but these are qualified with legal and parliamentary safeguards to eschew disproportionate action. In lieu of invoking the Act to deal with the coronavirus pandemic, the UK government instead created new legislation. The Coronavirus Act of 2020, however, was more lenient in its requirements for parliamentary oversight.

All tiers of government in the UK have machinery in place to respond to issues of (national) emergency. At the apex of UK government machinery is the Civil Contingencies Committee (COBRA), a coordinating and decision-making body that brings together relevant personnel and authorities depending on the nature of the emergency. Located in the cabinet rooms of Whitehall, COBRA is essentially an intra-governmental rather than intergovernmental body. Coordination with the devolved administrations takes place when required, but COBRA is not an intergovernmental forum. The UK does not have a specific intergovernmental emergency committee; during the coronavirus pandemic, traditional intergovernmental structures were shunned in favour of COBRA and newly created ministerial structures (see Section 8.4.5).

8.4 Rolling out measures to contain the pandemic

The announcement of a UK-wide lockdown on 23 March 2020 was supported by all major political parties in the UK. Opposition parties, including Labour, the Scottish National Party (SNP), and the Democratic Unionist Party, all of which were in government in the devolved territories, supported the UK government's lockdown. Among the public, there was 'almost universal support' for a full lockdown 'with 93% of the public saying they were in favour of the decision' (McDonnell 2020). As the lockdown was extended over April, both political and public support remained strong. In early May, however, as the UK government eased restrictions in England, divergence in approaches came to light in the devolved nations, with growing criticism among political parties that the lockdown in England was being eased too soon. The main opposition party, Labour, sought to balance its concern with the timeline for easing measures with consistent criticism that the government's plans were vague and entailed unnecessary risk for workers being urged to return to work. This had the backing of trade unions, smaller parties such as the Greens, as well as the devolved governments.

The divergence in approach to the easing of lockdown in May 2020 reinforced the status of the devolved administrations as autonomous governments. To the surprise of some, politicians and commentators alike, the Scottish, Welsh, and Northern Irish governments did not follow suit in lifting restrictions, precipitating criticism and concern about cross-border cooperation and revealing a lack of knowledge about the powers of the devolved governments to set their own agendas and route-maps vis-à-vis lockdown. The devolved governments criticised the UK government's approach to easing lockdown, which was pursued without significant consultation with the devolved leaders and thus did not take into consideration the impact that lifting restrictions would have on other parts of the UK. The confusion created by the easing of restrictions in England was compounded by the Prime Minister himself, who in a televised speech on 10 May addressed the population as 'the Prime Minister of the United Kingdom – Scotland, England, Wales and Northern Ireland', failing to mention that the lifting of measures applied to England only (Johnson 2020b).

8.4.1 Taking the initiative

The first Covid-19 case was identified in England on 31 January 2020, followed by confirmed cases in Northern Ireland (27 February), Wales (28 February), and Scotland (1 March). On 2 March, the UK government convened COBRA to discuss the UK response to the pandemic. Recognising the scale of the pandemic and the need for cooperation between the different governments, the first ministers of Scotland, Wales, and Northern Ireland also attended COBRA meetings. The involvement of the devolved administrations heralded the beginning of a collaborative approach to tackling the pandemic across the UK. This included a Coronavirus Action Plan jointly published by the four governments on 3 March, devolved support in the form of the Sewel Convention for the UK government's Coronavirus Act (receiving royal assent on 25 March), and parallel announcements of key decisions, such as the lockdown announced on 23 March.[2] The much-heralded 'four-nation approach' entailed unprecedented levels of cooperation and a degree of uniformity between the governments hitherto unknown. In a nod to the clear division of competences vis-à-vis policy jurisdictions such as health care and education, this was a decentralised response; uniformity did not entail centralisation.

As the government machinery reacted to increasing numbers of cases across the UK in early March, the UK government advised against 'non-essential' travel and gatherings in large groups and encouraged people to work from home. On 12 March, the Scottish government announced a ban on gatherings of more than 500 people, while elsewhere in the UK unnecessary social contact was discouraged. On 18 March, all four governments announced the closure of schools (to take effect from 20 March), while on 20 March bars, cafés, and restaurants were instructed to close. In a televised address on 23 March, the Prime Minister detailed further restrictions, including a stay-at-home order and the closure of non-essential shops as well as gyms, libraries, playgrounds, and places of worship (Johnson 2020a). Extra powers were rolled out to the police to enforce the strict measures. On 25 March, the Coronavirus Act of 2020 received royal assent and granted UK ministers broad legislative powers to respond quickly to the pandemic.

8.4.2 UK government action

Analysis of the role of the UK government in managing the coronavirus pandemic necessitates discussion of its role as the government of the UK as well as England. Prior to the roll-out of preventative measures such as the lockdown on 23 March, the UK government played a coordinating role between all four nations to respond to the pandemic. As noted earlier, this included using Whitehall machinery such as COBRA. Several COBRA meetings were convened prior to the widespread transmission of Covid-19 and increased in frequency throughout March and April 2020.

In early March, the government's advice was limited to self-isolation for seven days for individuals who developed Covid-19 symptoms such as a continuous cough or fever. By mid-March, the period of self-isolation was doubled to 14 days and extended to all individuals within a household in the event that one occupant tested positive for the virus. On 16 March, Boris Johnson announced further measures, including encouraging people to work from home and the cessation of non-essential contact and unnecessary travel. One week later on 23 March, in coordination with the devolved governments, he announced the lockdown. All non-essential businesses were closed, including bars, pubs, and restaurants (except for those that could offer food delivery and take-aways); places of worship were closed except for reduced-capacity funerals; nurseries, schools, colleges, and universities were closed; recreational activities were curtailed, including the closure of playgrounds, cinemas, museums, and art galleries; social events such as weddings and baptisms were prohibited; people were ordered to work from home where possible; and a stay-at-home order was issued.

To mitigate the economic damage caused by the pandemic, the government – which controls the lion's share of fiscal levers in the UK – played a leading role in supporting employers and employees affected by the pandemic. This included various schemes applicable across all four nations of the UK. On 20 March, Rishi Sunak, Chancellor of the Exchequer, announced the launch of the Coronavirus Job Retention Scheme to provide 80 per cent of employees' salaries up to GBP 2,500 a month for those unable to work due to the stay-at-home order, as well as the Coronavirus Business Interruption Loan Scheme to support small and medium-sized enterprises with 12 months of interest-free access to loans, overdrafts, and other financial assets. Further economic packages were rolled out, among them the Coronavirus Large Business Interruption Loan Scheme to support large businesses with finance up to GBP 50 million over three years; the Self-Employment Income Support Scheme to support self-employed individuals with grants; and value-added tax (VAT) and income tax deferrals (administered by Her Majesty's Revenue and Customs).

At an individual level, the UK government, which is responsible for employment rights and most benefits and social security, also implemented numerous measures: statutory sick pay was made available to people unable to work due to contracting Covid-19 or engagement in self-isolation or shielding; low-income self-employed people were given access to Universal Credit, a benefit to help with living costs; and Universal Credit and other Working Tax Credit benefits were increased.

Owing to competition between different NHS boards in the different parts of the UK in procuring necessary PPE, other medical equipment, and coronavirus testing kits, in early April the UK government took the lead in the coordination and distribution of PPE across the UK. The government also introduced various measures to ensure the mass roll-out of a vaccine if and when it became available, including research at the government's military research facilities at Porton Down.

On 10 May, after almost eight weeks of lockdown, the government announced a relaxation of restrictions in England. In a televised address to the whole of the UK, the Prime Minister announced a change in message from 'stay at home' to 'stay alert', unveiled a new Covid Alert System, and encouraged people with jobs that could not be done from home to return to work. In Scotland, Wales, and Northern Ireland, however, the devolved governments maintained the previous advice of 'stay at home' and kept lockdowns in force. The government announced plans for primary school pupils in England to return to school by 1 June 2020, but many local authorities took the decision to keep schools closed. Between June and July, rules for the retail and hospitality sectors were eased. From 15 June, non-essential shops reopened, while in early July, bars, restaurants, pubs, and hairdressers reopened, having to adhere to a one-metre-plus rule in line with social distancing.

The reopening of the hospitality and retail sectors marked a crucial moment in the government's economic-recovery phase. To spur on this recovery, on 8 July the Chancellor announced a cut in VAT from 20 per cent to 5 per cent for accommodation, hospitality, and tourism services. The government also launched the UK-wide 'Eat Out to Help Out' scheme from 3 to 31 August, offering diners a 50 per cent reduction in their bills at participating cafés, pubs, and restaurants. The scheme certainly boosted economic recovery, but with only a 2.1 per cent rise in gross domestic product (GDP) in August, it fell short of more optimistic expectations.

By September 2020, shoots of economic recovery were cut short by an increase in Covid case numbers and the looming threat of further local lockdowns. From 14 September, a 'rule of six' was introduced to limit gatherings of separate households. On 18 September, additional restrictions were announced in the North-east of England, including a ban on household mixing, and later rolled out to the Midlands, North-west of England, and West Yorkshire. By the end of the month, further restrictions applied across the rest of the UK, including a 22:00 closure for pubs and restaurants.

As case numbers continued to rise in October, the government introduced a new three-tier lockdown system in England to establish local and regional lockdowns and reopened several emergency hospitals constructed to deal with the first wave of the pandemic. By the end of the month, large parts of England (Greater Manchester, Lancashire, Liverpool city region, South Yorkshire, and

Warrington) were under the strictest tier 3 restrictions. On 31 October, the Prime Minister announced that the exponential growth in cases necessitated a further lockdown for an initial period of four weeks (until 2 December). The second lockdown was not as restrictive as the first (schools and universities, for instance, remained open), but pubs, restaurants, leisure facilities, and non-essential shops were closed.

In line with trends across the world (see Griglio 2020), there was a strong shift towards executive rule to manage the growing threat the pandemic posed. As mentioned, the Coronavirus Act granted UK ministers broad legislative powers to respond quickly to the pandemic. In addition, pre-existing powers, such as those in delegated legislation (legislation made other than by Parliament, but with the authority of Parliament), were also used. This was done mainly through statutory instruments (SIs), which at the end of October amounted to more than 282. As analysis by the Hansard Society (2020) has shown, 69 per cent of SIs used the 'made negative' procedure, which does not require parliamentary approval for the measure to come into force. The wide discretion given to the government to implement emergency measures came under greater scrutiny as the lockdown was eased, but, even so, further measures were introduced (e.g., the mandatory wearing of face masks), while the boundaries were blurred between what was law (and thus legally enforceable) and what was government guidance (Select Committee on the Constitution 2020).

With the resumption of parliamentary activities after the Easter recess on 22 April 2020, the House of Commons held its first virtual sitting. A hybrid model was adopted, with a limited number of parliamentarians present in the chamber and the majority following debate online. The hybrid parliament, however, was a short-lived endeavour and, in a controversial vote on 2 June, a majority of MPs supported the government's proposals to reinstate physical proceedings.

The shift to executive rule facilitated by the Coronavirus Act in effect side-lined Parliament during the pandemic, with there being limited opportunity for parliamentary oversight, and debate often occurring only after restrictions came into force. On 30 September, the House of Commons voted to extend the provisions of the Act for another six months, but the vote was preceded by uncomfortable accusations that in its use of emergency regulations the government had ridden roughshod over democratic procedures and undermined the role of Parliament in scrutinising legislation (HC Deb 30 September 2020).

Responding to pressure from parliamentarians to ensure Parliament would have a greater say in major rule changes and a vote on measures prior to implementation, the government capitulated somewhat in its position and agreed to do so, having secured the necessary parliamentary support for a six-month extension of the Act until March 2021 (HC Deb 30 September 2020).

As noted earlier, the response to the pandemic was driven not by the UK government but by a collective effort on the part of the UK and devolved governments. Many of the measures implemented by the UK government applied to England only, albeit the double role performed by the government created confusion when approaches diverged in the easing-of-lockdown phase. In the days after the initial lockdown in March, public approval of the government's handling of the pandemic reached a high of 72 per cent but gradually crumbled to 32 per cent at the end of October (YouGov 2020). The delayed response, weak communication, rising infection and death rates, and failure of government ministers and advisers to abide by the rules were oft-cited as contributing factors in the public's dwindling support for the government's handling of the pandemic (Waterson 2020).

8.4.3 Devolved government action

Working with the UK government, the devolved governments in Scotland, Wales, and Northern Ireland implemented a raft of measures within their competence jurisdictions. In early March, first ministers from the three administrations attended various COBRA meetings and the devolved governments had significant input in the creation of the four-nation Coronavirus strategy and Coronavirus Act. The Act conferred enhanced functions not only on UK government ministers but so too on ministers from the Scottish, Welsh, and Northern Irish governments. On 1 April 2020, the Scottish Parliament also passed its own legislation – the Coronavirus (Scotland) Act – to enshrine further provisions on various issues regarding housing provisions and evictions, judicial operations, and health-care regulations.

As at the national level, legislatures at the devolved level continued to operate. On 1 April, the Welsh Parliament was the first legislature to instate virtual proceedings, although a hybrid model was eventually rolled out. Akin to the House of Commons, the Scottish Parliament operated using a hybrid model of online and in-chamber debates and question times, while the Northern Irish Assembly continued to function in person, albeit with social distancing rules in place (Nicholson and Paun 2020).

In regard to preventative measures, the devolved governments took the lead in prohibiting gatherings, closing schools, and advising the use of face masks in public places, while the lockdown of 23 March was implemented in lockstep by all four governments. Despite limited financial resources, the devolved governments created financial support schemes for businesses, including loans and non-domestic rates relief. As early as 14 March, the Scottish government committed to a 75 per cent rates relief for the hospitality, leisure, and retail sectors from 1 April, as well as a GBP 80 million fund to provide grants to small businesses (Scottish Government 2020). Similarly, the Welsh government established the Economic Resilience Fund allowing small businesses to apply for rates relief as well as access to grants.

As discussed in the next section, the devolved governments also increased financial support for local authorities and worked with local stakeholders to harness local knowledge and innovation to curb the spread of the virus. Akin to the UK government, the devolved governments played a role in promoting advice and guidance related to preventing the spread of the coronavirus. The first ministers of Scotland and Wales, for instance, participated in daily press conferences broadcast on TV, while the first minister and deputy first minister of Northern Ireland held various joint and individual conferences.

Given the devolved governments' responsibility for health care, they were charged with ensuring that hospitals and health-care professionals were equipped with the necessary equipment. As noted, the UK government ultimately took the lead in securing PPE, but the devolved governments were responsible for the construction of field hospitals, conducting testing and tracing, and monitoring infection rates.

Despite the four-nation approach of March and April 2020, divergence appeared in May in the aftermath of the UK government's decision to ease the lockdown in England. In contrast with the jointly published Coronavirus Action Plan, each government published its own exit strategy for easing the lockdown. Divergence also emerged in regard to contact tracing and the adoption of digital approaches to making it more efficient. Both Northern Ireland and Scotland launched their own contact tracing apps in August and September, respectively, while a joint English and Welsh app was launched on 24 September.

As the second wave of Covid-19 began to rise in September, interaction between the UK and devolved governments increased, albeit it fell short of the unprecedented collaboration witnessed in March–April. The UK government's COBRA machinery was reconvened and localised restrictions followed in all four nations of the UK, as well as identical policies regarding the imposition on 22 September of a 22:00 curfew in bars and restaurants.

Divergence, however, appeared here too. The Scottish government was the first devolved administration to prohibit households meeting indoors in late September, and in early October, it introduced much tighter restrictions than any other government in the UK, including the closure of all bars, restaurants, and other social establishments in the central belt region for a period of three weeks. On 16 October, the Northern Irish government followed suit in closing pubs and restaurants for four weeks. It prohibited households from mixing, and went further by closing schools for a period of two weeks. Days later, on 19 October, the Welsh government announced a two-week lockdown from 23 October, requiring the closure of leisure facilities, places of worship and nonessential shops. By the end of October, restrictions remained in place in all three devolved territories.

The decentralised response to the pandemic in the UK unequivocally raised the profiles of the devolved governments. Responsibility for large swathes of public policy necessitated direct intervention by the Scottish, Welsh, and Northern Irish governments, each of which imposed and eased measures in their territories at their own pace. Tellingly, public perceptions of the handling of the pandemic saw the devolved governments repeatedly outpoll the UK government, including among inhabitants of England. In Scotland, despite the constitutional divide between pro- and anti-independence supporters, First Minister Nicola

Sturgeon's handling of the pandemic was repeatedly rated higher than Prime Minister Boris Johnson's among both pro-independence and pro-union supporters (Panelbase 2020).

The devolved governments presided over similar problems as the UK government, including PPE shortages, low testing capacity, and a large number of deaths in both hospitals and care homes, but perceptions of how the governments managed the pandemic were dramatically different, with the devolved governments consistently polling higher than the UK government (Ipsos Mori 2020).

8.4.4 Local government action

In the UK, local government is a devolved matter and the organisation of local government and relations between local authorities and the devolved governments vary in all four nations (Jeffery 2006). In England, Scotland, and Wales, local councils are responsible for several jurisdictions severely affected by the coronavirus, including education, housing, and social care.[3] Working and liaising with local authorities is thus the responsibility of each devolved government, and in the case of England, the UK government.

In all parts of the UK, governments issued guidance to local authorities and as such local government played an essential role in delivering and implementing measures endorsed by the respective governments. The essential role local government played in dealing with the impact of Covid-19 on education, social care, and protection for vulnerable people (such as the shielding initiative and food provision) necessitated significant increases in local government funding across all areas of the UK. Throughout the pandemic, governments in all four nations sought to address local government shortfalls and relieve financial pressures through multi-million-pound support packages for local authorities. By mid-August, the Welsh government had increased funding to local authorities to around GBP 500 million, while local authorities in Scotland benefited from additional spending powers and extra funding up to GBP 750 million. Likewise, the UK government increased local authority payments in England, but while financial packages of billions were rolled out to address local authority spending pressures, financial support for authorities in local lockdowns courted much controversy.

Introduced under Labour in 2009, but accelerated under the Conservative-Liberal Democrat coalition government (2010–2015), eight mayoral combined authorities exist in England, with responsibilities and powers over housing, social care, and transport. Recent research argues that the public profiles of directly elected mayors remain rather limited (Fenwick and Johnston 2020: 18), but the coronavirus pandemic undoubtedly raised the profile of some of these mayors. The relationship between these metro mayors and the central government, however, was fraught with difficulties, resulting in vehement opposition to aspects of the UK government's hyper-centralist approach in handling local outbreaks of the virus.

In early October, for instance, in a letter to the Health Secretary, council leaders from Leeds, Liverpool, Manchester, and Newcastle criticised the UK government's side-lining of local government input and described the ensuing measures as 'confusing' and 'counter-productive' (BBC News 2020). For several days in October, media headlines were dominated by a clash between the Mayor of Greater Manchester Andy Burnham and the government and a threat of legal action by the former over the imposition of further restrictions in the area without local authority agreement. While some government ministers dismissed the row as party political (Burnham is a Labour politician), some Conservative MPs were vociferous in their support for the demands of mayors and council leaders (Kenny and Kelsey 2020). Despite government rhetoric that alluded to a collaborative working relationship with local government (HC Deb 28 April 2020), actions rarely matched the rhetoric. Centre-local relations were marked by imposition, not coordination.

8.4.5 Intergovernmental relations

There are various processes and structures for IGR in the UK, but the UK's experience with intergovernmental interaction since devolution has been 'largely bilateral, vertical and informal' (McEwen et al. 2012: 189). Various forums have been developed at both a multilateral and bilateral level, such as the Joint Ministerial Committee (JMC) which brings together all four governments. The JMC is the main body for IGR between the UK and devolved governments, but its functions are limited largely to knowledge-sharing and maintaining communication between the different governments rather than co-decision-making (Anderson 2021a).

In recent years, intergovernmental interaction in response to the UK's withdrawal from the European Union (EU) has increased, including the establishment of a new JMC (European Negotiations) to secure a pan-UK approach to EU withdrawal. In lieu of managing communal tensions on Brexit, however, the prevalence of governmental incongruence and competing constitutional visions have rendered IGR a source of tension (McEwen 2017): no pan-UK approach was secured prior to triggering the withdrawal process in March 2017, nor by the official withdrawal in January 2020.

In contrast to the strained relations that characterised IGR in the UK since the vote to leave the EU in 2016, the phase of initial response to the pandemic was marked by unprecedented levels of intergovernmental interaction. This culminated in a coordinated approach to lockdown in late March, preceded by the Coronavirus Action Plan which had all the hallmarks of an intergovernmental report. Coordination and collaboration between the different governments was short-lived, though, and appeared to come to an end in the easing-of-lockdown phase. As the uniform approach dissipated, so did intergovernmental interaction.

Despite the JMC's location at the apex of IGR structures, it was side-lined during the pandemic in favour of COBRA and newly created Ministerial

Implementation Groups (MIGs). The first ministers of all three devolved nations participated in COBRA meetings, while MIGs, typically convened daily, brought together ministers and officials from all governments to respond to particular policy areas (health, public sector preparedness, economy, and international response) and serve as vehicles to facilitate communication and cooperation between the governments. This was also achieved through frequent meetings between officials from the various administrations and the chief medical officers and chief scientific advisers from different government departments and administrations.

The use of COBRA in lieu of formal IGR structures was easily justified given the emergency of the pandemic and the urgency of coordinating a response across the four parts of the UK. Tellingly, however, as the pandemic evolved and divergence in approach became apparent, COBRA was not convened, provoking criticism from the devolved governments that the UK government was seeking to 'sidestep difficult conversations' on diverging approaches (Savage 2020). In June 2020, the MIGs were disbanded and two new cabinet committees created: Covid-19 Strategy and Covid-19 Operations. Unlike MIGs, membership of the cabinet committees was not formally extended to the devolved governments, lending credence to the perception that intergovernmental interaction had returned to the strained relations of the pre-pandemic era.

Besides vertical interaction between the UK government and the devolved administrations, there was also evidence of horizontal relations between the three devolved administrations. This tended to focus on policy-specific issues, such as collaboration between the Scottish, Welsh, and Northern Irish finance ministers.

As has been pointed out elsewhere, even prior to the pandemic, IGR structures were in urgent need of 'a radical overhaul' (McEwen et al. 2020). Covid-19 nonetheless underlined the need for serious reflection at all levels of government on the importance of constructive relations and the efficacy of the UK's current institutional arrangements in facilitating them.

8.4.6 Intergovernmental fiscal relations

The UK economy was among some of the hardest hit of the world's developed countries as a result of the pandemic. In the period from April to June 2020, GDP contracted by 19.8 per cent and the UK economy fell by 21.5 per cent compared to 2019 (ONS 2020b). Since the easing of the lockdown in May, both GDP and the services, manufacturing and construction sectors saw significant improvement, even though the economy faces a long road to recovery, with unemployment levels forecast to increase with the cessation of the UK and devolved governments' economic intervention schemes and the prospect of continued disruption as a result of further lockdowns.

In a similar vein to the UK as a whole, the economic outlook for the devolved nations is also gloomy. A combination of limited economic activity and significantly increased public spending saw projections of a deficit in Scotland of 25–28 per cent of GDP, with potentially higher deficits in Northern Ireland and Wales due to their lower tax revenues and weaker economies (Phillips 2020). To ameliorate the economic impact of Covid, the UK Treasury increased funding via the Barnett formula (the block grant used to allocate funding to Scotland, Wales, and Northern Ireland) to all devolved governments. In March 2020, the Chancellor of the Exchequer announced a package of GBP 1.5 million of extra funding for the devolved administrations. As well as receiving increased Barnett funding, the devolved nations also benefited from increased funding under Barnett consequentials.[4] Increases in health-care spending and other policy ambits due to the pandemic therefore resulted in billions of pounds in increased funds for the devolved administrations.

Notwithstanding increased levels of funding to the devolved governments, the pandemic spotlighted the limited fiscal capacity of the devolved governments, particularly in terms of borrowing. Ministers in all three devolved governments subsequently called for the further devolution of more fiscal levers, yet calls for additional powers went unheeded (Bol 2020). In line with the decentralised approach to managing the pandemic, economic support on the part of the UK government was not given with strings attached: the devolved governments were able to prioritise the funding as they saw fit.

8.5 Findings and policy implications

Covid-19 proved not only to be a major health crisis across the globe, but also the greatest social, economic, and political challenge the UK has weathered in the two decades since the establishment of devolved institutions in Scotland, Wales, and Northern Ireland. The implications of the decisions made to curb the spread of the deadly coronavirus are thus likely to reverberate down the years and decades to come. In particular, the evolution of the UK's pandemic response – from coordinated strategy executed in lockstep to free-form, sometimes fractious, divergence of approach – focused attention among politicians and the public alike on the system of UK territorial governance, something which doubtless will shape future debates, not least on the constitutional future of the UK.

In analysing the UK's management of the pandemic, it is clear to see that the actions of the various governments underlined the decentralised nature of the system. The clear division of competences between the UK and devolved governments eschewed controversy vis-à-vis competence jurisdictions and thus avoided any (further) unnecessary delays in reacting to the crisis. The collaborative approach seen at the beginning of the pandemic illustrated, on the one hand, the respect that exists for the division of responsibilities between different tiers of government, and, on the other, the presence of shared recognition of the importance of working together when faced with a momentous cross-border crisis.

Nevertheless, despite rhetoric on the part of the UK government and Whitehall machinery around supporting the autonomy of the devolved governments to make their own decisions within their competence briefs, the easing of the lockdown revealed frustration and a lack of understanding amongst some Westminster parliamentarians about the permissibility of the devolved governments to diverge from UK government policy.

At a wider level, this hints at the precarious nature of the federal spirit in the UK and how this precariousness has served to sustain – notwithstanding the federal logic of devolution that has taken root over the last two decades – the unitary mindset and majoritarian thinking that often characterises UK government decision-making processes (Anderson 2021b). This is compounded by the absence of an English executive and thus the UK government's double role as both a UK-wide and English-only government. During the crisis, the Prime Minister himself at times rejected the notion that his authority extends only to England (HC deb 11 May 2020), a stance reinforcing the notion that while devolution has entailed much change in the devolved nations, very little has changed at the centre.

A second intriguing finding, linked with the above, concerns the importance of local government in England in the absence of a separate English executive and legislature. Across the world, governments at all levels have had to respond to the pandemic, but it is local governments that have played an essential role in taking initiatives both within and outside the scope of their responsibilities to curtail and manage the spread of the virus.

In the UK, local governments unequivocally played a leading role in responding to the pandemic, but this was overshadowed and marginalised in England by the over-centralised approach of the UK government in its engagement with local authorities. Elected mayors in England made significant interventions in the debate on responding to the pandemic, though these often focused on critique of the government and calls for a more constructive approach on the part of the UK government in its interaction with local authorities. There are clear lessons to be learnt about taking a more proactive approach to local government engagement, specifically in harnessing local knowledge and using this to advantage in times of emergency and crisis. Rescheduled elections for most of the local mayoralties will take place in 2021; it may well be that the pandemic is a catalyst to further the debate on the devolution and strengthening of more powers for England's metro-mayors.

The experience of IGR during the pandemic reveals the urgency of reforming extant machinery to enhance communication and collaboration between the different governments. Amidst crisis, all four governments in the UK showed maturity in responding collaboratively to the pandemic, putting aside partisanship and political issues to focus on the good of the country. This, as the evidence in this chapter attests, swiftly unravelled as the devolved governments diverged from the UK government approach and offers telling proof of the need to overhaul the Westminster-centric model of IGR.

The history of devolution has been marked by willingness in Westminster to cede responsibilities to the devolved legislatures but hesitance to share power and thus work together. As much in normal times as in times of emergency, a genuine commitment to work collaboratively, underpinned by mutual trust, recognition, and respect, is important, not least in a plurinational democratic state. The response to the pandemic in the UK has demonstrated not just that a cooperative approach to IGR is possible, but that working together need not compromise the decentralised structures and dynamics of the territorial system.

There is no doubt that the coronavirus pandemic itself as well as the way it has been managed by the different tiers of government in the UK will have short- and long-term implications for contemporary British politics. Opinion polls throughout the crisis repeatedly recorded higher support for the devolved governments' handling of the pandemic than the UK government's, with levels of trust in the latter depleted as the pandemic evolved (Ipsos Mori 2020).

In January 2020, the UK left the EU after almost four years of political wrangling in both the UK and Brussels, but the constitutional impact of withdrawal remains in the balance and is compounded by the pandemic. The passage of the UK government's Internal Market Bill – designed to ensure harmonisation in trading rules and regulations across the UK – between September and December 2020 triggered significant controversy and was interpreted by the devolved governments as an assault on devolution. In contrast with the Coronavirus Act, which was passed with the consent of all three devolved legislatures, legislative consent for the Internal Market Bill was refused by all three devolved legislatures. At the same time, polling on Scottish independence has begun to suggest that there may be a sustained majority in favour of independence, with evidence pointing to the Scottish government's handling of the pandemic as a key catalyst for growing support.

As has been pointed out elsewhere, there is evidence that nationalist forces around the globe have sought to 'weaponise' the coronavirus pandemic to further their aims (Woods et al. 2020). The UK is no exception. However, while there is no doubt that pro-independence supporters in Scotland are likely to point to the Scottish government's handling of the pandemic as proof of Scotland's ability to be an independent country (notwithstanding some complaints about its government's handling of the crisis), unionists have been equally proactive in underlining the might of the Union in responding to the pandemic. Covid-19 has not merely introduced new dynamics in contemporary British politics but has already begun to redefine well-entrenched territorial debates.

Notes

1 Figures on the overall death toll from Covid-19 vary and are counted in three different ways: deaths within 28 days of a positive result (this is used for government figures), death certificate mentions of Covid-19, and deaths over and above the usual number at a particular time of year. As of 31 October 2020, 46,555 deaths occurred within 28 days of a positive result, almost 59,000 death certificates stated Covid-19 as the cause of death, and more than 67,000 excess deaths had occurred over and above the yearly average.

2 The Sewel Convention states that the UK Parliament 'will not normally legislate with regard to devolved matters without the consent' of the devolved institutions.

3 Local governments in Northern Ireland have fewer responsibilities than elsewhere in the UK, with no policy responsibility for education or social care.
4 Barnett consequentials refer to the mechanism whereby any increase in public expenditure in England generates increased funding for the devolved administrations.

References

Anderson, Paul. 2021a. 'Plurinationalism, Devolution and Intergovernmental Relations in the UK', in Y. Fessha, F. Palermo and K. Kössler (eds), *Intergovernmental Relations in Divided Societies: A Comparative Analysis*. London: Palgrave MacMillan. Forthcoming.
Anderson, Paul. 2021b. 'Spain and the United Kingdom: Between Unitary State Tradition and Federalisation', in S. Keil and S. Kropp (eds), *Emerging Federal Models in the Post-Cold War Era*. London: Palgrave MacMillan. Forthcoming.
BBC News. 2020. 'Covid-19: Council Leaders Send Matt Hancock Action Plan', 7 October.
Bol, David. 2020. 'Kate Forbes Joins Forces with Welsh and Northern Irish Counterparts in Plea for Powers', *The Herald*, 8 July.
Fenwick, John and Lorraine Johnston. 2020. 'Leading the Combined Authorities in England: A New Future for Elected Mayors?', *Public Money & Management*, 40(1): 14–20.
Griglio, Elena. 2020. 'Parliamentary Oversight under the Covid-19 Emergency: Striving against Executive Dominance', *The Theory and Practice of Legislation*, 8(1–2): 49–70.
Hansard Society. 2020. Statutory Instrument Tracker, https://www.hansardsociety.org.uk/services/statutory-instrument-tracker (last accessed on 10 November 2020).
HC Deb. 11 May 2020, vol 676, col 33.
HC Deb. 19 March 2020, vol 673, col 1178.
HC Deb. 28 April 2020, vol 675, col 204.
HC Deb. 30 September 2020, vol 681, col 389.
Ipsos Mori. 2020. *COVID-19 Polling BBC Scotland*. 26 May.
Jeffery, Charlie. 2006. 'Devolution and Local Government', *Publius*, 36(1): 57–73.
Johnson, Boris. 2020a. Prime Minister's Statement on Coronavirus (COVID-19), 16 March.
Johnson, Boris. 2020b. Prime Minister's Statement on Coronavirus (COVID-19). 10 May.
Kenny, Michael and Tom Kelsey. 2020. 'Devolution or Delegation? What the Revolt of the Metro Mayors over Lockdown Tells Us about English Devolution', *LSE British Politics and Policy*. 12 November.
McDonnell, Adam. 2020. 'Public Support for a Two-week Lockdown Persists', *YouGov*, 30 October.
McEwen, Nicola. 2017. 'Still Better Together? Purpose and Power in Intergovernmental Councils in the UK', *Regional and Federal Studies*, 27(5): 667–90.
McEwen, Nicola, Wilfried Swenden and Nicole Bolleyer. 2012. 'Introduction: Political Opposition in a Multi-Level Context', *The British Journal of Politics and International Relations*, 14(2): 187–97.
McEwen, Nicola et al. 2020. 'Intergovernmental Relations in the UK: Time for a Radical Overhaul', *The Political Quarterly*, 91(3): 632–40.
Mitchell, James, 2009. *Devolution in the UK*. Manchester: Manchester University Press.
Nicholson, Elspeth and Akash Paun. 2020. 'Devolved Legislatures: How Are They Working in the Coronavirus Lockdown?', *Institute for Government*, 24 November.
Office of National Statistics (ONS). 2020a. *Population and Migration*.
Office of National Statistics (ONS). 2020b. 'Coronavirus and the Impact on Output in the UK Economy: June 2020'.
Panelbase. 2020. 'How have Johnson and Sturgeon Coped with Covid-19?', 11 July.

Phillips, David. 2020. 'Scotland's Implicit Budget Deficit could be around 26-28% of GDP in 2020-21', Institute for Fiscal Studies, 26 August.

Sandford, Mark. 2020. 'Giving Power Away? The "De-Words" and the Downward Transfer of Power in Mid-2010s England', *Regional and Federal Studies*, 20(1): 24–46.

Savage, Michael. 2020. 'Boris Johnson Has Not Hosted a Cobra Emergency Committee for over a Month', *The Guardian*, 14 June.

Select Committee on the Constitution. 2020. Constitutional Implications of Covid-19. 2 December.

Scottish Government. 2020. '£320 million Package of Support for Businesses'. 14 March.

Waterson, Jim. 2020. 'Public Trust in UK Government over Coronavirus Falls Sharply', *The Guardian*, 1 June.

Woods, Eric, et al. 2020. 'COVID-19, Nationalism, and the Politics of Crisis: A Scholarly Exchange', *Nations and Nationalism*. https://doi.org/10.1111/nana.12644 (accessed on 20 February 2021).

YouGov. 2020. 'Covid-19: Government Handling and Confidence in Health Authorities', 17 March.

9

RUSSIA'S FIGHT AGAINST COVID-19

Dealing with a global threat under crisis and stagnation

Viacheslav Seliverstov, Ivan Leksin, Nataliya Kravchenko, Vladimir Klistorin and Almira Yusupova

9.1 Introduction

The Russian Federation, covering 17.1 million km², is geographically the largest country in the world and, with its 146.7 million inhabitants, the ninth largest in population. It is a state with medium levels of urbanisation – in terms of urban population (74.4 per cent), it ranks 77th out of 218 countries – and it is sixth in a list of states by gross domestic product (GDP) based on purchasing-power parity.

Under the Constitution, the Russian Federation is a federal state made up of a complex system of 85 constituent units: republics, *krais*, oblasts, cities of federal significance, autonomous *okrugs*, and an autonomous oblast. Three federal cities – Moscow, St. Petersburg, and Sevastopol – have the status of a constituent unit, with their management systems and budgets consequently independent of the region where they are located; for example, the city of Moscow is in Moscow Oblast.

Since Russia's territory is so vast, it is divided into eight federal districts, each combining constituent units in a macro-region, namely the Central, North-western, Southern, North Caucasian, Volga, Urals, Siberian, and Far Eastern districts. They are not official administrative or territorial units but have authorised envoys who pursue the President's policies within the boundaries of their federal districts, as well as control and coordinate the work of the existing local bodies of federal executive power at the district level.

When Russia's first Covid-19 cases were reported on 31 January 2020, a number of economic, political, and social factors combined with one another to create a highly adverse background for efforts to combat the pandemic. First, the economy was in crisis: in the preceding seven years (2013–2019), economic stagnation had set in, with GDP per capita increasing by only 3 per cent (Aganbegyan 2020). Western sanctions, imposed on Russia in 2014 after the Crimea became

DOI: 10.4324/9781003166771-11

part of it, affected a few large Russian companies, among others, as well as the economy as a whole. Moreover, world oil prices dropped by half.

Secondly, the poor quality of public administration at the national and sub-federal level is compounded by a fairly high prevalence of corruption; within this context, constituent entities have been burdened heavily by social and economic inequalities (including in regard to their medical services). Thirdly, Russia has one of the longest land borders with China, the country where the virus originated.

Some favourable factors and conditions were nevertheless present. First, Russia has large gold and forex reserves that were accumulated in the past, in addition to a massive sovereign wealth fund (called the National Wealth Fund). Secondly, its enormous territory, combined with low population mobility, created natural barriers to the spread of the coronavirus. Thirdly, though much of it has been laid to waste, the system of public health care inherited from the Soviet era remains adequately functional.

The situation was further complicated by the political characteristics of contemporary Russia. Most notably, the state administration system is overcentralised, with the presidency playing a dominant role in it. The top-down command structure (consisting in what is known as 'the President's vertical power') was backed by presidential plenipotentiaries and their staff in eight federal districts established in 2002.

Furthermore, there is weak political competition. The ruling party, United Russia, dominates legislative and executive bodies at the federal and sub-federal levels: only 7 out of 85 governors represent opposition parties; two governors were elected as independent candidates; and another 20 were formally non-partisan but in actuality nominated or supported by the ruling party. Overall, United Russia wields power over 90 per cent of Russian governors.

To these considerations, one may add that, viewed geopolitically from the perspective of identifying sources of global-threat proliferation, Russia is an asymmetric federation with an excessively centralised and low-quality state administration system. Such conditions led to apprehensions that the Covid-19 pandemic would spread rapidly and uncontrollably in Russia, but, fortunately, these fears proved unjustified.

The country's first two Covid-19 cases, involving Chinese citizens visiting Russia, were recorded in Siberia on 31 January 2020. The first case in Moscow was identified on 2 March, which was a month later than happened in most countries in Europe and attributable to the quick closure of the border with China (on 31 January 2020) and then those with other countries. This bought some time in which to put in place the minimum necessary conditions for receiving patients in Moscow and the regions.

In the first wave of the pandemic, infections peaked on 11 May (11,600 people per day), and fatalities on 29 May 2020 (213 people per day). Over the summer (until the end of August), the infection rate decreased, then started to grow slowly. The second wave emerged in early October, with peak daily infection and mortality rates exceeding those of May. By 31 October, Russia was seeing 18,140 new cases per day; it had also recorded a total of 1.618 million cases, 1.215 million recoveries (i.e., 75 per cent of all cases), and 27,990 deaths.

Russia's constituent entities varied significantly in infection rates. The areas most affected by Covid-19 were those with high population density and mobility, namely the largest cities, North Caucasus, and regions in the north where people work primarily on a rotational basis.

This section has outlined some of Russia's distinctive features as a pandemic site and provided an overview of how Covid-19 spread through its territory in the course of 2020. The sections that follow examine how it responded to the crisis as a federation and what key actions it took in terms of its constitutional and legislative framework and within the context of its intergovernmental relations (IGR) between the centre and the regions.

9.2 The federal constitutional and legislative framework

The Constitution of the Russian Federation of 1993, as amended in 2020 (RF Constitution), contains general provisions that are applicable to a wide variety of disaster situations. These provisions include ones that set out the federal structure, declare the autonomy of local governments, specify the jurisdictions of government orders, and define the powers of the federal president and federal government.

In terms of articles 71 and 72 of the RF Constitution, governmental powers are divided into two categories: those under federal jurisdiction and those under the 'joint jurisdiction' of the federal and 85 regional governments. Many of the constitutional formulas in the respective lists are equivocal and thus open to varying interpretations, making the distribution of powers quite flexible and leaving a small degree of latitude for exclusive regional legislation. As far as pandemics are concerned, two jurisdictional areas are relevant, disaster management and health care, both of which used to be regarded as matters of 'joint jurisdiction'.

The joint jurisdiction of the Russian Federation and its constituent units is not 'joint' in the proper sense. Some intergovernmental coordination is provided for when it comes to implementing federal statutes on matters within joint jurisdiction, but the RF Constitution does not put federal and regional law-making at a par with each other or set any limits on federal law-making within the area of joint jurisdiction. In fact, this area is concurrent, with the federal legislator enjoying overwhelming predominance (Leksin and Seliverstov 2017). It was by means of federal statutes that, within less than two decades after the adoption of the 1993 Constitution, Russia evolved from a loose, semi-confederate arrangement into a highly centralised federal state (Leksin 2016).

With regard to local government, article 12 of the RF Constitution asserts that local self-government constitutes a separate form of governance; however, local governments' powers do not cover an exclusive sphere of jurisdiction that could be separated from the powers mentioned in articles 71, 72, and 73 of the

RF Constitution. The constitutional assertion that municipalities enjoy self-government means no more than that they execute federal and regional laws.

Detailed statutory provisions dealing with the allocation of powers are found in several federal statutes. According to the statutes regarding a pandemic, the federal and regional governments are both responsible for issues that include protecting human rights in health care, organising medical care and licensing certain types of activities in health care, and facilitating medical treatment by medical institutions. The federal government deals mostly with policy-making, law-making, administrative regulation, and supervision, while the regional governments deal mostly with the practical issues of health protection; local governments fulfil auxiliary functions. The single-tier and upper-tier municipalities participate in health protection activities in several ways: they are responsible for, among other things, creating the conditions for providing medical care to the population, preventing diseases, ensuring the provision of medical care in municipal health-care institutions, warning the population about epidemic threats, raising awareness about healthy lifestyles, and promoting blood donation.

The jurisdiction over disaster management is more decentralised. Every level of government is responsible for dealing with emergencies, depending on the scale of the latter. As such, federal, regional, and local governments are entitled to declare a 'regime of emergency situation' or a 'state of heightened preparedness' in order to mobilise the necessities for (1) protecting the population; (2) evacuations and emergency rescues; (3) keeping stocks of material, including food and medical supplies, for purposes of civil defence; and (4) informing the population in the emergency zone about the status of the situation and the measures taken in response to it. However, only federal and regional governments are entitled to make laws on population-protection measures and to maintain public order during emergencies.

Because disaster management falls within 'joint jurisdiction', federal statutes play the leading role. Federal legislation since the 1990s used to distinguish between three legal regimes related to emergencies. The first was called the 'regime of emergency state'. According to the 1993 RF Constitution, the President can introduce this regime in the entirety of the Russian Federation or in certain parts only. Having introduced it, he immediately has to inform the chambers of the Federal Assembly (the State Duma and the Federation Council). The Federation Council is entitled to confirm the presidential decree. The RF Constitution does not go into detail about the nature of this regime but refers instead to a special statute (a federal constitutional law) that should establish the rules for it. This special statute was enacted finally in 2001 but has never been used. States of emergency were declared several times between 1992 and 1995, though not on epidemiological grounds.

Along with the 'regime of emergency state', two other legal regimes applicable in the case of a national disaster are provided for in the federal law, On the Protection of Population and Territory against Natural and Technogenic Emergency Situations (1994). These are the 'regime of emergency situation' and a 'state of heightened preparedness'. While they are little different in content, the first refers to the period after the emergency has occurred, whereas the second can be introduced when there is the threat of an emergency.

All three regimes can be introduced to address natural or man-made emergencies, including epidemics. However, the primary objectives of the 'regime of emergency state' are restoring law and order and ensuring safety during armed rebellion; attempts of violent overthrow of the regime; terrorist attacks; and national, confessional, and regional armed conflicts; the two other regimes are focused on disaster management.

9.3 Preparedness for a national disaster: The institutional framework

The Russian Federation has a huge network of institutions dealing with disaster management. The most relevant of them are as follows:

- The Federation Ministry of Health Care, and, under it, the Federal Health Care Surveillance Service with its regional departments.
- The Federal Service for Surveillance on Consumer Rights Protection and Human Wellbeing and its regional subdivisions. This institution played a leading role in administering the 'state of heightened preparedness' during the pandemic in 2020, even though it had been regarded previously as of minor importance.
- The Federation Ministry of Emergency Situations and its regional departments. These used to be the leading problem-solvers during natural and made-made disasters but played only a supporting role in the response to Covid-19.
- Regional ministries and agencies performing administrative and supervisory functions in the areas of health care and disaster management.

In the past decades, Russia's system for managing disasters has undergone changes in regard to the executive branch. With natural disasters having become more common due to climate change, the Federal Ministry of Emergency Situations, along with similar departments of the regional governments and local administrations, had to be enhanced significantly. The federal executive bodies governing health-care issues (and similar departments of the regional governments), as well the ones tasked with supervision of hospitals and other medical institutions, evolved mainly in terms of their functions, which were altered in the course of updates to legislation and health-care standards.

Subordination between the federal and regional ministries, agencies, and the like does not exist in a formal sense. However, federal ministries issue standards and other regulations that are to be followed by regional hospitals and organisations for which regional governments are responsible. Thus, indirectly, regional executives are influenced significantly by the Federal Ministry of Health Care and similar bodies when it comes to preparedness for disasters.

9.4 Rolling out measures to contain the pandemic

The unprecedented crisis caused by the pandemic changed the way in which state power and governance in Russia are organised, primarily by affecting relationships and functions among the central, regional, and local levels of the federal structure. Three stages may be identified.

In the first (January to February 2020), federal authorities took preventative measures to contain outbreaks (for instance, closure of borders) and make medical preparations. In the second stage (March to early April 2020), they continued combating the pandemic, but one region exercised its own judgment, Moscow (as Moscow metropolis is a separate constituent unit in the federation). In the third (from April 2020 onwards), the foci of decision-making moved to the regions. Simultaneously, federal agencies carried out large-scale hospital construction and, among other things, secured equipment and specialist supplies.

Notably, from the outset, Russia's efforts to combat the pandemic did not involve interparty conflict. The entire parliamentary opposition – that is, the three parties called the 'systemic opposition' – supported the President and the government in the measures they took. The non-systemic opposition – in other words, the parties which are excluded from the political system and absent in state government agencies and which are strongly opposed to the ruling party and status quo – did not consider it appropriate either to capitalise on the hardship the pandemic brought to the country. As mentioned, the ruling party's rigid discipline, adhered to by most of the governors, reinforced its dominance.

9.4.1 Taking the initiative

Before the first cases of Covid-19 were recorded on 31 January 2020, the federal government, in response to events in China, moved into action. On 27 January an operational headquarter ('task force') was established for the prevention of Covid-19, with Deputy Prime Minister Tatiana Golikova appointed as its chief. Later, similar 'task forces' appeared under the governments in all Russian regions and large cities. As measures to prevent the coronavirus from entering Russia, borders with China were closed on 31 January and later with other countries, while rail traffic was suspended and most flights cancelled.

After Moscow reported its first case of infection on 2 March 2020, the city government imposed lockdown measures on 5 March. In a national televised address on the same day, President Vladimir Putin announced a stay-at-home period (called 'non-working days' in Russia) from 30 March to 3 April 2020. Then, in a national address on 2 April, the President extended this until 30 April. On 30 March, Prime Minister Mikhail Mishustin asked regional authorities to consider the measures taken in Moscow and explore whether they could follow the capital's example. As a result, 26 regions had declared a lockdown (the 'self-isolation regime') by 31 March. On 8 April, President Putin instructed regional leaders to take measures independently from Moscow in line with the epidemiological situation.

Although federalism in Russia has tended towards centralisation since the early 2000s (Leksin 2008; Seliverstov 2015), the pandemic managed to shake the division of powers between the centre and the regions to a certain extent. From April 2020, restrictions and other measures aimed at fighting the pandemic, ensuring the health of the population, and supporting local economies were entrusted fully and personally to the governors of the regions (Presidential Decree No. 239 of 2 April 2020). At the same time, President Putin maintained strict control over the regional authorities and what they did; presidential plenipotentiary representatives in eight federal districts served this purpose. The federal government also retained management over the powers transferred to constituent units by, for example, issuing standard guidelines for regional governments and setting criteria for lifting restrictions and switching to softer measures.

The role and importance of several federal structures changed with the roll-out of pandemic response measures. For instance, the Federal Service for Surveillance on Consumer Rights Protection and Human Wellbeing (*Rospotrebnadzor*) and its regional departments came to the fore. From March 2020, this authority collected and processed all operational information on the spread of the virus, as well as drafted decisions and recommendations for other federal executive bodies.

In the complex system of measures to manage the pandemic nationwide and locally, we should note the President's role. Putin was well aware that the pre-existing crisis in Russia's economy would be compounded by negative public reaction to the pandemic's consequences and affect his popularity. Therefore, especially in the first stages, he took the initiative, showed himself demonstrably in control of the situation, and interacted continually with federal and regional authorities. As part of this, he delivered numerous televised addresses, and between April and May 2020, held almost weekly live-broadcast videoconferences with governors. Clearly, the President's actions were taken with an eye to the anticipated summer constitutional amendment referendum, a matter that received his special attention.[1]

9.4.2 Federal action

The actions taken by federal authorities fall into three main categories: situational monitoring and raising public awareness, coordinating devolved powers, and undertaking planning and economic support.

9.4.2.1 Monitoring and raising public awareness

In the face of extreme uncertainty, a panic epidemic can be as harmful as a viral epidemic: a rising flow of spontaneous information about the spread of disease increases societal tension and frustration. Accordingly, the State Centre for Information of Citizens about the Coronavirus, established in mid-March 2020, created an official public website covering these issues to advance public education.

9.4.2.2 Coordination and devolving powers

Between 2 April and 30 May 2020, President Putin issued three decrees granting extended powers to the top officials in the constituent units. These legal instruments enabled them to take a range of response measures to Covid-19 depending on the particular circumstances within their jurisdictions.

The Amendment Law No. 1-FKZ of 14 March 2020 introduced an additional matter under exclusive federal jurisdiction, namely, 'setting the common legal basis for the healthcare system'. At the same time, the matter of joint jurisdiction, referred to in article 72 of the RF Constitution as 'coordination of the health-care issues', was supplemented by provisions, inter alia, for widely available and high-quality medical care and the promotion of healthy living.

Several structures were established at the federal level for developing and implementing measures to combat Covid-19 and support the economy: operational headquarters for cooperation between the relevant executive authorities (which included the heads of federal ministries); a government commission (comprising heads of federal ministries and two heads of constituent units) to ensure sustainable economic development; a government coordination council (comprising heads of federal ministries and two heads of constituent units) to control the incidence of coronavirus infection; and a state council working group (consisting of federal and regional heads) to counter the spread of the virus.

There was also coordination of procedures for lifting Russia's nationwide restrictions after a first wave of coronavirus infections abated. The date 11 May 2020 marked the end of the 'non-working days' that had been in effect since 28 March. The federal government announced a three-stage plan for easing restrictions, one in which governors were given the right to decide when and how to lift them, albeit subject to the mandatory requirement that they comply with federal health regulations. Phase 1 allowed walks and open-air exercise, and small shops and service providers were permitted to reopen. Phase 2 permitted the opening of schools, large shops, and service companies, while Phase 3 extended this to parks, hotels, restaurants, and all shops. The criteria for easing restrictions in certain regions included infection rates, the availability of hospital beds, and testing for Covid-19.

9.4.2.3 Planning and economic support

The most important outcomes of the governmental commissions and coordinating bodies mentioned above were the Plan of Priority Measures (Actions), approved by the federal government on 17 March 2020, for ensuring sustainable economic development in the face of a worsening situation due to the spread of infections, followed by a plan, approved on 20 April, to address the pandemic's economic consequences. Within a few weeks in April and May, the government announced three packages to combat the pandemic and support the economy and population.

An important task for the federal authorities during the first months was to rectify shortages of personal protective gear, medicine, and equipment. Between March and April 2020, the number of tests for the virus increased ninefold; by mid-October, 200 test systems were being used to diagnose for Covid-19, of which more than 80 were of domestic origin. This fact places Russia among the world leaders in coronavirus test coverage (as of 31 October 2020, 60.4 million tests had been performed). In addition, by that date the number of hospital beds available for infected patients had quadrupled to 200,000.

In this regard, the Ministry of Defence made a significant contribution. Within a short period, it built 20 inpatient hospitals (on average, two months per hospital) in various regions of the country. Field hospitals were also set up in particularly disadvantaged constituent units, such as the Republic of Dagestan and the Transbaikal Region, while military personnel provided health treatment in some of the most affected areas.

The first package of federal economic support included credit holidays for small- and medium-sized businesses and certain categories of citizens, financial support for affected industries, and a preferential loan programme for paying wages. The most significant measure was a reduction – from 30 per cent to 15 per cent – in social insurance payment rates for small and medium-sized businesses. The second package, to the value of about 1 per cent of GDP, sought to assist strategically important companies, support regional budgets, and provide increased pay for health workers.

Both of the packages were criticised for being insufficient, focused on businesses rather than citizens, and lacking in cash transfers to beneficiaries. The third package, however, was larger, amounting to about RUB 800–900 billion, and provided for direct payments for families with children, for those recently unemployed due to business interruption, and for other socially vulnerable groups. Nevertheless, experts (Aganbegyan 2020) deemed these measures as inadequate, maintaining that the country's gold and forex reserves, along with the Russian National Wealth Fund, made it possible to (at least) double support for people and businesses affected by the pandemic.

On 23 September 2020, the federal government approved the National Action Plan to ensure the recovery of employment and income, economic growth, and long-term structural reform to the economy. Although morbidity had increased notably by then, the document did not mention this second wave of infection but spoke rather of restoring employment, supporting entrepreneurship, launching a new investment cycle, and improving the business climate. Other topics dealt with accelerating technological development, boosting exports, and encouraging import substitution.

9.4.3 Regional action

The decentralisation of decision-making during the pandemic highlighted how vastly different Russian regions are in terms of socio-economic development and the availability of tangible and intangible resources. Experts emphasise that this often happens when, in the face of unmanageable crises like Covid-19, the federal centre seeks to shift responsibility for tough or unpopular measures to regional authorities (Smyth et al. 2020); as a result, the task, say, of making trade-offs between the need to preserve citizens' health, on the one hand, and to sustain economic activity, on the other, is ultimately transferred to regional governments. Thus, it was that in the Russian Federation, it was the governors, not the President, who closed down business operations and imposed restrictions on people's movement.

During the pandemic, the jurisdiction of the federation's constituent units was increased. In terms of Federal Law No. 98-FZ (1 April 2020), the regional governments received one – though highly significant – power, namely, the power to determine the rules of conduct during the 'regime of emergency situation' and the 'state of heightened preparedness', rules that were binding on citizens and organisations. Regional legislatures and executives made avid use of this innovation, imposing limitations on rights that hitherto had been possible only under either martial law or a federal state of emergency.

9.4.3.1 Pandemic control measures

The regions actively engaged in the fight against the pandemic. In March 2020 alone, the heads of regions issued more than a thousand regulations that imposed restrictions of varying degrees of severity. These were based on Federal Law No. 68-FZ (21 December 1994) On Protection of Civilians and Territories from Emergencies Caused by Natural and Man-made Disasters, on Federal Law No. 52-FZ (30 March 1999) On Sanitary and Epidemiological Well-being of the Population, and on regional laws for protecting civilians and territory during emergencies.

The speed with which regions managed to respond to the coronavirus depended more on central government directives than on the epidemiological situation in any given region. The Russian Federation itself did not declare a national state of emergency. Instead, some of the first restrictions were introduced by the Moscow government on 5 March 2020. While the Republic of Buryatia was the only constituent unit to declare a state of emergency – which it did on 18 March, a point when no cases of Covid-19 had been recorded there yet – the majority of the regions (a total of 45 constituent units) imposed a 'state of heightened preparedness', with the rest operating under variants of the 'restriction state', which is less than 'a state of heightened preparedness' to enable them to respond promptly to outbreaks (Garant 2020).

Research by the St. Petersburg Policy Foundation divided the constituent units into three groups according to the severity of their restrictions (the so-called viral sovereignty index) (St. Petersburg Policy Foundation 2020). The toughest ones were adopted in 14 regions; 33 units were classified as average; and another 36 introduced relatively soft restrictions. Kalabikhina and Panin (2020) also identified three levels of lockdown measures (strict, medium, and low). The tighter the restrictions, the greater the possible economic losses and social tensions.

Moscow adopted the strictest measures, among which was QR (quick response) code contact tracing to control citizens' mobility. Some constituent units also introduced so-called digital passes but later abandoned this practice. A few regions kept a tight hold on visitors from Moscow, St. Petersburg, and other major cities. Many tried to introduce strict traffic control (Nizhny Novgorod), while the Chechen Republic and the Republic of Crimea first closed entry completely but then retracted the measure. When Ramzan Kadyrov, the head of the Chechen Republic, closed the region's borders entirely, his actions drew harsh criticism from Prime Minister Mikhail Mishustin, who warned the Chechen leader not to confuse the regional with the federal scope of authority.

Although Putin announced 12 May 2020 as the end of 'non-working days', the decision as to when to start lifting the specific Covid-19 restrictions was up to the governors who imposed them. Russian regions began easing quarantine restrictions starting from May 2020, almost immediately after the number of cases had peaked. In Moscow, most restrictions were significantly eased or lifted as early as June, but in other regions, they remained in place for longer and fell markedly by 1 September.

Regional government measures to combat the pandemic led not only to a gradual reduction in the number of people falling ill, but also to sharp drops in economic demand and household income, the curtailment of a large part of the service sector, and the virtual collapse of several industries, for example, tourism and the hotel and restaurant trade. Governmental restrictions were particularly devastating for small and medium-sized enterprises (SMEs).

9.4.3.2 Support for regions

At the end of April 2020, about a month after the restrictions were introduced, the federal government developed the Corona Crisis Action Plan, in terms of which all 85 constituent units adopted economic measures to stimulate local business: 84 regions had non-tax-support measures (e.g., subsidies and reductions in rental rates), while 80 also had tax-support measures (such as tax deferrals and abatements). It is estimated that, all in all, the regions deployed 839 economic measures, 45 per cent of which were tax-related and 55 per cent, non-tax-related. The most common ones were tax incentives, deferred rent for small businesses and companies from affected sectors, and subsidies to SMEs (Mavrina 2020).

According to rankings by the National Rating Agency (2020), Moscow, the Republics of Buryatia and Crimea, Perm Krai, Chukotka Autonomous Okrug, Tula, Irkutsk, and Chelyabinsk Oblasts took the most measures to support businesses affected by the pandemic. Support from local authorities may have buffered regional economic decline, but in the pandemic situation, it simply harmed many regional budgets. Regional economies that were the most affected by the restrictions suffered primarily due to regionally specific circumstances rather than the pandemic itself. Therefore, the search for a balance between economic well-being and health in these regions shifted, quite predictably, towards economic well-being. As survey data show, support measures were not available to everyone who needed them (Chamber of Commerce and Industry of the Russian Federation 2020).

Our analysis suggests that the downturn in economic activity was likely to have a negative impact on regional development and increase regional disparities in terms both of economic indicators and of social well-being. Experts have underlined that transferring authority and responsibility for the fight against Covid-19 to regions where resources are scarce would, first of all, increase regional expenses: indeed, it is estimated that budget expenditure increased by 30 per cent over six months and that more than half of the regions experienced increased budget deficit (Komin and Poltoratskaya 2020; Trunova and Zemlyanski 2020).

The arrangement in turn would have made disadvantaged regions lacking in resources of their own even more dependent on the centre and its financial support. Given that the capacity to support people and businesses depends on regional economic and social development (primarily in the health-care system), more advanced and wealthier regions would be able to fight the pandemic more effectively than poorer ones, leading to greater inequality. Possible long-term negative consequences include deferred problems in the economy (including those resulting from reduced private sector investment) and increased social tensions.

9.4.3.3 Federal-regional dynamics

The need for prompt solutions and the high level of diversity in living and working conditions across the country inevitably led to decision-making on specific measures being delegated to the regions. This process, as noted, exacerbated existing problems and created new ones.

During the pandemic, the centre exercised supervision over the situation in the regions, with the President or the federal government intervening in certain cases to enable regions to carry out their devolved functions. Due to the existence of multiple channels for transmitting information requiring action and difficulties in coordinating individual agencies, sometimes only the centre's direct intervention could clear the red tape.

After the Federal Service for Surveillance on Consumer Rights Protection and Human Wellbeing criticised them for the inadequacy of their measures to combat Covid-19, several regional heads (those of Kamchatka Krai, Arkhangelsk Oblast, and the Komi Republic) handed in resignation letters to the RF President (RBK Information Agency News 2020). The Governor of Khabarovsk Krai was dismissed by the President for loss of trust and confidence (TASS Information Agency News 2020).

In a few cases involving abnormal outbreaks and inadequate health-care systems in constituent units, the federal government provided improved capacity at federal medical centres, ambulance services from neighbouring regions, and hospital construction by the defence ministry.

The Covid-19 crisis again illustrated a fundamental problem with Russian federalism: the gap between how much responsibility regional (and municipal) authorities have in comparison to the resources and powers available to them and their capacity to fulfil their responsibilities.

9.4.4 Self-government in cities and municipalities

One well-known feature of Russian federalism is the relatively weak role that cities and municipalities play in the administration (Chikhladze et al. 2020). Their subordinate place in intergovernmental and fiscal relations is due largely to the limited possibilities for drawing up local budgets. In the fight against the coronavirus, this all became clearly apparent when major decisions and concrete measures were taken at the national and regional levels, while cities and municipalities worked with whatever funds they had. While there is no doubt that city authorities did not take a passive stance in combating Covid-19, their actions were limited by their powers, on the one hand, and, on the other, their physical and financial resources.

For example, the mayor's office in Novosibirsk (the third-most populous city in Russia) monitored the availability of drugs in pharmacies across the city and, in case of shortages, negotiated with manufacturers and suppliers. Similarly, a shortage of personal protective equipment (PPE) was eliminated swiftly with its help. Considerable effort was also put into supporting municipal hospitals and medical institutions. As a second wave of infection started to emerge, the city authorities began well in advance to retool individual hospitals, health centres, and social assistance centres in their jurisdiction for treating coronavirus patients.

Moscow City, as a unit of the federation, made the most effective and innovative governance decisions. Among other things, the local administration used CCTV and facial recognition to control patient mobility; devised special schedules for Muscovites to go out and get groceries during the first wave of infection; used QR code contact tracing; and deployed systems to control travel using personal transport. The city authorities also paid great attention to improving remote learning for schoolchildren and students. Crucially, the mayor, Sergey Sobyanin, was personally and constantly engaged in resolving issues and in direct contact with the population.

The effectiveness of Moscow's management of the pandemic meant that the rest of the country could avoid economic collapse and social instability. Moscow may yet become a kind of laboratory for testing managerial solutions within the digital economy.

9.4.5 Intergovernmental relations

In Russia, intergovernmental relations (IGR) are facilitated via various institutions, officials, and procedures (Leksin 2018). First of all, the President and the two chambers of the Federal Assembly, namely, the State Duma and Federation

Council, are important instruments of IGR. Under the RF Constitution, the President ensures coordinated functioning of the country's governing bodies. In fact, he is the key IGR instrument, albeit influencing regional governors mainly through informal meetings and consultations. The State Duma also enables informal IGR, but it interacts directly and formally with regional legislatures and executives, which are entitled to make submissions on federal bills on matters of joint jurisdiction. The Federation Council's relations with regional governments are the closest of all, given that every regional legislature and executive has a representative in the Federation Council.

Furthermore, specialised institutions exist for enhancing the interaction between orders of government. These are advisory bodies, including the RF State Council, the Council of Legislators under the Federal Assembly's chambers, and the councils under plenipotentiary representatives of the President in the federal districts. Such institutions were not explicitly designed to deal with disasters; they were designed to enable discussion and cooperation, not to make orders or execute them. However, all of these structures were involved in disaster management during the pandemic. For instance, a specialised working group on pandemic issues operated within the RF State Council.

The intergovernmental structures designed to face a wide variety of challenges, including national disasters, are primarily the above-mentioned Federation Council, the State Council, and the councils under the President's plenipotentiary representatives in the federal districts. The State Council of the Russian Federation is an advisory body chaired by the President and consisting of the leaders of all the constituent units, as well as of a number of federal officials. Similar bodies exist under the plenipotentiary representatives of the President in the eight federal districts.

The IGR structures of a technical nature are provided for in the federal law, On the Protection of Population and Territory against Natural and Technogenic Emergency Situations (1994). This statute entrusts coordination of emergency prevention and response activities to a system of specialised bodies. The system consists of commissions that can comprise officials representing two orders of government, the ministries and other governmental structures designed to deal with emergencies, as well as the national control centre at the federal level and crisis management centres at the interregional and regional levels.

In addition, during the pandemic, governments at all levels established bodies designated as 'task forces'. At the federal level, separate ministries and agencies created their bodies of this type. According to the regulations establishing these bodies, they perform coordinating and advisory functions. However, their recommendations are generally taken as mandatory guidelines for governmental bodies and legal entities. These institutions also provide for intergovernmental coordination, given that their informal nature permits them to constitute an organic hierarchy. At a minimum, 'task forces' at the lower levels convey information upwards and follow directions from above.

Apart from these institutions, other informal means of enhancing inter-governmental cooperation are relatively common. These include councils and meetings of officials responsible for various health-care and disaster management issues.

Horizontal cooperation among regional and local governments did not bur-geon during the pandemic, seeing as every government was responsible for taking measures within its own territory. However, coordination and sharing best practices were common occurrences. For one thing, because Moscow was the first to experience mass contagion, most regional governments followed the broad pattern laid out in the policies it adopted; for another, adjacent regions occasionally employed coordinated lockdown measures. For instance, during the most restrictive period, driving in vehicles without having a digital pass was banned in many regions – because each region issued its own passes, it was incon-venient to travel through several regions using this kind of system. However, the e-government platforms of Moscow City and Moscow Oblast (Moscow prov-ince) issued passes valid in both regions.

The pandemic also led to instances of interregional discord, especially during the first months. For instance, various regional governments arbitrarily decided to impose a 14-day quarantine on visitors from regions with high infection rates (particularly Moscow), with some even closing their borders to entry. The fed-eral government responded with verbal criticism, but no punitive measures were exacted, as the disputes were settled informally.

It should be noted that many problematic issues in IGR during the pandemic were resolved through hands-on management (common in Russia). Several gov-ernors sought a personal meeting with the President, where they asked for special federal support due to crisis in their regions. Such informal arrangements, for instance, ensured the construction of field hospitals for Covid-19 in Dagestan and inpatient hospitals in other territories.

9.4.6 Intergovernmental fiscal relations

At present the share of regional and local budget revenues in the consolidated budget of the Russian Federation is 34.7 per cent. Moreover, there is a signifi-cant asymmetry in the distribution of federal support – 16 regions do not receive transfers from the federal budget while in some regions the share of transfers in their budget revenues is higher than 70 per cent, for example, in the republics of the North Caucasus and the Republic of Crimea.

In the first half of 2020, the intergovernmental fiscal transfers provided to the regions amounted to RUB 1.4 trillion, which was 1.6 times higher than in the first half of 2019. However, a low level of expenditure is observed – on subsidies (29 per cent) and other transfers (30.6 per cent) on non-Covid related activities.

As of 1 July 2020, the federal government had adopted about 80 resolutions on the allocation of funds to address the following: supporting measures to ensure that the worsening situation did not impact on economic sectors and their development; preventing and eliminating the consequences of the pandemic; and protecting the population's health and treating the ill, along with other pandemic-related support to citizens. All this amounted to RUB 1.3 trillion. The most significant support measures were social spending on benefits to families with children under 16 years (RUB 496.5 billion) and grants to the constituent units allowing them to balance their budgets while providing medical care to Covid-19 patients (RUB 168.2 billion).

In general, the revenues of the consolidated budgets of constituent units for January–June 2020 were 2.1 per cent higher than in the corresponding period in 2019, amounting to RUB 6.3 trillion. However, the expenditure during the first half of the year increased by 18.9 per cent and amounted to RUB 6.5 trillion. Such a ratio of income to expenditure growth rates is due to the fact that during the first half of 2019, the regions' total budget resulted in a surplus of RUB 695.7 billion, while 2020 showed a deficit of RUB 213.7 billion.

The growth in expenditure was mostly covered by uncompensated receipts from the federal budget. A decrease in revenue of the consolidated budgets of constituent units was observed in 16 regions, with the largest ones in the Yamal-Nenets Autonomous District (19.2 per cent) and Tyumen region (17.2 per cent). However, due to higher transfers, an increase in income was observed in 69 regions, with the largest ones in the Jewish Autonomous region (39.3 per cent) and the Republic of Ingushetia (35.2 per cent).

In most units of the Russian Federation, business support was provided from regional budgets regardless of the size of their own-source revenues and deficits since a basic source of resources were federal transfers and budget loans provided by the federal Ministry of Finance. Commercial loans were generally less significant for closing gaps in regional and local budgets.

The federal government allocated RUB 300 billion as transfers and grants, and it restructured budget loans for RUB 69.5 billion. Moreover, the government mitigated measures of responsibility for the fulfilment of obligations under the agreement with the regions and eased requirements for the parameters of the debt load on commercial loans. Experts estimated that the shortfall in regional budget revenues was about three times higher, and believed the support from the centre was still insufficient (St. Petersburg Policy Foundation 2020).

With more financial resources allocated to them, constituent units became accountable for their response measures to Covid-19 and the socio-economic impact of the pandemic. The federal centre also imposed stricter control on spending and policy efficiency. Based on these conditions, one can conclude that centralisation in public administration has strengthened in Russia.

9.5 Findings and policy implications

Several conclusions can be drawn from this case study of the Russian Federation.

First, Russia's success in pandemic response was due to the joint efforts of the central and regional authorities. These efforts were facilitated to a large extent by strong presidential vertical power and the ruling party's dominance over regional and municipal administrations. As a result, Russia avoided centre-region confrontation, interparty competition, tensions between national autonomies and the central government, and interreligious conflicts.

Secondly, despite the increasing centralisation of Russian federalism in recent decades, a certain balance of interests between the centre and regions was achieved during a crisis-ridden 2020. In view of Russia's vast size, the inequality among its constituent units, and the significant regional disparities it saw in the spread as well as control of the coronavirus, a decentralised approach to countering the pandemic was the only viable option.

Delegating powers to the units to combat the pandemic from April 2020 onwards generally strengthened federative principles in Russia, albeit that it did not result in new formalised structures for IGR. In some cases, inter-state and inter-budgetary relations were nevertheless either inadequate or only semi-formal in nature. As such, one of the implications of the crisis the federal system faced in 2020 is that Russia should make provision for a more consolidated form of decentralisation, for stronger centre-region bonds, and better institutional support for IGR processes – all of which improved immensely during the fight against the pandemic.

Thirdly, most constituent units and urban settlements in Russia coped adequately with the pandemic at its onset, with some, such as Moscow and Novosibirsk Oblast, employing particularly innovative models of crisis management. However, when the authority to make decisions was given to the regions, they were often reluctant or unprepared to leverage their newfound powers due to poor regional governance. In several regions, the federal centre was forced to intervene in the fight against Covid-19, allocate additional resources, and impose strict control measures.

Fourth, in this regard, a lesson for the future is that there is a need to find an equilibrium and compromise between Russia's competitive federalism and the cooperative form prevalent in certain European countries. On the one hand, the fight against global threats will require, as noted, widespread solidarity based on the understanding that these are common rather than private or sectarian issues. On the other hand, the inevitable growth of the digital economy and, with it, phenomena such as telework and telemedicine, will lead to greater 'digital inequalities' among Russian regions and thus to even greater asymmetry and competition among them for qualified personnel, new technologies, personalised medicine, and more.

Special measures will hence be needed in intergovernmental and inter-budgetary relations to smooth out such asymmetry in the future. Although one of the dominant features of 'wild' Russian federalism during the deep economic and political crisis of the 1990s – namely, political loyalty by regional elites in exchange for federal resources – is a thing of the past, the next goal is finally to eliminate elements of this system that make it necessary to rely on hands-on management of federative relations by the President alone.

As 2020 showed us, the current high centralisation of executive power in Russia's federal system is likely to have reached its limit and can hardly intensify any further. The joint fight against the Covid-19 pandemic triggered decentralisation processes in relations between the Russian federal centre and regions. Moreover, we may consolidate this fairly successful experience and expand it not only to other crises but also the general development of federalism in Russia.

Note

1 The national constitutional referendum was held in Russia between 25 June and 1 July 2020. The proposed amendments included various social guarantees and human rights; changes to certain powers held by the Federal Assembly; granting the President extended authority and reducing that of the government; and judicial reforms establishing the supremacy of Russian law over international law. A major amendment concerned nullifying the number of presidential terms served, thereby allowing Vladimir Putin to remain in power after his term ends in 2024. In the referendum, 78 per cent of voters supported these amendments, with the percentage varying from 44 per cent to 98 per cent across the constituent units.

References

Aganbegyan, A. G. 2020. 'Crisis as a Window of Opportunity for Socio-economic Development', Moscow Economic Academic Forum, 14 May, https://www.ieie.su/assets/files/news/2020/statya-aganbegyana.pdf (accessed on 11 October 2020).

Chamber of Commerce and Industry of the Russian Federation. 2020. 'Business Barometer First Stage', http://ngtpp.ru/wp-content/uploads/2020/04/Prilozhenie_ITOGI-BBS-1-939160-v1.pdf (accessed on 2 October 2020).

Chikhladze, L. T., A. A. Larichev and E. N. Khazov (eds). 2020. *Local Government in a Unified System of Public Administration: Vector and Consequences of the Constitutional Reform in the Russian Federation*. Moscow: YUNITI-DANA.

Garant. 2020. 'Legal Information System', http://base.garant.ru/77398959/ (accessed on 8 October 2020).

Kalabikhina, I. and A. Panin. 2020. 'Spatial Choreography of the Coronavirus', *Population and Economics*, 4(2): 123–52.

Komin, M. and V. Poltoratskaya. 2020. 'Responsibility Instead of Rights: Did the Pandemic Lead to the Federalisation of Russia', *RBC*, 4 April, https://www.rbc.ru/opinions/politics/04/04/2020/5e87291b9a7947054c55500f (accessed on 12 September 2020).

Leksin, I. 2016. 'Constitutional Federalism and Public Administration: Russia', in A. Farazmand (ed.), *Global Encyclopaedia of Public Administration, Public Policy, and Governance*. Cham: Springer International Publishing.

Leksin, I. 2018. 'The Dialectic between the BRICS Partnership and Multilevel Government in the Russian Federation', in Nico Steytler (ed.), *The BRICS Partnership: Challenges and Prospects for Multilevel Government*, pp. 20–31. Cape Town: Juta.

Leksin, I. and V. Seliverstov. 2017. *Concurrency of Powers in the Russian Federation*, in Nico Steytler (ed.), *Concurrent Powers in Federal Systems: Meaning, Making, Managing*, pp. 164–206. Leiden: Brill Nijhoff.

Leksin, V. 2008. *Federativnaya Rossiya I ee regional'naya politika (Federal Russia and its Regional Policy)*. Moscow: INFRA.

Mavrina, L. 2020. 'The Regions Used the Potential of Business Support to the Maximum', *Vedomosti*, 15 September, https://www.vedomosti.ru/economics/articles/2020/09/14/839894-regioni-podderzhki (accessed on 15 October 2020).

National Rating Agency. 2020. 'Between Scylla and Charybdis: How Russian Regions Deal with Pandemic Economic Consequences', https://www.investinregions.ru/analytics/a/materials-71332/ (accessed on 28 August 2020).

RBK Information Agency News. 2020. 2 April, https://www.rbc.ru/rbcfreenews/5e85f9499a7947051649bb27 (accessed on 13 September 2020).

Seliverstov, V. E. 2015. 'Genesis of Federalism, Regional Development and Regional Policy of Post-Soviet Russia', in F. Palermo and E. Alber (eds), *Federalism as Decision-making: Changes in Structures, Procedures and Policies*, pp. 148–66. Leiden: Brill Nijhoff.

Smyth, R. et al. 2020. 'The Russian Power Vertical and the Covid-19 Challenge: The Trajectories of Regional Responses', *PONARS Eurasia Policy Memos*, 646, https://www.ponarseurasia.org/memo/russian-power-vertical-covid-19-challenge-trajectories-regional-responses (accessed on 18 September 2020).

St. Petersburg Policy Foundation. 2020. 'Rating', https://davydov.in/politics/rejting-fonda-peterburgskaya-politika-za-avgust-2020-goda/ (accessed on 23 September 2020).

TASS Information Agency News. 2020. 20 July, https://tass.ru/politika/9007027 (accessed on 13 September 2020).

Trunova, N. and D. Zemlyanski. 2020. 'What Did the Sudden Onset of "Crisis" Federalism in Russia Lead to?', *Forbes*, 28 May, https://www.forbes.ru/finansy-i-investicii/401625-k-chemu-privel-vnezapno-nastupivshiy-krizisnyy-federalizm-v-rossii (accessed on 28 August 2020).

PART II

North America

10

AMERICAN FEDERALISM AND COVID-19

Party Trumps policy

John Kincaid and J. Wesley Leckrone

10.1 Introduction

Although the United States (US) ranked first among 195 countries on the 2019 Global Health Security Index, it responded poorly to the pandemic, mainly because President Donald Trump did not forge a coordinated response with the states' governors and because political party polarisation often thwarted cooperative state-federal, inter-state, and state-local relations. Near the end of November 2020, among federal countries only Belgium (136.7 deaths per 100,000 population), Spain (91.2), Argentina (83.2), Brazil (80.8), and Mexico (80.6) had worse outcomes than the United States (78.5).

However, because of the dualist structure of US federalism and the states' constitutionally reserved police power, the states were able to respond to the pandemic in ways that ranged from strict to lax, thus reducing Covid-19 deaths below what is likely to have prevailed if the federal government had controlled the pandemic response but higher than would likely have prevailed under a cooperative-federalism response. Nevertheless, the federal government performed a crucial role by providing financial support for the development of vaccines against Covid-19. Overall, the pandemic has not, to date, wrought significant changes in the constitutional or operational features of American federalism.

The US has 331 million people, with a median age of 37.9 years and a 79.1-year life expectancy. Levels of urbanisation and density vary from Maine (38.7 per cent urban) to California (95.0), and from Alaska (1.3 people per square mile) to New Jersey (1,210.1). Of persons most susceptible to Covid-19, 16.5 per cent are aged 65 and over. They experienced 79 per cent of all Covid-19 deaths. People (mostly elderly) in long-term care facilities accounted for about 8 per cent of coronavirus cases but 45 per cent of all Covid-19 deaths.

DOI: 10.4324/9781003166771-13

Additionally, 13.4 per cent of Americans are black (108.4 deaths per 100,000), totalling 20.7 per cent of all US deaths; 2.4 per cent are American Indian (90.0), totalling 1 per cent of deaths; 16.7 per cent are Latino (73.5), totalling 21.3 per cent of deaths; 60.1 per cent are white (54.4), totalling 51.4 per cent of deaths; and 5.6 per cent are Asian (45.4), totalling 4.1 per cent of all deaths.

Public health is mainly a state responsibility, which most states decentralise in varying degrees to their county governments (which exist in 48 states). The federal government's public health duties apply to foreign and inter-state travel and commerce and to providing support to the states, such as research, data collection and dissemination, pharmaceutical approvals, expertise, health guidelines, financial aid, supplies, and emergency field hospitals. Health care and insurance are mostly private, but the federal Medicare programme insures citizens aged 65 and over; two intergovernmental programmes, Medicaid and the Children's Health Insurance Program, cover low-income people of all ages (about 18 per cent of the US population being enrolled in these programmes); and the intergovernmental Affordable Care Act subsidises private health insurance for another 23 million citizens. However, about 28 million non-elderly remain uninsured.

The first laboratory-confirmed Covid-19 case occurred on 20 January 2020 and was reported to the US Centers for Disease Control and Prevention (CDC) on 22 January. The first announced Covid-19 death was on 29 February in Washington state (although several deaths were later discovered to have occurred earlier). The country experienced its first Covid-19 surge in late March to early April, with a peak of 34,904 cases on 9 April, a second surge in July with a peak of 79,086 cases on 24 July, and a third surge in October and November with a peak of 200,447 cases on 20 November.

As of 23 November 2020, the US had recorded 12,778,467 reported infections, equating to 3,906 cases per 100,000 people. Daily deaths peaked at 2,702 on 15 April, dropping sharply thereafter. However, deaths began to increase in late fall, with an increase from 898 to 1,929 between 31 October and 19 November, making for a total of 263,198 deaths since January. Together, the commuter-connected states of Connecticut, New Jersey, and New York, with 9.6 per cent of the US population, had 27.2 per cent of US deaths on 18 September (dropping to 22.0 per cent by 21 November 2020).[1]

The initial epicentre was New York City, with a second centre on the West coast. Covid-19 entered California, Oregon, and Washington from China but entered the New York region from Europe. During the summer, Covid-19 spread to more urbanised areas in the Midwest and South but spread into all states and rural areas during September through November.

The federal government reacted first when President Trump restricted travel from China on 31 January and Congress enacted a USD 8.3 billion emergency supplemental appropriation signed by Trump on 6 March. State and local governments began reacting substantially on 11 March. Yet despite efforts to contain the coronavirus, the country was experiencing its third and largest case surge in late November 2020.

10.2 The federal constitutional and legislative framework

The US federal system was established upon ratification of the US Constitution in 1788. It is a congressional-presidential federation with 50 states and seven territories and a dualist structure in which the states delegated certain limited powers to the federal (i.e., national) government and reserved all other powers to themselves. The powers delegated to the federal government chiefly involve international and interstate commerce, national defence, and foreign affairs, although in the 20th century, the federal government assumed substantial responsibility for national social welfare and enforcement of civil rights and liberties. Tax powers to raise revenue are also delegated, as a consequence of which the federal government is not dependent on the states for revenue as was the confederal government under the prior Articles of Confederation of 1781. The major federalist innovation of the US Constitution, according to Alexander Hamilton, is the authority of the federal government to legislate directly for individuals within its sphere of authority (i.e., levy taxes and conscript men into the military) (Kincaid 2014). Each state has its own constitution and complete government, consisting of an elected legislature, elected governor and often other elected executives, and a supreme court (whose members are elected in many states). The federal system operates with two political parties: Democrats, which are left-oriented, and Republicans, right-oriented. Other parties exist but have little political impact.

The states have primary responsibility for public health because they possess the police power, which is the authority to legislate for the health, safety, welfare, and morals of their citizens. The states did not delegate this power to the federal government. It is a key reserved power of the states under the US Constitution's Tenth Amendment (1791). Historically, state and local governments have managed epidemics with little or no federal assistance, as was the case in the last major epidemic in 1918 (Barry 2004).

Responsibility for managing other matters affected by a pandemic are divided and shared between the federal and state governments. The federal government commands monetary policy and can enact laws to stimulate the economy by altering federal taxes and engaging in deficit spending to aid persons and jurisdictions. Most social welfare programmes are intergovernmental, with the federal government paying half or more of the cost. Child care, education, policing, emergency medical services, and small businesses, among other matters, come under the states' purview. They have the authority to close and reopen schools and businesses. They might also have authority to close their borders, but no state has done so. Instead, many states have required out-of-state arrivals to quarantine for 14 days, although it has been difficult to enforce the quarantines. The authority of county and municipal governments to take drastic measures varies among the states, but many local governments issued stay-at-home orders (SAHOs) before their state government (see below).

The US Constitution contains no explicit provision for any federal branch to exercise emergency powers. However, Congress and presidents have found ways to assert some emergency powers. The National Emergencies Act of 1976 terminated all previous emergencies and authorises the President to exercise 136 specific emergency powers defined in the law and within procedural limits. A presidential emergency declaration can be ended by a joint resolution of Congress. In addition, the Public Health Service Act of 1944 includes some emergency powers.

Since the enactment of the Federal Disaster Relief Act of 1950, presidents have had authority to declare disasters. The currently significant federal disaster statutes are the Stafford Act of 1988 and Homeland Security Act of 2002. The leading federal agency is the Federal Emergency Management Agency (FEMA), created in 1979.

Ordinarily, governors must request disaster declarations from the President; however, under exigent circumstances, the President can issue a disaster declaration without a gubernatorial request. This unilateral presidential authority is somewhat unusual in the American system because many presidential decisions require consent or consultation with other officials. A disaster declaration authorises the dispatch of sometimes substantial personnel, material, and financial aid to the affected jurisdictions. On 13 March 2020, Trump issued 57 disaster declarations for all states, Washington, D.C., and US territories – the first all-state declaration in US history. Past declarations have covered only one state or a group of states affected by a disaster such as a hurricane.

To date, the federal courts have placed few constraints on states' emergency powers and on the federal government's pandemic responses. The principal US Supreme Court ruling upholding state emergency responses to public health crises is *Jacobson v. Massachusetts* (197 US 11, 1905), which upheld the authority of states to enforce compulsory vaccination laws.

10.3 Preparedness for a national disaster: The institutional framework

Compared to other countries, the US was well prepared for a pandemic; however, the President was initially slow to deploy resources and less than efficient in doing so later. He generally prioritised maintenance of the economy over suppression of the virus. In addition, money for federal, state, and local public health programmes had been cut for decades.

The leading federal agency for pandemic responses is the US Department of Health and Human Services, which houses the CDC, National Institutes of Health, Food and Drug Administration, and National Vaccine Advisory Committee. The US Department of Homeland Security plays a role because FEMA and some other relevant agencies are located there. The US Department of Defense performs such response functions as accelerating delivery of medical supplies to states and localities. The US Department of the Interior is responsible for public health on 500 million acres of federal land and Indian reservations. All these agencies mobilised at varying speeds, and Dr Anthony Fauci, director of the National Institute of Allergy and Infectious Diseases since 1984, soon became the most televised and trusted voice on the pandemic. Trump and Dr Fauci had a tense relationship because Fauci sometimes contradicted the President's messaging (Cathey 2020).

Avian flu outbreaks and a lack of national strategy to deal with a pandemic led President George W. Bush to push for new federal policies (Homeland Security Council 2005). The Public Readiness and Emergency Preparedness Act of 2005 authorised more than USD 3 billion for pandemic preparedness. A Pandemic and All-Hazards Preparedness Act was enacted in 2006, providing for development of a National Health Security Strategy and a Biomedical Advanced Research and Development Authority. However, funding for most of the Act's programmes expired in 2018. A reauthorisation of the Act was signed by President Trump in June 2019.

In 2016, President Barack Obama's administration developed a Playbook for Early Response to High-Consequence Emerging Infectious Disease Threats and Biological Incidents (Diamond and Toosi 2020). The Trump administration apparently did not use it, relying instead on its own plans: a National Biodefense Strategy (2018), which is mostly goals rather than plans, and two plans generally viewed as flawed, a Biological Incident Annex (2017) and Pandemic Crisis Action Plan (2018) (Johnson 2020). In an effort to coordinate federal-agency responses, Trump organised a White House Task Force on the Coronavirus headed by Vice President Mike Pence.

None of the federal agencies or the taskforce are formally intergovernmental, although most have advisory committees that include state and local officials. Agencies such as the CDC in particular have regularised channels of communication with state and local public health officials. The CDC also relies on those governments to report data regularly, such as Covid-19 cases, deaths, hospitalisation rates, and testing rates. All of the states and many counties have public health agencies, although they vary in their capacities and levels of expertise.

10.4 Rolling out measures to contain the pandemic

Most of the major federal, state, and local government responses occurred from mid-March to late April 2020 after the gravity of Covid-19 had become apparent to public officials and citizens. Details of these responses are discussed below.

Most notable was sharp political party polarisation over Covid-19 among politicians and citizens. Generally, Democrats supported stern measures to suppress Covid-19 and encouraged such personal behaviours as mask-wearing; generally, Republicans supported living with the coronavirus so as to maintain jobs and the economy and resisted state governments' mask-wearing mandates as violations of individual freedoms. This party polarisation affected all aspects of intergovernmental relations and weakened pandemic responses. The roles of the parties confirm long-standing theories about the importance of parties in federal systems (e.g. Grodzins 1960; Riker 1964; Detterbeck et al. 2015).

Otherwise, the US is not marked by deep multicultural or multinational diversity; however, as noted above, blacks, Latinos, and indigenous peoples were affected more severely by Covid-19 than whites and Asians. This difference led to controversy, though conflict was channelled through the party system given that blacks, Latinos, and indigenous peoples are key voting blocs within the Democratic Party.

10.4.1 Taking the initiative

Early in the pandemic, there was little conflict over which order of government should go first because governments acted largely independently within their spheres of authority. The Trump administration declared a Public Health Emergency on 31 January 2020 that allowed for travel restrictions from China (2 February), Iran (28 February), and Europe (12 March), as well as other mitigation efforts to prevent people infected with Covid-19 from entering the US. Trump declared a National Emergency on 13 March, which authorised USD 50 billion to address the pandemic.

State and local governments were simultaneously acting to prevent Covid's spread within their jurisdictions. San Francisco was the first locality to declare a local emergency on 15 February and joined with surrounding local governments to enact the first order closing businesses and schools. California was the first state to declare an emergency and on 19 March became the first to issue a statewide SAHO. By 1 April, 33 other states had followed suit. However, conflict between the federal and state governments emerged in March and early April, as the Trump administration proved unwilling to coordinate distribution of medical supplies and testing equipment, while at the same time pushing states to open their economies while Covid cases were increasing. Despite the histrionics between Trump and some governors, intergovernmental coordination began to develop, particularly among federal, state, and local bureaucrats.

10.4.2 Federal action

Following the President's restrictions on international travel, his emergency, and disaster declarations, and his signing of Congress's emergency supplemental appropriation on 6 March, and following the World Health Organization's declaration of a global pandemic on 11 March, Congress passed four relief bills by huge bipartisan margins:

- Families First Coronavirus Response Act, signed by Trump on 18 March, providing USD 95 billion;
- Coronavirus Aid, Relief, and Economic Security (CARES) Act (27 March), providing USD 2.2 trillion;
- Pay Check Protection Program and Health Care Enhancement Act (23 April), providing USD 484 billion; and
- Pay Check Protection Program Flexibility Act (5 June).

Altogether, Congress provided about USD 360 billion in aid to state and local governments to fight the pandemic. Further, the Federal Reserve (the US central bank equivalent) initiated many stimulus programmes, including USD 2.3 trillion in lending to support households, employers, financial markets, and state and local governments as well as a Municipal Liquidity Facility (MLF) for the state-local bond market. Although USD 500 billion was pledged to the MLF, few states and localities participated in the programme, in part because they obtained better or equivalent borrowing terms in the regular markets.

The President conferred frequently with governors (although Vice President Mike Pence became the preferred contact for many governors) and invoked the Defense Production Act (1950) on 2 April, which enabled the federal government to expedite purchase contracts and loans for private companies to produce medical equipment and supplies needed for the pandemic. The President also expedited supply deliveries to states and localities and fast-tracked production of a Covid-19 vaccine. The CDC issued voluntary SAHOs and other preventive guidelines for state and local officials. In taking these actions, the President did not substantially enhance executive powers or marginalise Congress, although he did issue a few executive orders that raised concerns about power enhancement and circumvention of Congress. One controversial measure was signed by Trump in early August when he unilaterally suspended payroll taxes and announced USD 400 weekly payments for the unemployed when talks on larger Covid relief legislation broke down with Congress (Haberman et al. 2020).

By April, moreover, the President was at loggerheads with many governors, especially Democrats, because he wanted them to end their SAHOs and reopen their economies. He called resistant governors 'mutineers' and tweeted such messages as 'LIBERATE MICHIGAN.' By late June, gridlock settled in between the Democratic House and Republican Senate and between the President and congressional Democrats and some congressional Republicans.

Even so, President Trump's most consequential action was his 15 May 2020 announcement of Operation Warp Speed, a public-private partnership funded with USD 10 billion in federal money, to develop an anti-Covid-19 vaccine by the end of 2020. By late November, three corporations – Pfizer, Moderna, and AstraZeneca-Oxford University – announced successful vaccine trials. Pfizer and AstraZeneca each received more than USD 1 billion from Operation Warp Speed; Pfizer received a USD 1.95 billion advance-purchase agreement from the initiative. Distribution of the vaccine was expected to start in late December and be carried out mostly through the states.

The federal government did not use the pandemic to augment intrusions into state and local domains. The federal government lacks constitutional authority to command a national response, and the President largely left response responsibilities to the states. On 13 April 2020, Trump claimed 'total' power to reopen states' economies, but he retreated the next day under heavy criticism. The state-local aid packages enacted by Congress contained the usual conditions and structures of accountability attached to federal aid but no unusual regulatory leaps.

The federal courts largely deferred to the pandemic responses undertaken by the federal, state, and local governments. There was considerable litigation by religious groups against state SAHOs, but the US Supreme Court was initially unsympathetic. For example, in *Calvary Chapel Dayton Valley v. Sisolak* (No. 19A1070) in July 2020, the Court upheld Nevada's restrictions on worship services that were stricter than rules governing casinos and restaurants, leading one dissenting justice to quip, 'There is no world in which the Constitution permits Nevada to favour Caesars Palace [a casino] over Calvary Chapel.' In a series of decisions, the Court also held that in litigation over the 3 November presidential election, federal courts should uphold changes in voting procedures, such as mailed ballots and deadline extensions, enacted by state legislatures or decided by state agencies and courts. The Supreme Court also rejected intervention by lower federal courts attempting to loosen state voting restrictions due to Covid-19 in a number of cases. However, on 14 September, a US district court judge ruled that the Pennsylvania governor's March SAHO violated various rights, including property rights, guaranteed by the US Constitution (*County of Butler v. Wolf*, 2:20-cv-677, 2020). The ruling is on appeal.

There was no supranational governance dimension to pandemic policy-making, except that, at the time of this writing, the US borders with Canada and Mexico had been closed since 23 March. Many states along the Canadian border wanted to reopen the border, but Canada was refusing to do so until the US had Covid-19 under greater control (Wamsley 2020).

10.4.3 State action

Many governors, county officials, and mayors reacted to Covid-19 by mid-March 2020, usually without legislative approval. In 38 states, the governor can suspend certain laws during a disaster, but in 25 states, the legislature can terminate a governor's emergency declaration, and in six states, an emergency declaration ends within 2–60 days. Nonetheless, as of October, 24 legislatures were considering bills to limit their governor's emergency powers.

Few legislatures constrained their governor's pandemic policies, and in some cases, governors vetoed legislative constraints. For example, Pennsylvania's Democratic governor vetoed seven bills passed by the Republican-majority legislature to reverse some of his policies (Scolforo 2020) and announced his intention to veto two more bills at the time of this writing (Levy 2020).

From 19 March, when California issued the first SAHO, to 7 April, 43 governors issued SAHOs of varying scope and stringency. Of the first ten governors issuing SAHOs, nine were Democrats. The seven states having no SAHO had Republican governors. SAHOs required most residents to stay at home, except for essential travel, and closed businesses deemed non-essential as well as some public functions, such as mass transit. Had governors and local officials not issued SAHOs in March, Covid-19 cases and deaths would have been higher.

Most SAHO-issuing governors enjoyed high public approval, although support ebbed as SAHOs endured (Solender 2020).

Most state courts did not intervene in gubernatorial policy-making, although the supreme courts of Michigan and Wisconsin, which had Republican majorities, overturned most of their Democratic governor's SAHO, while Pennsylvania's Democratic Supreme Court upheld the Democratic governor's SAHO. Thirty-eight states elect their supreme courts in partisan or non-partisan elections, with the rest being appointed. The party affiliation of judges is generally known, even among those chosen by non-partisan election (Ballotpedia n.d.).

Table 10.1 arrays the states by party control. A trifecta means the governorship and both legislative houses were controlled by one party. In the other two categories, different parties controlled the governorship and one or two legislative houses. Given partisan differences among the states, the table's purpose is to summarise key state policy and outcome differences and illustrate how differently the groups of states experienced Covid-19, not to assert causal relationships.

All the states with a Republican governor and Democratic legislature had a SAHO by March 30. They were followed by states with a Democratic governor and Republican legislature on April 1 and Democratic trifectas on April 2.

TABLE 10.1 United States: selected Covid-19 statistics and dates, by state party control

Statistics and dates	Democratic trifecta	Democratic Gov/ GOP Leg	GOP Gov/ Dem Leg	GOP trifecta
Date of last SAHO[a]	April 2 (100%)	April 1 (100%)	March 30 (100%)	July 31 (67%)
Date of last reopening[b]	June 9 (100%)	June 1 (100%)	May 18 (100%)	May 12 (100%)
Date of last mask mandate[c]	July 17 (100%)	August 1 (100%)	August 1 (60%)	August 4 (43%)
Death rate per 100k population (through 1 Sep)[d]	55.4	39.3	47.6	34.2
Death rate per 100k population (through 21 Nov)[d]	75.3	64.6	56.2	66.2
Unemployment rate, March 2020[e]	4.4%	4.4%	3.5%	4.0%
Unemployment rate, April 2020[e]	15.0%	13.8%	14.0%	12.2%
Unemployment rate, May–July 2020[e]	12.7%	10.0%	11.9%	8.8%
Unemployment rate, August–October 2020[e]	8.9%	6.8%	6.6%	6.0%
Public sector job loss (February–October)[f]	−7.3%	−5.8%	−7.6%	−4.2%

[a]   Mervosh et al. (2020).
[b]   Lee et al. (2020).
[c]   Compiled from Fernandez (2020); Kim et al. (2020); Markowitz (2020); Roberts and Mitroff (2020).
[d]   Centers for Disease Control (n.d.). Rates are for deaths since 21 January 2020.
[e]   Herman (2020); US Bureau of Labor Statistics (2).
[f]   Compiled from US Bureau of Labor Statistics (1).

Only 67 per cent of Republican trifectas had SAHOs, and only by July 31. Republican trifectas began reopening the earliest; Democratic trifectas reopened last. However, a few states reasserted SAHO measures in response to case surges in October. Democratic trifectas issued a mask mandate much earlier than the other state groups, although only 60 per cent of states with a Republican governor and Democratic legislature and 43 per cent of Republican trifectas mandated masks.

As the pandemic progressed, the difference in death rates for Democratic and Republican trifectas narrowed, though Democratic trifectas still had the highest death rates. The most common explanations for this is that Democratic states are more urbanised, have higher numbers of people of colour with underlying health conditions, and are more likely to have metropolitan areas that serve as major travel hubs conducive to spreading Covid (Brown 2020; Medina and Gebeloff 2020). Unemployment and public sector job losses were consistently highest in the Democratic trifectas since the pandemic's outbreak. This is probably due to SAHOs being stricter and more prevalent in Democratic states.

This difference contributed to gridlock in Congress over more relief. On 15 May 2020, the House passed a USD 3 trillion bill, which included about USD 950 billion for state, local, and tribal governments. The Republican Senate refused to consider the bill, arguing in part that it would bail out mostly Democratic states whose economic and fiscal straits are due to their own policy choices (Cole 2020).

States used their own funds and federal funds to ameliorate some of the economic and social consequences of their SAHOs, such as providing more unemployment benefits, subsidising small businesses, and postponing evictions for rent or mortgage non-payments. States also worked to mobilise private-sector resources for food banks and other welfare services.

States were laboratories for some innovative policies, and some innovations diffused among some states, albeit party polarisation limited diffusion. For example, the Republican governors of North and South Dakota refused to institute a SAHO and other anti-Covid-19 policies employed by most other states, in part because the two states had few cases during the first half of 2020. However, cases soared in both states during October, such that by 31 October, North Dakota had 813.2 weekly new cases per 100,000 people and South Dakota had 767.4 – both being far higher than the peaks of any other state since the pandemic's start. Yet a senior advisor to South Dakota's governor said, 'We feel pretty good about where we're at. The governor is not going to change any of her approach' (Findell 2020).

Otherwise, many states cooperated with each other to coordinate policies, share medical equipment, engage in collective purchasing, and the like. Cooperative agreements among the states were primarily regional, although Democratic governors were more likely than Republicans to participate. The three most formal cooperative ventures included three states in the west, seven in the northeast, and seven in the Midwest (Strauss 2020). Many states also loosened medical licensing standards to allow out-of-state medical personnel to practise in the state during case surges.

10.4.4 Local action

Most local governments did not undertake policies substantially different from their state's policies, though many large urban counties and municipalities acted somewhat independently. San Francisco was the first US jurisdiction to act by banning large gatherings on 11 March 2020. It joined five neighbouring counties to issue the first US SAHO on 16 March. Between then and 1 April, 136 counties (out of 3,031 counties) nationwide, accounting for 66.9 million people, imposed SAHOs before their states (Brandtner et al. 2020).

County officials and mayors did not stray far from their legal powers or suspend customary accountability measures. Counties and big cities had primary responsibility for implementing state policies and providing direct services such as testing and contact tracing. Many local governments helped mobilise resources for food banks and other services and provided grants and loans to small businesses. Many municipalities permitted restaurants to offer outdoor dining and closed streets to vehicular traffic for restaurants to do so. Most states also allowed municipalities to decide whether or how children could trick-or-treat on Halloween (31 October).

In some states, schools were closed and reopened by the governor; in others, decisions were left to local school districts. During the initial outbreak of Covid in March and April, 48 states mandated or recommended school closures, while the western states of Montana and Wyoming deferred to individual school districts (*Education Week* 2020a). As the new school year started in the fall, most schools were closed during case surges, and many schools were operating entirely online or with a mixture of online and in-person instruction. However, the 'digital divide' between children with and without access to technology impelled most school districts to provide technology to minority and low-income children needing equipment.

The majority of states provided guidance or allowed counties or school districts to determine when in-person instruction had to cease due to Covid infection levels. Arkansas, Florida, Iowa, and Texas, all with Republican governors, mandated that schools be open five days a week for in-person instruction unless cases spike (*Education Week* 2020b). Most states also allowed universities and colleges to decide whether to welcome students on campus for the fall and spring semesters.

Conflict occurred between governors and local officials, especially those of different parties. Most big cities are governed by Democrats, including those in states having a Republican governor and/or legislature. County and municipal Democrats resisted efforts by Republican state officials to end SAHOs, reopen the state economy, and overturn local mask mandates. Georgia was particularly contentious, as Republican Governor Brian Kemp moved to reopen the economy in late April. Atlanta Mayor Keisha Lance Bottom and other Democratic mayors were not consulted by the governor and opposed reopening high-risk businesses (Forgey 2020). In turn, local Republican officials, such as county sheriffs, refused to enforce mask mandates and other measures emanating from Democratic state officials. Governors retaliated by threatening fund cut-offs and other punitive measures against local governments and license revocations for non-compliant businesses. For example, when faced with county sheriffs and local law enforcement officials who refused to enforce state mask orders, California governor Gavin Newsom (D) threatened to withhold federal and state Covid relief funding from non-compliant local governments (Koseff 2020).

One state-local conflict, however, had catastrophic consequences for US Covid-19 cases and deaths. In New York, Governor Andrew Cuomo and New York City Mayor de Blasio, both Democrats, had clashed frequently before the pandemic. On 17 March, de Blasio advised city residents to prepare to shelter in place, but Cuomo's office accused the mayor of 'scaring people' (Vielkind et al. 2020). Cuomo pre-empted the mayor and delayed a state SAHO until 22 March. He also ordered elderly Covid-19 hospital patients relocated to nursing homes. On 11 June, New York, with 5.9 per cent of the US population, had 6.0 per cent of the world's Covid-19 deaths and 22.8 per cent of US deaths. As of 23 November 2020, New York City still had 288 Covid deaths per 100,000 population, one of the world's highest rates.

The property tax is the main own-source revenue for counties, municipalities, townships, and school districts. These entities have not been eager to defer payments or reduce tax rates in mid-year because tax payments on due dates are crucial to their ability to provide services. A few states authorised some deferrals, and a few more states extended deadlines for people to apply for existing property tax relief benefits. Eighteen states already had a property-tax circuit breaker that limits the tax to a certain percentage of household income, and 13 states offer property-tax credits based on income.

Since the pandemic's start, 45 states and 56 per cent of big cities implemented moratoriums on housing evictions; 40 per cent of big cities and 54 per cent of states provided rent relief; 66 per cent of states and 19 per cent of large cities enacted a foreclosure moratorium; 33 per cent of big cities and 58 per cent of states offered mortgage relief; and 30 per cent of states and 37 per cent of large cities provided some property-tax relief (Einstein et al. 2020). Michigan enacted a 'Pay to Stay' law that allows local governments to lower delinquent-tax amounts, making it easier for owners to stay in their homes. Connecticut enacted a law allowing local governments to reduce interest rates on delinquent taxes; a few states allow localities to delay or waive late payment penalties (Collins 2020). Economists expect property-tax declines to be smaller than sales and income tax declines (McClelland 2020).

Counties, municipalities, townships, and school districts each have their own organisations (e.g., state municipal leagues) for fostering cooperation, communications, innovation sharing, and collective pressure on their state government and the federal government. These continued to function as usual, in part because most local governments shifted fairly quickly to working online. In some cases, online council and school-board meetings increased citizen attendance.

10.4.5 Intergovernmental relations

State-federal relations were contentious in the political arena given that President Trump jousted with the country's 24 Democratic governors and a few Republican governors. Democratic state and local officials, along with some Republican officials, believe Congress and the President were uncooperative in refusing to enact a second relief stimulus, although, as of late October, many states had not spent all their federal aid from the March stimulus. On 21 December, however, Congress enacted a USD 920 billion relief stimulus, which included money for various state and local functions, such as education, health, and transportation.

In the bureaucratic arena, cooperation largely continued as usual, such as close cooperation between the CDC and state and local public health officials. Also, for example, the US Army Corps of Engineers was praised for quickly constructing field hospitals to handle case overloads in Covid-stressed localities (Williams 2020). Since the demise of the US Advisory Commission on Intergovernmental Relations in 1996, there has been no overarching intergovernmental institution, but intergovernmental mechanisms of varying types and robustness among federal, state, and local administrators as well as relevant private-sector stakeholders exist in virtually every policy field. It is unlikely that Covid-19 adversely affected these mechanisms. These mechanisms are also important for communicating and sharing ideas and are likely to have helped officials across policy fields respond and adapt to Covid-19, such as in developing new protocols for ambulance personnel, firefighters, and the police.

States cooperated with each other in many ways, especially on regional bases, although there was a period of intense competition for medical equipment and supplies during March–May 2020 when the President told the states to fend for themselves (Nicholas and Gilsinan 2020). The office of Michigan's governor dubbed the competition 'the hunger games' (Mahler 2020). Some states sought to alleviate the competition by forming joint purchasing arrangements. State officials also relied on their national associations, such as the National Governors Association, to share ideas, formulate policies, and lobby the federal government.

However, the rise of remote working generated tax conflict and competition between a few states where workers employed by an entity in one state were working remotely from their homes in other states. In October, New Hampshire, which does not tax earned income, filed suit in the US Supreme Court against Massachusetts, arguing that Massachusetts' tax on the incomes of New Hampshire residents working remotely in New Hampshire is unconstitutional. Many commuter-connected states already had reciprocal tax agreements that resolve this issue, but a victory for New Hampshire would encourage many workers employed in or living in high income-tax states to work remotely from states with no income tax or a lower tax.

To date, there is little information on how Covid-19 affected inter-local relations; however, many central cities were losing revenue because state SAHOs reduced the number of daily commuters and visitors. In late October, conflict arose between the mayor of San Francisco and the independent San Francisco Unified School District, which was ignoring the mayor's pleas to reopen schools.

10.4.6 Intergovernmental fiscal relations

The principal federal aid response to Covid-19, the USD 2.2 trillion CARES Act, is extremely complex and allocated funds to governments, for-profit and non-profit entities, and citizens. CARES provided USD 150 billion directly to state, local, tribal, and territorial governments. This aid was distributed on the basis of population, though direct aid to local governments was limited to jurisdictions having more than 500,000 residents. States could use some of their CARES funds to help smaller local governments. No direct aid was in the form of a block grant, although USD 5 billion of local aid was funnelled through the 47-year-old Community Development Block Grant programme.

CARES also infused neglected public health institutions with new money. For instance, the CDC's annual budget for emergency public-health preparedness had declined from USD 1.4 billion in fiscal 2002 to USD 675 million in the 2020 fiscal year (adjusted for inflation). Funds for hospital preparedness had dropped by 62 per cent from USD 723 million in fiscal 2004 to USD 275.5 million in 2020. It is also estimated that the 2007–2009 recession, associated with the global financial crisis, resulted in the loss of 50,000 state and local public health jobs that were not recovered after the recession (Johnson 2020).

Most of the CARES funds were distributed through existing intergovernmental mechanisms and formulas, such as the federal-state unemployment insurance programme. Little of the money was allocated according to Covid-19 case levels. New mechanisms were managed by extant institutions, such as new aid for hospitals that was distributed by the US Department of Health and Human Services based on each hospital's total net patient revenue. CARES provided USD 1,200 to each adult citizen (USD 500 for children) earning less than USD 75,000 per year. The money was distributed by the 86-year-old Social Security Administration. Some of the CARES money was in the form of loans, mostly for private-sector businesses, and some loans were forgivable under certain conditions. Otherwise, all the CARES money was accompanied by the usual spending and accountability rules and regulations attached to federal aid. A downside of such rules is that they can delay the actual expenditures by recipients; consequently, Congress delivered most of the money through established channels having established rules.

The CARES Act and other spending resulted in a federal budget deficit of USD 3.1 trillion in fiscal year 2020 – 15.2 per cent of gross domestic product (GDP) – out of USD 6.6 trillion in total spending, and total debt reached 102 per cent of the nation's GDP (Committee for a Responsible Federal Budget 2020).

Policy responses to the pandemic, especially SAHOs, reduced state and local revenues. States might experience a USD 555 billion revenue shortfall through to fiscal year 2022 (Center for Budget and Policy Priorities 2020). However, fiscal 2021 losses will vary from about 1 per cent in Idaho to perhaps 30 per cent in New Mexico (National Conference of State Legislatures 2020). At the close of fiscal 2019, states had only USD 74.9 billion of reserve funds (called rainy-day funds) to compensate for revenue losses. An analysis of 150 cities predicted revenue loses between 5.5 and 9.0 per cent (Chernik et al. 2020). A National League of Cities survey of mayors estimated a 13 per cent revenue drop (McFarland and Pagano 2020). Revenue declines will likely be largest in Democratic jurisdictions, partly because of stricter SAHOs.

A few states might increase aid to local governments, but most will not do so due to their own budget shortfalls. State and local governments are typically required to balance their annual budgets. In the absence of an influx of federal funding, they resort to spending cuts or tax increases, both of which can exacerbate the effects of an economic downturn. Draw-downs on reserve funds, government employee layoffs, benefit reductions, postponed spending on capital projects, underfunding public pensions, and cuts to programmes such as education are all tools used to adapt state and local budgets to market conditions. The level of austerity will depend on how hard individual states and localities are hit by Covid and the level of economic disruption caused by closures. By mid-November 2020, however, revenues in many states were rebounding at higher levels than projected several months earlier (Editorial Board 2020).

10.5 Findings and policy implications

The US response to Covid-19 has been highly non-centralised, largely because President Donald Trump, despite his alleged autocratic proclivities, left most of the response duties to the states and because party polarisation generated sharply different pandemic policy preferences across states and localities. This response pattern departed, therefore, from the tradition of cooperative federalism whereby federal and state officials work more closely to forge common guidelines and policy actions. There was an initial burst of cooperative federalism from about early March to late April 2020 when the President and Congress acted vigorously to support the states in a largely bipartisan fashion through established intergovernmental channels, but this cooperative spirit was undercut by partisan polarisation that induced gridlock, delayed enactment of a second major federal fiscal relief measure and negotiation of a more coordinated and cooperative state-federal response, and prevented full and more effective mobilisation of the system's federal, state, and local institutional capacities.

The model of dual federalism thus seems to fit the US response best: that is, pandemic-relevant federal agencies performed most of their customary public health functions, but each state acted independently to formulate and implement its own Covid-19 policies. The states' possession of the police power is a key feature of the federal system's dualist structure. State governors in particular used this power in unprecedented ways. There is no precedent in US history for the SAHOs instituted by the states to combat Covid-19. This expression of dual federalism also highlighted the continuing limits of federal power despite the centralisation that has occurred in the federal system since its founding (Kincaid 2019).

The major liability of this response pattern is that the US has had one of the world's highest levels of cases and deaths. A cardinal rule for responding to a disaster is issuing clear, consistent, and trustworthy messaging. Such messaging proved impossible due to the fact that partisan polarisation generated often diametrically opposed Covid-19 messages and that the diversity of state and local policy responses conveyed mixed messages to citizens. Furthermore, the high levels of mistrust Americans evinced towards governments and each other before the pandemic were exacerbated by mixed and combative messaging during the pandemic. President Trump set the tone for Republicans by downplaying Covid-19's severity and focusing on opening the economy; Democratic governors in states hit hard early in the pandemic framed the response for their own party. Federal, state, and local officials, and citizens, fell in line behind their party's narrative, and the fight against Covid-19 became a partisan battle throughout the federal system.

The US response illustrates the potent role of political parties in a federal system. There has been no profound change in the federal system, either constitutionally or bureaucratically, but party combat has thwarted the effective operation of the system. Perhaps aggravating the conflict was Covid-19's arrival during President Trump's first impeachment trial and during a year when he was running for re-election against a Democratic Party eager to unseat him.

As 2020 drew to a close, President-elect Joe Biden was signalling a more bipartisan approach to fighting Covid-19 and pledging greater cooperation with governors and between federal, state, and local health officials. The blueprint is for a centralised, coordinated plan coming from the CDC to determine when and how Covid-related economic and health restrictions should be put in place, including school and business closures, limits on the size of gatherings, and when SAHOs should be issued. Biden was championing a national mask-wearing mandate while acknowledging that the federal government lacks the constitutional authority to impose a mandate directly. A national mandate would apply to federal property and inter-state transportation. Biden was proposing to convince governors to impose mask mandates, but partisanship may thwart that goal. His intent was to increase federal planning to help states acquire and distribute rapid Covid testing, vaccines, and personal protective equipment. In sum, the incoming Biden administration signalled more reliance on cooperative federalism and less on dual federalism.

Note

1 Real-time data on Covid-19 cases and deaths are available on the CDC's website at https://covid.cdc.gov/covid-data-tracker.

References

Ballotpedia. n.d. 'State Supreme Court Elections, 2020', https://ballotpedia.org/State_supreme_court_elections,_2020 (accessed on 19 November 2020).

Barry, J. 2004 *The Great Influenza*. New York: Penguin.

Brandtner, C. et al. 2020. *Creatures of the State? Metropolitan Counties Compensated for State Inaction in Initial US Response to Covid-19 Pandemic.* Chicago: Mansueto Institute for Urban Innovation Research Paper, University of Chicago.

Brown, M. 2020. 'Fact Check: Comparison of COVID-19 Case Data Based on State Politics is Wrong', *USA Today*, 5 June, https://www.usatoday.com/story/news/factcheck/2020/06/05/fact-check-comparison-covid-19-data-state-politics-false/5252816002/ (accessed on 19 November 2020).

Cathey, L. 2020. 'Tracking Trump and Fauci's Tense Relationship', *ABC News*, 15 July, https://abcnews.go.com/Politics/tracking-trump-faucis-tense-relationship/story?id=71771514 (accessed on 17 November 2020).

Center for Budget and Policy Priorities. 2020. 'Needed: Federal Aid to Reverse Deep Public-Sector Job Cuts, Including in Education', 10 September, https://www.cbpp.org/blog/needed-federal-aid-to-reverse-deep-public-sector-job-cuts-including-in-education (accessed on 17 October 2020).

Centers for Disease Control. n.d. 'CDC COVID Data Tracker', https://covid.cdc.gov/covid-data-tracker/#cases (accessed on 21 November 2020).

Chernik, H., D. Copeland and A. Reschovsky. 2020. 'The Fiscal Effects of the COVID-19 Pandemic on Cities: An Initial', *National Tax Journal* 73(3): 699–732.

Cole, B. 2020. 'Pelosi Accuses Senate Republicans of "Political Retribution" by Refusing to Consider HEROES Act', *Newsweek*, 21 May, https://www.newsweek.com/nancy-pelosi-heroes-act-trump-republicans-1505628 (accessed on 21 November 2020).

Collins, C. 2020. *Property Tax Trends 2019 and 2020*. Cambridge, MA: Lincoln Institute of Land Policy, https://www.lincolninst.edu/sites/default/files/pubfiles/property_tax_trends_report_2019-2020.pdf (accessed on 2 November 2020).

Committee for a Responsible Federal Budget. 2020. 'A Closer Look at the Record $3.1 Trillion Deficit in FY 2020', http://www.crfb.org/blogs/closer-look-record-3-1-trillion-deficit-fy-2020 (accessed on 1 November 2020).

Detterbeck, K., W. Renzsch and J. Kincaid (eds). 2015. *Political Parties and Civil Society in Federal Countries*. Don Mills: Oxford University Press.

Diamond, D. and N. Toosi. 2020. 'Trump Team Failed to Follow NSC's Pandemic Playbook', *Politico*, 25 March, https://www.politico.com/news/2020/03/25/trump-coronavirus-national-security-council-149285 (accessed on 17 November 2020).

Editorial Board. 2020. 'State Tax Revenue Rebound', *Wall Street Journal*, 16 November, https://www.wsj.com/articles/state-tax-revenue-rebound-11605568517 (accessed on 16 November 2020).

Education Week. 2020a. 'Map: Coronavirus and School Closures in 2019–2020', 6 March (updated 16 September), https://www.edweek.org/ew/section/multimedia/map-coronavirus-and-school-closures.html (accessed on 21 November 2020).

Education Week. 2020b. 'Map: Where are Schools Closed?', 28 July updated 20 November, https://www.edweek.org/ew/section/multimedia/map-covid-19-schools-open-closed.html (accessed on 21 November 2020).

Einstein, K. L., P. Maxwell and S. Fox. 2020. 'COVID-19 Housing Policy'. *Initiative on Cities*, Boston University, https://www.bu.edu/ioc/files/2020/10/BU-COVID19-Housing-Policy-Report_Final-Oct-2020.pdf (accessed on 18 November 2020).

Fernandez, Marisa. 2020. 'The States Where Face Coverings are Mandatory', AXIOS, https://www.axios.com/states-face-coverings-mandatory-a0e2fe35-5b7b-458e-9d28-3f6cdb1032fb.html%20accessed%207/30/20 (accessed on 30 July 2020).

Findell, E. 2020. 'Dakotas, Once a Haven, Now See Infections Surge', *Wall Street Journal*, 2 November, 7.

Forgey, Q. 2020. '"There's Nothing about This That Makes Sense": Georgia Democrats Rail against Kemp's Move to Reopen State', *Politico*, 21 April, https://www.politico.com/news/2020/04/21/atlanta-mayor-blindsided-georgia-governor-reopening-state-197937 (accessed on 21 November 2020).

Grodzins, M. 1960. '"The Federal System" in American Assembly', in M. Grodzins (ed.), *Goals for Americans*, pp. 265–82. Englewood Cliffs: Prentice-Hall.

Haberman, M., E. Cochrane and J. Tankersley. 2020. 'Sidestepping Congress, Trump Signs Executive Measures for Pandemic Relief', *The New York Times*, 8 August, https://www.nytimes.com/2020/08/08/us/politics/trump-stimulus-bill-coronavirus.html (accessed on 20 November 2020).

Herman, Z. 2020. 'State Unemployment Rates, September 2020', NCSL, 26 October, https://www.ncsl.org/research/labor-and-employment/state-unemployment-update.aspxhttps://www.ncsl.org/research/labor-and-employment/state-unemployment-update.aspx (accessed on 21 November 2020).

Homeland Security Council. 2005. 'National Strategy for Pandemic Influenza.' October. https://www.cdc.gov/flu/pandemic-resources/pdf/pandemic-influenza-strategy-2005.pdf (accessed on 17 November 2020).

Johnson, M. 2020. 'The US Was the World's Best Prepared Nation to Confront a Pandemic. How Did It Spiral to "Almost Inconceivable" Failure?' *Milwaukee Journal Sentinel*, 14 October, https://www.jsonline.com/in-depth/news/2020/10/14/america-had-worlds-best-pandemic-response-plan-playbook-why-did-fail-coronavirus-covid-19-timeline/3587922001/ (accessed on 29 October 2020).

Kim, Allen, Scottie Andrew and James Froio. 2020. 'These are the States Requiring People to Wear Masks When out in Public', CNN, https://www.cnn.com/2020/06/19/us/states-face-mask-coronavirus-trnd/index.html (accessed on 30 July 2020).

Kincaid, J. 2014. 'The Federalist and V. Ostrom on Concurrent Taxation and Federalism', *Publius: The Journal of Federalism* 44(2): 275–97.

Kincaid, J. 2019. 'Dynamic De/Centralization in the United States, 1790–2010', *Publius: The Journal of Federalism* 49(1): 166–93.

Koseff, A. 2020. 'Newsom Threatens California Counties that Defy Coronavirus Rules as Cases Spike', *San Francisco Chronicle*, 25 June, https://www.sfchronicle.com/politics/article/Newsom-pleads-with-Californians-as-cases-spike-15363884.php (accessed on 21 November 2020).

Lee, Jasmine C. et al. 2020. 'See How All 50 States Are Reopening (and Closing Again)', *New York Times*, 29 July, https://www.nytimes.com/interactive/2020/us/states-reopen-map-coronavirus.html (accessed on 20 November 2020).

Levy, M. 2020. 'Pennsylvania Gov. Tom Wolf to Veto Bills On Carrying, Selling Guns during Disasters', Associated Press, 19 November, https://www.mcall.com/news/pennsylvania/mc-nws-pa-gun-sales-bills-20201119-dbvhk5lgdbbnpaz4fishzk75ou-story.html (accessed on 23 November 2020).

Mahler, J. 2020. 'A Governor on Her Own, with Everything at Stake', *New York Times Magazine*, 25 June, https://www.nytimes.com/2020/06/25/magazine/gretchen-whitmer-coronavirus-michigan.html (accessed on 20 November 2020).

Markowitz, Andy. 2020. 'State-by-State Guide to Face Mask Requirements', AARP, 14 September, https://www.aarp.org/health/healthy-living/info-2020/states-mask-mandates-coronavirus.html (accessed on 20 November 2020).

McClelland, R. 2020. 'Will COVID-19 Cause a Decline in Property Taxes?', Washington, DC: Tax Policy Center, https://www.taxpolicycenter.org/taxvox/will-covid-19-cause-decline-property-taxes (accessed on 1 November 2020).

McFarland, C. and M. A. Pagano. 2020. *City Fiscal Conditions 2020.* Washington, DC: National League of Cities, https://www.nlc.org/sites/default/files/users/user57221/City_Fiscal_Conditions_2020_FINAL.pdf https://www.nlc.org/resource/city-fiscal-conditions-2020 (accessed on 9 October 2020).

Medina, J. and R. Gebeloff. 2020. 'The Coronavirus is Deadliest Where Democrats Live', N, *New York Times*, 25 May, https://www.nytimes.com/2020/05/25/us/politics/coronavirus-red-blue-states.html (accessed on 19 November 2020).

Mervosh, Sarah, Denise Lu and Vanessa Swales. 2020. 'See Which States and Cities Have Told Residents to Stay at Home', *New York Times*, 20 April, https://www.nytimes.com/interactive/2020/us/coronavirus-stay-at-home-order.html (accessed on 20 November 2020).

National Conference of State Legislatures. 2020. 'Coronavirus (COVID-19): Revised State Revenue Projections', https://www.ncsl.org/research/fiscal-policy/coronavirus-covid-19-state-budget-updates-and-revenue-projections637208306.aspx (accessed on 9 October 2020).

Nicholas, P. and K. Gilsinan. 2020. 'The End of the Imperial Presidency', *The Atlantic*, 2 May, https://www.theatlantic.com/politics/archive/2020/05/trump-governors-coronavirus/611023/ (accessed on 20 November 2020).

Riker, W. H. 1964. *Federalism: Origin, Operation, Significance*. Boston: Little, Brown.

Roberts, Caroline and Sarah Mitroff. 2020. 'Where are Face Masks Required? The Rules for All 50 States and D.C.', *CNET.com*, 16 July, https://www.cnet.com/health/where-are-face-masks-required/ (accessed on 20 November 2020).

Scolforo, M. 2020. 'Wolf Vetoes Bill to Let Restaurants Operate at Full Capacity', Associated Press, 16 October, https://apnews.com/article/virus-outbreak-business-public-health-pennsylvania-legislation-b7f8a1a06d75ac4d8c3243ae9493d7bc (accessed on 19 November 2020).

Solender, A. 2020. 'Governors Who Took Strict COVID-19 Measures Enjoy Highest Approval, Survey Shows', *Forbes*, 15 September, https://www.forbes.com/sites/andrewsolender/2020/09/15/governors-who-took-strict-covid-19-measures-enjoy-highest-approval-survey-shows/?sh=5b82fc8a340b (accessed on 19 November 2020).

Strauss, D. 2020. 'The US States Uniting to Combat Coronavirus amid Leadership Vacuum', *The Guardian*, 27 April, https://www.theguardian.com/us-news/2020/apr/27/us-states-councils-pacts-coronavirus-trump (accessed on 21 November 2020).

US Bureau of Labor Statistics (1). n. d. 'State and Metro Area Employment, Hours, and Earnings', https://www.bls.gov/sae/data/ (accessed on 21 November 2020).

US Bureau of Labor Statistics (2). n. d. 'Unemployment Rates for States', https://www.bls.gov/web/laus/laumstrk.htm (accessed on 20 November 2020).

Vielkind, J., J. Palazzolo and J. Gershman. 2020. 'In Worst-Hit Covid State, New York's Cuomo Called All the Shots', *Wall Street Journal*, 11 September, https://www.wsj.com/articles/cuomo-covid-new-york-coronavirus-de-blasio-shutdown-timing-11599836994?mod=hp_lead_pos6 (accessed on 16 September 2020).

Wamsley, L. 2020. 'US Borders with Canada and Mexico Will Stay Closed another Month', *NPR*, 19 October, https://www.npr.org/sections/coronavirus-live-updates/2020/10/19/925479699/u-s-borders-with-canada-and-mexico-will-stay-closed-another-month (accessed on 19 October 2020).

Williams, P. 2020. 'Urgent Care', *The New Yorker*, 3 and 10 August, pp. 26–33.

11

FACING THE CORONAVIRUS PANDEMIC IN THE CANADIAN FEDERATION

Reinforced dualism and muted cooperation?[1]

Johanne Poirier and Jessica Michelin

11.1 Introduction

To begin with the obvious, size matters – and Canada is a large country. Second only in size to the Russian Federation, its area of 9,984,670 km² is bordered by three oceans and the longest land frontier in the world to the south. With a population of 38 million, it is one of the world's least densely populated countries, although its largest city, Toronto, hosts 5 million people. There are 5.5 time zones in Canada. Although viruses, like pollution and people, do travel, what happens out west does not immediately affect what happens in the centre, the east, or the north. Geography matters and the coronavirus pandemic has underscored the huge regional diversity of the Canadian federation. Infection rates and deaths differed radically across the country, with the Atlantic provinces having fared better than New Zealand, and Québec having been similar to France, Belgium, or Spain. This reinforces the importance of looking beyond aggregate national statistics in comparative analysis.

Beyond geography lies another obvious element: federalism impacts on the fight against the microscopic enemy; conversely, fighting the virus impacts on the dynamics of federalism. In other words, when it comes to combating a pandemic, federalism – like size, population density, and regional diversity – matters.

The Canadian federation is composed of ten provinces and three northern territories of widely different sizes. Canada, a country of immigration, is deeply multicultural and known for its 'complex diversity'. A federation founded by two groups of European descent, it is officially bilingual, and for a long-time was considered, at least in Québec, as 'bi-national'. With the – very belated – recognition of the place of indigenous peoples in the complex polity, few today would challenge the idea that Canada is multinational. Throughout its history,

DOI: 10.4324/9781003166771-14

Canadian federalism has had a differential impact on key actors (Gagnon and Poirier 2020). Unsurprisingly, the same is true in the context of the pandemic.

To use somewhat simplistic labels, Canadian federalism is officially 'dualist', pragmatically 'cooperative', multipolar, multicultural, multinational, symmetric in some ways, and asymmetric in others. The official division of powers is still outlined in a Constitution Act adopted by the Parliament of Westminster in the middle of the 19th century. Consequently, courts have played a major role in determining 'who can do what' in the Canadian federal system. Periods of decentralisation and centralisation have succeeded one another, with the last few decades heralding overlapping jurisdictions that challenge the dualist nature of the formal institutions. The Covid-19 pandemic underscored several of these paradoxes and grey zones.

This chapter examines the initial outbreak and first wave of infection (March–June 2020), the partial lull that occurred during the summer, and the beginning of the second wave, up to October 2020. In all three phases, the federal and provincial/territorial (P/T) governments acted largely in parallel, in keeping with the dualist nature of the federation; however, a fair degree of congruence in provincial action at the start gave way to differentiation in the later stages. Meanwhile, the federal order sought to keep the economy afloat by setting up financial aid packages and income replacement strategies. Although welcomed across the country, these costly initiatives were likely to generate the country's highest federal deficit in decades, and there were concerns that P/T (and future generations) would eventually pay the price in the search for balanced budgets.

By the end of October 2020, about 235,000 cases and over 10,000 deaths had been reported. The vast majority of cases (77.2 per cent) and deaths (92.6 per cent) occurred in Ontario and Québec, which make up slightly more than 60 per cent of Canada's population. More remarkable – and rather hard to explain – was Québec's initial inordinate proportion both of cases and deaths. With only 23 per cent of the Canadian population, it accounted in the early stages for slightly less than half of all cases and slightly more than half of all deaths (Table 11.1).

By October 2020, Ontario and Québec faced a massive rise in infections. The Atlantic provinces were generally spared, and there were increases in the west. The situation was asymmetrical from the outset and remained so. The same is true of the country's responses to the pandemic. These facts and figures reflect the first six months of the pandemic and had to be taken with caution, as federal and provincial responses were in constant evolution.

Overall, the story of the federation's initial 'pandemic era' is one of parallel action by various orders of government, with cooperation taking place quietly and largely behind the scenes. There were hardly any jurisdictional turf battles. Provinces came out as 'real actors' alongside Ottawa. Unlike the situation in some federations that saw either centralisation or the creation of formal multi-lateral bodies under federal leadership, in Canada intergovernmental relations (IGR) did occur, particularly at the operational level, but were muted.

TABLE 11.1 Canada: Covid-19 cases and deaths by province/territory (31 October 2020)

Region	Cases (total)	Deaths (total)	Rate of cases (per 100,00 population)	Rate deaths (per 100,00 population)
British Columbia	14,733	263	290.52	5.19
Alberta	28,245	323	646.14	7.39
Saskatchewan	3,144	25	267.7	2.13
Manitoba	5,723	67	417.9	4.89
Ontario	75,730	3,136	519.89	21.53
Québec	106,016	6,246	1,249.46	73.61
Newfoundland and Labrador	291	4	55.8	0.77
New Brunswick	343	6	44.15	0.77
Nova Scotia	1,109	65	114.17	6.69
Prince Edward Island	64	0	40.78	0
Yukon	23	1	56.3	2.45
Northwest Territories	10	0	22.31	0
Nunavut	0	0	0	0
Total	235,431	10,136	617.19	26.9

Source: Public Health Agency of Canada (2020a)

11.2 The federal constitutional and legislative framework

Despite the 'pragmatically' cooperative nature of Canadian federalism on a day-to-day basis, the fundamental structure of the federation remains dualist (Poirier 2020). Each order of government has its own legislative and executive – and to a certain extent, judicial – branch. The delegation of administrative and regulatory functions is possible between orders of government, but generally P/T are not seen as implementers of federal law or programmes. The management of the Covid-19 crisis was no exception.

Innumerable policy areas were implicated in the fight against the pandemic. They ranged from public health and health-care delivery, elderly care and schools, and medical research to policing, prisons, fiscal and financial arrangements, relations with indigenous nations, emergency measures, border closures, and more. The following discussion focuses though on health and disaster management.

The relevant constitutional provisions are vague and have been interpreted broadly. Particularly in the recent past, the Supreme Court of Canada has invoked 'cooperative federalism', not in order to impose cooperation (or any form of loyalty) on members of the federation, but to facilitate jurisdictional overlap (Gaudreault-DesBiens and Poirier 2017). This allows all orders of government to intervene in matters of health and disaster management, increasing the possibility of public action. It also leaves the responsibility for sorting out 'who should do what' to the political branches, which coordinate – or not – the various interventions.

Coordination takes place through a plethora of means that have no constitutional – and hardly any legislative – grounding. There is little official input by constitutive units into federal law- or decision-making, particularly since the Canadian Senate is inadequate as a body of provincial or regional representation – Canada's model is the archetype of 'inter-state' federalism (Broschek 2020). Consequently, in the context of Covid-19, a significant degree of informal consultation regularly occurred through pre-existing as well as ad hoc intergovernmental channels.

11.2.1 Public health, health-care delivery, and elderly care facilities

As the Supreme Court noted, health 'is an amorphous topic which can be addressed by valid federal or provincial legislation, depending [on] the circumstances' (*Carter v. Canada (AG)* 2015 SCC 5: paragraph 53). While in theory each order's action finds its constitutional grounding in an exclusive power, there is, in practice, a substantial degree of de facto concurrency (Steytler 2017: 7). This generates both interdependence between orders of government and confusion about who can do what.

11.2.1.1 Federal constitutional authority and legislation

Ottawa's explicit powers over health are limited to 'quarantine', 'marine hospitals', and 'patents', including those for pharmaceuticals (Constitution Act of 1867 [CA, 1867], section 91(11) and 91(22)). Of increasing relevance is reliance on the federal 'criminal law' power to intervene in matters of public health (CA, 1867, section 91(27); Klein 2017). Explicit federal authority over certain classes of people, such as indigenous peoples and immigrants, extends to their health care and is exercised in conjunction with provinces. Ottawa has an important department of health and an arm's-length public health agency.

Numerous federal statutes address health matters. The Quarantine Act of 2002, for example, enables the federal administration to prohibit entry into Canada or subject it to strict conditions. It foresees some intergovernmental collaboration, including mandatory notification to provinces of suspected infected persons. It also authorises delegating the administration and enforcement of quarantine measures to provinces.

11.2.1.2 Provincial constitutional authority and legislation

Provinces bear the brunt of the burden of health-care delivery. Provincial power over health is rooted in one explicit section regarding hospitals and the very broad powers over 'property and civil rights' and 'matters of a merely local or private nature' (CA, 1867, section 92(7), 92(13) and 92(16)). In practice, provinces are responsible for hospitals, and structuring public health care, among other things. They are also responsible for long-term care for the elderly – the population segment in which, in the first wave, most of the cases and deaths occurred.

Each province and territory has its own legislative and regulatory health scheme. Moreover, certain indigenous communities exercise a degree of self-government, including in regard to health matters. The overall public character of the health-care system depends largely on targeted federal financial transfers to provinces, with a loose conditionality set out in the Canada Health Act of 1985. These transfers have decreased significantly over the last several decades, a trend which provincial leaders have decried for years and which became acute during the Covid-19 pandemic.

11.2.2 Disaster and emergency management

As with health care, jurisdiction over disaster and emergency prevention and management is not explicitly provided for in the Constitution. In practice, it is a shared responsibility, with each order acting pursuant to some of its – officially – exclusive powers. In the Covid-19 context, it is mostly provincial emergency powers that have been mobilised.

11.2.2.1 Federal constitutional authority and legislation

Courts have grounded the federal emergency power in the 'peace, order and good government' clause (CA, 1867, section 91, preamble). The effect of invoking the federal emergency power is a temporary federal take-over of provincial jurisdiction. The potential political fallout of such drastic action is a key limiting factor in the federal government's decision to invoke this power (Deschenes 1992). A number of federal statutes provide legislative grounding for federal action in dealing with health emergencies. In the context of Covid-19, the Emergencies Act of 1988 and Emergency Management Act of 2007 stand out.

The former identifies four types of emergencies: public welfare, public order, international, and war. The classification affects permissible actions and the duration of the emergency declaration. Noteworthy, the Act subjects these measures to the Canadian Charter of Human Rights and Freedoms and provides for detailed parliamentary oversight mechanisms. It also explicitly recognises provincial jurisdiction over emergencies, imposes consultations, and invites concerted intergovernmental action. Parliament has thus strongly limited the conditions under which a 'federal take-over' could occur.

For its part, the companion Emergency Management Act addresses emergency preparedness. It outlines the responsibilities of the federal minister of public safety. These include supporting – not overseeing – provincial or local emergency initiatives, establishing intergovernmental arrangements for consulting cabinet with respect to declarations of emergencies, and providing assistance – including financial – to provinces on request. As with the Emergencies Act, a federal institution may not respond to a provincial emergency unless the province requests assistance.

Read in this way, both Acts seem like models of federalism of the type based on respect for provincial autonomy. The Emergencies Act was not activated in response to Covid-19, but the Emergency Management Act gave rise to some degree of intergovernmental preparation prior to the outbreak, steps which were initiated in March 2020.

11.2.2.2 Provincial constitutional authority and legislation

In parallel with the federal order's powers in the context of emergencies, provinces also have jurisdiction over disaster management and emergencies in areas that fall within their own sphere of competence (Deschenes 1992). This is not pursuant to any explicit constitutional provision but rather to provinces' authority over 'local matters' and the administration of justice (which includes the police) (CA, 1867, sections 92(13)–(14)). In some P/Ts, governmental departments have emergency response plans similar to federal ones.

The 'real' federal emergency power needs to be activated through a formal declaration by the governor-general, which did not occur. In a way, provincial emergency powers are the baselines, with the federal one understood as the exception. Later, in Section 11.4.2, we address the question of why a federal emergency was not declared.

11.3 Preparedness for a national disaster: The institutional framework

A number of intergovernmental committees and agreements were already in place at the beginning of the pandemic. Many of these structures were developed in the wake of Canada's poor response to the outbreak in 2003 of SARS (severe acute respiratory syndrome), a response characterised by a lack of coordination between Ontario's provincial authorities and the federal order (Fierlbeck and Hardcastle 2020).

The Public Health Agency of Canada (PHAC) is a federal institution, not a multilateral one, yet its mandate includes promoting intergovernmental collaboration on public health policy and planning. Meanwhile, the Pan-Canadian Public Health Network is the primary intergovernmental body dealing with public health. It is governed by a council composed of federal and P/T government officials and is accountable to another group of civil servants, the federal and P/T deputy ministers of health. The network has developed a number of intergovernmental agreements establishing frameworks for information-sharing and assistance with health resources during health emergencies.

The key intergovernmental agreement is the Federal/Provincial/Territorial Response Plan for Biological Events (Pan-Canadian Public Health Network 2018a). It sets out a governance structure and articulates a complex response-pathway from notification of potential threats to post-incident review. It also outlines possible responsibilities for each order of government, including areas of overlap.

When a coordinated response is deemed necessary, a special advisory committee is established to advise the deputy ministers of health. The Plan also anticipates a plethora of working groups to address technical issues, logistics, and communications (McNeill and Topping 2018).

In addition to this general response plan, the network developed a specific pandemic flu guidance framework, articulated in the document, Canadian Pandemic Influenza Preparedness: Planning Guidance for the Health Sector (Pan-Canadian Public Health Network 2018b). Intended to guide the development of a consistent and coordinated F/P/T pandemic response, it – again – seeks to clarify responsibilities for each order of government regarding laboratory services, public health measures, vaccines, and so on.

Four other intergovernmental agreements are worth noting. The Multilateral Information Sharing Agreement (Pan-Canadian Public Health Network 2014) sets out the terms for sharing information relevant for routine surveillance, case management, and responses to infectious diseases. The Memorandum of Understanding on the Provision of Mutual Aid in Relation to Health Resources during an Emergency Affecting the Health of the Public (Pan-Canadian Public Health Network 2009) establishes a framework for interjurisdictional sharing of health resources during public health crises. This led to the development of the Operational Framework for Mutual Aid Requests (OFMAR), a non-binding mechanism to operationalise the general framework and allow P/Ts to identify and share healthcare professionals and assets across jurisdictional boundaries during public health events (Framework for Mutual Aid Requests (OFMAR) n.d.). Even more specifically, in August 2020, PHAC released the collaboratively developed F/P/T Public Health Response Plan for Ongoing Management of Covid-19 (Public Health Agency of Canada 2020b). It uses epidemiological modelling to predict different scenarios and anticipate various responses until vaccines or treatments are in place.

In short, while the Response Plan for Biological Events sets out the governance structure, at least four intergovernmental agreements anticipate operational responses to a pandemic; the Covid-19 Plan detailing respective responsibilities for the current crisis. None of these agreements have statutory force, however. They are intergovernmental executive instruments, often written in rather hortatory language, and probably even lacking in contractual force between the executive branches party to it (Poirier 2004).

11.4 Rolling out measures to contain the pandemic

A federal election in the autumn of 2019 saw the incumbent Liberal Party retain power, though as a minority government. Partisan politics are never hugely relevant in IGR in Canada (Adam et al. 2015). They barely played a role in the initial response to Covid-19, either in the intergovernmental context or within orders of government. In fact, political leaders who did not get along particularly well, or had distinct political agendas, showed remarkable respect for one another during the first six months of the pandemic.

While there was some later fracturing of this united front, criticism was directed less at the health crisis management and more at deficit-creating spending (federally) and at needs for greater funding (from provinces). Regardless of political affiliation, Canadians expressed high levels of satisfaction with the initial government responses (Harell 2020). With time, greater opposition was voiced through party politics, but it remained moderate and cordial (Noël 2020).

11.4.1 Taking the initiative

The measures set out in the Response Plan for Biological Events were activated by the federal PHAC in early January 2020 and a special advisory committee was established. By early March, the virus was spreading exponentially in certain regions. This asymmetrical impact saw some provinces mobilising more quickly than others. That being said, in contrast to the more disjointed reopening schemes that were implemented as the pandemic progressed, these first initiatives took place in relatively close concert with each other.

On 13 March 2020, Québec became the first of Canada's governments to declare a public health emergency, in the process shutting down schools, universities, and day-care centres and forbidding indoor gatherings of more than 250 people. Subsequent provincial orders prohibited all indoor and outdoor gatherings and proscribed visits to hospitals and seniors' residences. Interregional travel was also banned and enforced by road blockades. An executive order gave Québec's Minister of Health and Social Services enhanced powers, including the authority to contract without public tender. Legal prescription periods were suspended, as courts were closed for all but urgent matters. In short, the declaration of a public health emergency thrust Québec into a full-on pandemic response.

Four other provinces (Prince Edward Island, Ontario, British Columbia, and Alberta) all declared public health emergencies prior to significant federal response, which occurred on 18 March. Saskatchewan, Newfoundland, Labrador, and the three territories declared an emergency on the day the federal government closed the border with the United States, while New Brunswick, Manitoba, and Nova Scotia declared public health emergencies in the days thereafter (Breton and Tabbara 2020).

A federal response group was convened at the end of January 2020 to monitor the virus. Initial actions had an international focus, first with travel warnings and then repatriation of Canadians stranded abroad. In March, a special cabinet committee was established to ensure a whole-of-government response. From mid-March, all foreign nationals were banned from entering Canada (with limited exceptions) and anyone entering the country, including Canadians, had to quarantine. While public authorities take note of World Health Organization decisions, their actions do not seem to have been directly influenced by any supranational considerations.

11.4.2 Federal action

Federal actions can be broadly classified into five categories. The first were measures taken pursuant to various areas of federal jurisdiction. Regulations and orders were issued addressing quarantine, air, rail and marine travel, drug safety, financial administration, federal prisons, indigenous services, and immigration and justice matters. In tandem with the provinces, Ottawa scaled up its procurement of medical supplies and personal protective equipment (PPE) and negotiated with pharmaceutical companies to procure an eventual vaccine.[2]

Secondly, responding to provincial requests, the Canadian armed forces sent personnel to 54 long-term care homes (47 in Québec and 7 in Ontario). In the first wave, 80 per cent of deaths occurred in these institutions, which were woefully ill-prepared compared to hospitals. Soldiers were also deployed to remote areas, notably to support indigenous communities (National Defence 2020).

A third set of initiatives provided direct financial support to citizens, organisations, and interest groups. Two 'omnibus' bills (Covid-19 Emergency Response Act Nos. 1 and 2, 2020) dealt with tax deferrals, insurance, the housing mortgage industry, student loans, farm credit, and the like. A wage subsidy programme for businesses, along with temporary income benefits for workers and students unable to work, were rapidly introduced. Funding was also mobilised to support scientific industry research, including vaccine development.

Fourth, Ottawa supported provincial initiatives, much in the way it does in non-pandemic times. Pursuant to the multilateral Safe Restart Agreement, concluded in September 2020, Ottawa would transfer CAD 19 billion to provinces and territories for a range of measures, with P/Ts specifying their respective needs (Intergovernmental Affairs 2020). These included testing, tracing, health care, long-term care support, PPE procurement, child care, and support for municipalities. Additional funding targeted, inter alia, homelessness, gender-based violence, indigenous communities, and schools.

The fifth category of federal action includes the issuance – often in an intergovernmental setting – of guidance frameworks in a flurry of domains, often within provincial jurisdiction, such as virtual health-care delivery, schools, long-term care, and funeral homes. Ottawa also developed a smartphone tracing app into which provinces could co-opt.

Perhaps strikingly from a comparative perspective is what the federal order did *not* do: declare a full-on pan-Canadian state of emergency. While there is no doubt that the Emergencies Act could have been invoked, it was not, for at least five reasons. To begin with, it was not truly necessary. The federal government could close borders, impose quarantine, and assist provinces – including deploying the army – under existing legislation. Secondly, every P/T rapidly declared 'health emergencies'. Given that the pandemic affected regions differently – as noted, geography matters – a wholesale, one-size-fits-all solution was not warranted, particularly in that the P/T generally all adopted restrictive measures, at any rate in the early stages.

Thirdly, the Emergencies Act requires provincial buy-in, mostly in the form of consultation and, where it is the case that an emergency is localised, actual provincial consent. Ottawa chose to heed the provinces' express reluctance to see the Act invoked. Fourth, the Emergencies Act places the executive branch under strict parliamentary scrutiny. Parliamentary sittings were reduced as of mid-March and used mostly to adopt specific legislation (introducing financial aid packages, for instance). The executive was even authorised to circumvent the need for appropriations bills (An Act to amend the Financial Administration Act (special warrant), 2020; MacDonnell 2020). Parliament was in fact suspended between mid-August and 23 September 2020. Meanwhile, the Senate, including its committees, resumed sitting in any regular manner only in October. Overall, Parliament was less mobilised than it would have been under the Emergencies Act. Hence, paradoxically, not invoking it probably increased the federal executive's room for manoeuvre (Leuprecht 2020).

Finally, for reasons unrelated to the pandemic, there was political reluctance in Ottawa, at least under Liberal leadership, to invoke federal emergency powers. The last time these were put into action was in the 1970 October Crisis when a foreign diplomat was kidnapped and a provincial minister killed, in the context of claims for Québec's independence. At the request of the Québec government, Ottawa had sent the army to Montreal, civil liberties were suspended, and nearly 500 people imprisoned, most of them without being charged. The federal prime minister at the time, Pierre Elliott Trudeau, was the father of the current Prime Minister, Justin Trudeau. It is likely that the latter sought to avoid rekindling that saga 50 years later, even if in very different circumstances.

In brief, emergency powers were in place as of March 2020, but only within provincial and territorial legal orders. Federal action was grounded instead in other – less politically sensitive and constraining – legislation. As the third wave of infection began to spread, it remains to be seen whether the federal government might change its strategy in favour of a more centrally driven response. But this, in our view, is unlikely.

11.4.3 Provincial and territorial action

It will be apparent by now that there were (at least) 13 different pandemic regimes in Canada, each corresponding to the circumstances of a P/T (and in some cases, those of indigenous communities). Nonetheless, there was initially a degree of convergence. The following is a partial survey of the measures taken.

Between March and September 2020, all 10 provinces declared a state of emergency. At different points, they all closed schools, restaurants (except for take-out), and bars, radically restricted visits to long-term care centres, prohibited residential evictions, and limited gatherings indoors and outdoors. Moreover, most constitutive units closed day-care centres, sport facilities, and cultural centres (Breton and Tabbara 2020). All P/T legislative assembly meetings were temporarily suspended (Sahota 2020).

Extraordinary measures affecting labour and employment law were taken. Just within Québec, executive orders suspended the terms of some collective agreements, allowing forced overtime for health-care staff, preventing them from taking vacation, and permitting compulsory reassignment. The latter measure led to health-adjacent personnel such as speech therapists being sent to fill staffing shortages in long-term care homes. While many drastic measures were lifted during summer, some were re-implemented in autumn.

In addition to federal initiatives, some provinces introduced financial support measures, such as grants and loan-forgiveness for small businesses, investment programmes for hard-hit industries (e.g., restaurants and the arts), and bonuses for essential workers (Lee and Hamidian 2020). However, certain provinces were criticised for clawing back federal assistance payments (Béland et al. 2020a).

Given the significantly divergent impact of the pandemic in the first wave, there was noticeably greater variation in reopening protocols than observed in the initial shutdown. In some provinces, students returned to classes in the spring, while others waited until autumn. Ontario offered a choice between virtual classrooms or in-class teaching, while Québec favoured in-person schooling until it opted for limited 'alternate days' for some students when the second wave expanded. There was a patchwork of mandatory mask mandates, with some provinces leading the charge and others leaving the decision to local authorities. At least four provinces (Manitoba, New Brunswick, Québec, and Ontario) created a colour-coded system to introduce measures of variable intensity in different intra-provincial regions. The strict approach taken by the territories may be explained in part by their particular geographic situation as remote Northern communities, where accessing health resources is a challenge. This is compounded by demographics, as territories have significant indigenous communities, often marginalised in the Canadian health-care system.

Particularly fascinating was the asymmetrical closure of interprovincial borders. The Atlantic provinces created an 'Atlantic travel bubble' whereby anyone entering from the rest of the country had to self-isolate for 14 days upon arrival, with some exceptions made for the eastern parts of Québec. This paid dividends – the region was spared the high death rates and resurgent infection rates observed elsewhere. Nunavut and the Northwest Territories created a two-unit travel bubble. Manitoba required self-isolation for anyone entering the province from the east, but not the north or west (where infection rates were lower). Saskatchewan, Québec, and Manitoba limited intra-provincial travel to protect certain regions or indigenous communities regarded as vulnerable.

Canadians enjoy a constitutional right to move across the country, subject to limitations deemed justifiable in a 'free and democratic society' (CA, 1982, sections 1, 6(2)). While Ottawa could limit or prohibit inter- and intra-provincial travel under the Emergencies Act, whether provinces have constitutional jurisdiction to take similar actions is unclear. A court in Newfoundland ruled that the province's severe travel restrictions (before the creation of the Atlantic bubble) were valid exercises of provincial power and constituted reasonable limitations on mobility rights, given the nature of the pandemic (*Taylor v. Newfoundland and Labrador*, 2020 NLSC 125). This decision was being appealed, and other challenges targeting travel restrictions were also making their way through the courts.

By and large, few courts have issued decisions assessing the legality of government decisions in response to Covid-19 in general. In addition to challenges to interprovincial travel bans, legal action has targeted occupational safety regulations regarding the use (or not) of PPE, confinement and social distancing, mandatory masks, and return to school protocols. In any event, it is doubtful that judicial review can compensate for shortcomings in political accountability, given the courts' deferential attitudes to valid delegations of authority (Daly 2020a).

Parliamentary scrutiny of executive action also varied across provinces. As with the federal parliament, several provincial legislatures adapted their schedules, often with virtual options (Sahota 2020). Much of the regulatory activity related to the Covid-19 response occurred through subordinate legislation, in the form of ministerial orders, which are not subject to legislative debate (Daly 2020b).

11.4.4 Local government actions

Under Canadian law, municipalities do not constitute a third order of government. Local authorities only enjoy powers delegated through provincial legislation. That said, while their autonomy is formally limited, they have a wide range of responsibilities, all of which the health crisis put to the test (Flynn 2020). For example, many cities reimagined urban spaces to facilitate social distancing and distributed free masks to citizens even in the absence of province-wide mask mandates. The limitations of municipal authority were also evident. For instance, Toronto's health director lacked power to implement enhanced public health measures at the beginning of the second wave and issued a call for Ontario's top health officer to take action.

Municipalities raised concerns about the strain the crisis was putting on their budgets. The misalignment of revenue and expenditure responsibilities was the greatest for municipalities, with the Federation of Canadian Municipalities calling for CAD 10 billion in emergency federal funding (Béland et al. 2020c). This pan-Canadian organisation created a Covid-19 website highlighting available municipal resources and local innovation. That apart, there did not seem to be any ground-breaking sharing of best practices to maximise the 'laboratory' potential of decentralisation, albeit information-sharing certainly took place, nor was there systematic coordination between regional and municipal authorities.

11.4.5 Intergovernmental relations

There is a general consensus that federal and P/T intergovernmental communication during the first wave of the pandemic response was fairly effective (Schertzer and Paquet 2020a). Governments avoided undermining each other's public health directives, in stark contrast with the situation south of the border.

Federal and P/T leaders publicly committed to ongoing collaboration when restarting the economy and de-escalating public health measures.

The fact that Ottawa did not invoke federal emergency powers probably set a positive tone of respect between orders of government. Nonetheless, certain measures that were announced at the opening of Parliament in September 2020 potentially altered that sentiment. For instance, Ottawa suggested that it might impose 'national standards' on long-term care homes. As it does not have constitutional authority in this area, it could act only through its spending power. This announcement annoyed some provinces, which reaffirmed their jurisdictions and called for increased – and unconditional – federal funding.

By contrast to Belgium's National Security Council, or Australia's 'National Cabinet', there was very little structured or visible interaction between governments. Federal press conferences were held in parallel with those of the provinces. The public was simply told that regular phones calls were being made among the top leadership. Informal discussions with senior civil servants reveal that a lot of intergovernmental communication and consultation took place in a wide range of contexts. These were grounded in existing emergency preparation plans but also emerged spontaneously as the need arose.

The pandemic generated creative forms of horizontal cooperation, particularly between provinces with regional and economic ties. The eastern provinces have a history of regional cooperation, including in the health sector, which may explain the fact that they managed to forge the 'Atlantic bubble'. Québec and Ontario premiers and several members of their cabinets held joint meetings. That being said, provinces generally acted with a great deal of autonomy, with calls made for greater interprovincial action and pooling of best practices.

The degree to which pre-existing intergovernmental arrangements were effected in practice is also unclear. The detailed three-layered coordination frameworks set out in the Response Plan for Biological Events, the Pandemic Influenza Preparedness Plan, and the specific Covid-19 plan seem to have been mobilised, although the extent to which they were followed, or were effective, remains difficult to ascertain. Similarly, while the federal government made billions of dollars in funding available to the provinces, little information was publicly available about the details of the funding agreements. Formal sources of horizontal cooperative arrangements, such as the Atlantic bubble, are also difficult to access. What one saw were the results, but not the processes or legal mechanisms on which they were built.

In short, IGR remain executive-led. They are apparently widespread, relatively effective, and quietly innovative – and as opaque as ever.

11.4.6 Intergovernmental fiscal relations

Canadian fiscal federalism faced major criticism prior to the pandemic – the economic challenges created by Covid-19 only exacerbated some of these tensions. While provinces enjoy substantial taxing powers, the federal order has much greater fiscal capacity; meanwhile, the cost for provinces of meeting their responsibilities continues to rise. This imbalance was reinforced by the fact that key areas impacted on by the pandemic – such as health care, long-term care, education, housing, and most social assistance programmes – are provincial responsibilities. Although Ottawa announced major financial transfers to P/Ts in response to the pandemic, securing the funding was likely to prove challenging, given the politics of negotiating bilateral transfer agreements. Québec in particular has been a vocal opponent of conditional federal funding.

Scholars have suggested that Covid-19 might provide the momentum for significant structural changes in Canadian fiscal federalism or certain federal redistribution programmes such as (un)employment insurance (Béland et al. 2020b; Noël 2020). Political actors were certainly trying to seize the opportunity, with Québec and Ontario advocating for increased health-related transfers. Alberta, which has been a net contributor to fiscal equalisation for decades but has been facing a major economic crisis since the prices of fossil fuel crashed, also pushed for reforms to fiscal federalism, even calling for a referendum to launch a constitutional reform of fiscal equalisation across the federation.

11.5 Findings and policy implications

11.5.1 Effectiveness of the federal system

Mixed conclusions are drawn from the Canadian response to the first wave of Covid-19. At one end of the spectrum, some maintain that Covid-19 underscores the strength of a decentralised system in that it allows for effective asymmetrical responses (Mathieu and Guénette 2020). Diversity in epidemiological and geographical realities calls for localised solutions. High infection rates in some provinces did not lead to widespread outbreaks in neighbouring ones. This might be explained in part by the high degree of convergence in initial provincial responses and the unprecedented closure of domestic borders. Indeed, some provinces were modelling solutions based on other provinces' experiences. Migone notes that compared to the SARS outbreak, there was greater cooperation, a trend she attributes to Canada's tradition of executive federalism, including the interjurisdictional bodies and agreements specifically designed to palliate policy fragmentation and jurisdictional turf wars (Migone 2020). We see subsidiarity as well as 'cooperative' and 'laboratory federalism' at play.

At the other end of the spectrum, critics argue that Canada's Covid-19 response was bungled due to a weak federal presence. Notably, they criticise the Multilateral Information Sharing Agreement, which allows provinces to limit the publication of data otherwise needed to craft effective responses (Attaran and Houston 2020). The extent to which Ottawa could impose health-data-sharing on provinces is, however, uncertain from a constitutional perspective. Others also called for greater federal action, not through the Emergencies Act – which only justifies federal temporary intervention – but through the initiation of pan–Canadian policy responses to address social problems arising from (or exacerbated by) the pandemic (Lee and Hamidian 2020). This would likely generate jurisdictional battles.

Somewhere in the middle, others reject greater centralisation but also deplore ad hoc mechanisms activated only during a crisis and the lack of sustained, coordinated actions. This contributes to thin intergovernmental trust (Schertzer and Paquet 2020b). In response to this intergovernmental weakness, Da Silva and Saint-Hilaire call for a new multilateral intergovernmental agreement to clarify roles and responsibilities and increase vertical and horizontal coordination (Da Silva and Saint-Hilaire 2020). They suggest that an intergovernmental agreement would ease provincial concerns about federal intrusion, as intervention conditions would be outlined and agreed upon. Unfortunately, they do not identify precise failings of the current intergovernmental bodies and agreements – a failure which only serves to underline the opacity of IGR alluded to previously.

11.5.2 Impact on the federation's multinational character

It is generally admitted that systemic issues make indigenous populations more vulnerable to Covid-19, with such issues including overcrowded housing, homelessness, high incarceration rates, inadequate health services, food insecurity, lack of clean water, and the remoteness of northern, fly-in communities (Carling and Mankani 2020). In addition to the differential impacts of urban/rural and on-reserve/off-reserve divides, the tug-of-war between Ottawa and provinces regarding services to indigenous peoples is bound to have an impact in crisis situations (Poirier and Hedaraly 2020). Some indigenous communities adopted self-isolation measures, such as putting up road blocks to prevent visitors from entry. For outside observers, what is striking is that indigenous peoples seemed to be largely absent from public media as interlocutors or decision-makers; the narrative instead was mainly about 'protecting' these communities. This seems to contrast with the place which reconciliation and the call for indigenous self-government occupied in public discourse just prior to the pandemic.

Unsurprisingly, a new chapter in the Québec-Canada story was also unfolding. At least since the 1960s, Québec has considered itself a distinct nation within Canada. Yet appeals by the premier to the special solidarity that Québécois are supposed to share with each other did not appear to resonate strongly with the population. Health care and old-age housing – under provincial jurisdiction – proved to be dramatically inadequate. Initially at least, infection and death rates were initially – inexplicably – higher in Québec than in the rest of the country. Sociologists will have much to reflect upon in considering the impact of the pandemic on Québec's sense of 'distinctiveness' and how this played out in its commitment to, or rejection of, the federal system.

The Québec government's decision to request military assistance in staffing long-term care homes was undoubtedly difficult for what is not an officially independentist but nationalist government. When Québec requested that the military remain until autumn, the federal government refused. Québec replied that its tax contributions help fund the military (National Assembly 2020). As a compromise, the Canadian Red Cross stepped in to fill personnel shortages ... with federal funding!

French-speaking minorities in other provinces saw their linguistic rights abridged during the pandemic. Since the outbreak, respect for linguistic obligations in certain public institutions and governments gradually diminished (Chouinard and Normand 2020). For example, Ottawa exempted certain products from bilingual labelling. In New Brunswick, the only officially bilingual province, the premier refused simultaneous interpretation services during briefings and even ignored questions from French-speaking journalists. In contrast, Québec authorities conduct a (limited) part of all briefings in English, and key communications were available in both languages on government websites (as it is for the federal order).

The extent to which public messaging reached immigrant communities was also of concern, particularly given that some of these communities were hard-hit by the virus. Several provinces, notably British Columbia, disseminated information in a number of languages other than French and English.

11.5.3 Looking to the future: Quo vadis, the federal spirit?

The impact of federalism on pandemic management is a trade-off (Migone 2020). The Canadian model's strength is its ability to tailor responses to different needs; the cost is a lesser degree of coordination, even when it would be beneficial. This, of course, is a textbook instance of the advantages and disadvantages of federalism.

A main thread in the story is that both provinces and the centre remained strong actors during the pandemic in 2020. Despite the absence of constitutionalised and structural inputs into federal law-making, several key federal acts do call for consultation and coordination with provinces. Ottawa's decision not to invoke the Emergencies Act – particularly in the face of provincial resistance – suggests that it did not seek to play a dominant role. Federal action, especially of such a pronounced kind, would have required serious provincial buy-in.

Also noteworthy during the Covid-19 crisis: orders of government did not raise jurisdictional obstacles to each other. When Québec sent officials to the Montreal airport prior to federal action on Ottawa's part, the latter did not flinch, nor did it object to provinces closing internal borders. Despite the absence of any recognised principle of subsidiarity in Canadian constitutional law, the federal order was probably only too relieved to leave these difficult decisions to provinces. In turn, the Québec government called upon the army and allowed Ottawa to set up new – emergency – income replacement programmes. In a federation where governments use courts fairly regularly to clarify federal issues, it is striking that basically no challenges to actions taken by any order of government seem to have been considered. Whether this constitutional truce will last was, of course, an open question.

In the landscape of Canadian federalism, the real test moving forward will be managing the aftermath of Covid-19. Numerous economic response measures have generated the highest federal deficit since the 1960s. This is bound to have a major impact on equalisation and transfer payments. The resultant social problems are likely to fall in the provinces' backyards, as they did in the 1990s during a period of federal fiscal austerity, apart from the issues of *who* will pay for the required measures, and *how*, the situation risks increasing fiscal inequality between provinces (Noël 2020). These concerns are exacerbated by serious budgetary problems in British Columbia and Alberta, which are historically net contributors to equalisation.

Interprovincial solidarity is thus both reinforced and tested. Regional blocs have emerged to improve public health measures but so too for maximising bargaining power and political pressure on the federal government. Meanwhile, solidarity has also been strained for non-pandemic reasons, such as environmental policy and fiscal redistribution. Vertical and horizontal friction will be heightened in the course of events as orders of government attempt to recover from the economic impact of Covid-19. In their reading of Canada's experience in 2020, Schertzer and Paquet see complex intergovernmental problems being met initially in a collaborative manner, only to give way to subsequent conflict (Schertzer and Paquet 2020b). This suggests that we should anticipate that rising intergovernmental tensions will partly displace the current cooperation and interjurisdictional respect as the pandemic and its aftermath unfold.

Notes

1 We thank Atagün Kejanlioglu, Félix Mathieu, Dave Guénette, André Lecours, and Christian Leuprecht for their helpful comments, as well as Melisande Charbonneau-Gravel for superb research assistance on intergovernmental agreements. We are also grateful for the financial support of the Research Support Programme of the Québec Secretariat for Canadian Relations and of the Centre de recherche interdisciplinaire sur la diversité et la démocratie (CRIDAQ).
2 The Canadian Armed Forces coordinated PPE stocks and flew them across the country to ensure that all P/Ts had adequate supplies.

References

Adam, Marc-Antoine, Josée Bergeron and Marianne Bonnard. 2015. 'Intergovernmental Relations in Canada: Competing Visions and Diverse Dynamics', in Johanne Poirier, Cheryl Saunders and John Kincaid (eds), *Intergovernmental Relations in Federal Systems: Comparative Structures and Dynamics*, pp. 135–73, Don Mills: Oxford University.
Attaran, Amir and Adam R. Houston. 2020. 'Pandemic Data Sharing: How the Canadian Constitution Has Turned into a Suicide Pact', in Colleen M. Flood et al. (eds), *Vulnerable: The Law, Policy and Ethics of COVID-19*, pp. 91–104, Ottawa: University of Ottawa Press.
Béland, Daniel et al. 2020a. 'Social Policy Responses to COVID-19 in Canada and the United States: Explaining Policy Variations between Two Liberal Welfare State Regimes', *Social Policy & Administration*, 55(2): 280–94.

Béland, Daniel et al. 2020b. 'A Critical Juncture in Fiscal Federalism?: Canada's Response to COVID-19', *Canadian Journal of Political Science*, 53: 239–43.

Béland, Daniel et al. 2020c. 'COVID-19 Will Force a Change to Canada's Fiscal Arrangements', *Policy Options*, https://policyoptions.irpp.org/magazines/may-2020/covid-19-will-force-a-change-to-canadas-fiscal-arrangements/ (accessed on 7 May 2020).

Breton, Charles and Mohy-Dean Tabbara. 2020. 'How the Provinces Compare in Their COVID-19 Responses', *Policy Options*, https://policyoptions.irpp.org/magazines/april-2020/how-the-provinces-compare-in-their-covid-19-responses/ (accessed on 22 April 2020).

Broschek, Jörg. 2020. 'Bicameralism and the Consequences of Political Structuring in Canada: Lost Alternatives, Future Options', in Alain G. Gagnon & Johanne Poirier (eds), *Canadian Federalism and Its Future: Actors and Institutions*, pp. 53–83, Montréal/Kingston: McGill-Queen's University Press.

Carling, Amanda and Insiya Mankani. 2020. 'Systemic Inequities Increase Covid-19 Risk for Indigenous People in Canada', *Human Rights Watch*, https://www.hrw.org/news/2020/06/09/systemic-inequities-increase-covid-19-risk-indigenous-people-canada (accessed on 9 June 2020).

Chouinard, Stéphanie and Martin Normand. 2020. 'Talk COVID to Me: Language Rights and Canadian Government Responses to the Pandemic', *Canadian Journal of Political Science*, 53(2): 259–64.

Da Silva, Michael and Maxime St-Hilaire. 2020. 'Pandemic Preparedness and Responsiveness in Canada: Exploring the Case for an Intergovernmental Agreement', *Centre for Constitutional Studies Blog*, https://ualawccsprod.srv.ualberta.ca/2020/06/pandemic-preparedness-and-responsiveness-in-canada-exploring-the-case-for-an-intergovernmental-agreement/ (accessed on 15 June 2020).

Daly, Paul. 2020a. 'Governmental Power and COVID-19: The Limits of Judicial Review', in Colleen M. Flood et al. (eds), *Vulnerable: The Law, Policy and Ethics of COVID-19*, pp. 211–22, Ottawa: University of Ottawa Press.

Daly, Paul. 2020b. 'Regulating the Covid-19 Pandemic: Forms of State Power and Accountability Challenges', *Centre for Constitutional Studies*, https://ualawccsprod.srv.ualberta.ca/2020/05/regulating-the-covid-19-pandemic-forms-of-state-power-and-accountability-challenges/ (accessed on 7 May 2020).

Deschenes, Michel. 1992. 'Les pouvoirs d'urgence et le partage des compétences au Canada', *Cahiers de droit*, 33(4): 1181–1206.

Fierlbeck, Katherine and Lorian Hardcastle. 2020. 'Have the Post-SARS Reforms Prepared Us for COVID-19? Mapping the Institutional Landscape', in Colleen M. Flood et al. (eds), *Vulnerable: The Law, Policy and Ethics of COVID-19*, pp. 31–48, Ottawa: University of Ottawa Press.

Flynn, Alexandra. 2020. 'Municipal Power and Democratic Legitimacy in the Time of COVID-19', in Colleen M. Flood et al. (eds), *Vulnerable: The Law, Policy and Ethics of COVID-19*, pp. 127–38, Ottawa: University of Ottawa Press.

Framework for Mutual Aid Requests (OFMAR). n.d. http://publications.gc.ca/collections/collection_2018/aspc-phac/HP45-13-2017-eng.pdf (accessed on 13 November 2020).

Gagnon, Alain G. and Johanne Poirier (eds). 2020. *Canadian Federalism and its Future: Actors and Institutions*, Montreal and Kingston: McGill-Queen's University Press.

Gaudreault-DesBiens, Jean-François and Johanne Poirier. 2017. 'From Dualism to Cooperative Federalism and Back? Evolving and Competing Conceptions of Canadian Federalism', in Peter Oliver, Patrick Macklem and Nathalie Desrosiers (eds), *The Oxford Handbook of the Canadian Constitution*, pp. 391–413, New York: Oxford University Press.

Harell, Allison. 2020. 'How Canada's Pandemic Response is Shifting Political Views', *Policy Options*, http: policyoptions.irpp.org/magazines/april-2020/how-canadas-pandemic-response-is-shifting-political-views/ (accessed on 8 April 2020).

Intergovernmental Affairs. 2020. 'Safe Restart Agreement', *Government of Canada*, https://www.canada.ca/en/intergovernmental-affairs/services/safe-restart-agreement.html (accessed on 16 September 2020).

Klein, Alana. 2017. 'Jurisdiction in Canadian Health Law', in Joanna Erdman, Vanessa Gruben and Erin Nelson (eds), *Canadian Health Law and Policy*, 5th ed, pp. 29–50, Toronto: LexisNexis.

Lee, Marc and Armand Hamidian. 2020. 'Comparing Provincial Economic Responses to COVID-19', *Policy Note*, https://www.policynote.ca/provincial-responses-covid/ (accessed on 23 April 2020).

Leuprecht, Christian. 2020. 'COVID's Collateral Contagion: Why Faking Parliament Is No Way to Govern in a Crisis', *MacDonald Laurier Institute Commentary*, https://macdonaldlaurier.ca/files/pdf/MLICommentary_June2020_Leuprecht_FWeb.pdf (accessed on 15 June 2020).

MacDonnell, Vanessa. 2020. 'Ensuring Executive and Legislative Accountability in a Pandemic', in Colleen M. Flood et al. (eds), *Vulnerable: The Law, Policy and Ethics of COVID-19*, pp. 141–62, Ottawa: University of Ottawa Press.

Mathieu, Félix and Dave Guénette. 2020 'Quebec, Canada and the Covid-19 Crisis: Making Federalism Work Again?', *UACES Territorial Politics*, https://uacesterrpol.wordpress.com/2020/06/16/quebec-canada-and-the-covid-19-crisis-making-federalism-work-again/ (accessed on 16 June 2020).

McNeill, R. and J. Topping. 2018. 'Federal, Provincial and Territorial Public Health Response Plan for Biological Events', *Canadian Communicable Disease Report*, 44(1): 1–5.

Migone, Andrea. 2020. 'Trust, but Customize: Federalism's Impact on the Canadian COVID-19 response', *Policy & Society*, 39(3): 382–402.

National Assembly. 2020. *Débats de l'Assemblée nationale*, 45(120), 12 June P 8270.

National Defence. 2020. 'Operation LASER', *Government of Canada*, https://www.canada.ca/en/department-national-defence/services/operations/military-operations/current-operations/laser.html (accessed on 10 July 2020).

Noël, Alain. 2020. 'COVID-19 et tensions intergouvernementales?', *Policy Options*, https://policyoptions.irpp.org/magazines/may-2020/covid-19-et-tensions-intergouvernemen-taleschronique-dalain-noel/ (accessed on 4 May 2020).

Pan-Canadian Public Health Network. 2009. Memorandum of Understanding on the Provision of Mutual Aid in Relation to Health Resources during an Emergency Affecting the Health of the Public, http://www.phn-rsp.ca/pubs/mou-ma-pe-am/index-eng.php (accessed on 1 October 2020).

Pan-Canadian Public Health Network. 2014. Multilateral Information Sharing Agreement, http://www.phn-rsp.ca/pubs/mlisa-emer-eng.php (accessed 1 October 2020).

Pan-Canadian Public Health Network. 2018a. *Federal/Provincial/Territorial Response Plan for Biological Events*. Catalogue No. HP45-20/2018E-PDFR. Ottawa: Minister of Health.

Pan-Canadian Public Health Network. 2018b. *Canadian Pandemic Influenza Preparedness: Planning Guidance for the Health Sector*. Catalogue No. HP40-144/2018E-PDF. Ottawa: Minister of Health.

Poirier, Johanne. 2004. 'Intergovernmental Agreements in Canada: At the Crossroads between Law and Politics', in Peter Meekison, Hamish Telford, and Harvey Lazar (eds), *Reconsidering the Institutions of Canadian Federalism*, pp. 425–62. Kingston: Institute of Intergovernmental Relations.

Poirier, Johanne. 2020. 'The 2018 Pan-Canadian Securities Regulation Reference: Dualist Federalism to the Rescue of Cooperative Federalism', *Supreme Court Law Review*, 94 (2): 85–123.

Poirier, Johanne and Sajeda Hedaraly. 2020. 'Truth and Reconciliation Calls to Action across Intergovernmental Landscapes: Who Can and Should Do What?', *Review of Constitutional Studies*, 24(2): 171–206.

Public Health Agency of Canada. 2020a. *Data on COVID-19 in Canada*, https://open.canada. ca/data/en/dataset/261c32ab-4cfd-4f81-9dea-7b64065690dc (accessed on 31 Oct 2021).

Public Health Agency of Canada. 2020b. *Federal/Provincial/Territorial Public Health Response Plan for Ongoing Management of COVID-19*. Ottawa: Minister of Health.

Sahota, Ruby. 2020. *Parliamentary Duties and the COVID-19 Pandemic: Report of the Standing Committee on Procedure and House Affairs*. Ottawa: House of Commons.

Schertzer, Robert and Mireille Paquet. 2020a. 'How Well is Canada's Intergovernmental System Handling the Crisis?', *Policy Options*, https://policyoptions.irpp.org/magazines/ april-2020/how-well-is-canadas-intergovernmental-system-handling-the-crisis/ (accessed on 8 April 2020).

Schertzer, Robert and Mireille Paquet. 2020b. 'COVID-19 as a Complex Intergovernmental Problem', *Canadian Journal of Political Science*, 53(2): 343–7.

Steytler, Nico. 2017. 'The Currency of Concurrent Powers', in Nico Steytler (ed.), *Concurrency Powers in Federal Systems: Meaning, Making, Managing*, pp. 1–11. Leiden/ Boston: Brill Nijhoff.

12

MANAGING THE CORONAVIRUS PANDEMIC IN A CENTRALISED FEDERAL SYSTEM

The case of Mexico

José María Serna de la Garza

12.1 Introduction

According to its most recent census, taken in 2010 (the 2020 census was suspended due to the pandemic), Mexico has a population of 120 million people. Of this count, 25.694 million (21.5 per cent of the total) consider themselves members of the indigenous population, with 7.3 million people over the age of 3 years speaking a Native-American language – of them, 12 out of every 100 do not speak Spanish. Around 77.8 per cent of Mexicans live in urban areas, and the balance of 22.2 per cent in rural areas (INEGI 2010), yet in spite of this high rate of urbanisation, the population is dispersed across a territory almost 2 million km^2 in size and characterised by great geographical diversity, as a result of which there are important regional differences in cultural and political identity. These differences, however, have not led any subnational community to claim recognition as a 'nation within the nation' (as happened, for example, with Catalonia in its relationship with Spain), nor does any component of the Mexican union demand secession.

Mexico's rather centralised federation consists of 31 states, Mexico City (which has a different status), and 2,457 municipalities. The origins of its centralisation lie in the hegemonic party system that prevailed between 1929 and 2000. In this system, an all-powerful president led a party that controlled most of the political positions at national and subnational level, subordinated state and municipal authorities to his will, and centralised the federal arrangement by way of formulas for allocating powers and sharing fiscal revenue (Cabrero Mendoza 2013). To this day, the logic of centralisation persists in the institutional and normative design of what is otherwise a competitively multiparty federal system.

Mexico's first case of Covid-19 – a 35-year-old man who had travelled from Italy to Mexico – was reported on 28 February 2020 in Mexico City, and its first

DOI: 10.4324/9781003166771-15

fatality, on 18 March. During 2020, there were more than 90,000 deaths from Covid-19. States and municipalities were the first to take steps to combat the pandemic; as for the federal government, it espoused a policy of denialism until it became evident that Mexico (and the rest of the world) was facing a global health crisis. After numerous social and economic activities were placed under lockdown, a gradual reopening began in June of the year, though the pace and rhythm of the lockdown and reopening were a matter of dispute between the federal and state governments.

This chapter examines the actions and decisions that federal, state, and municipal actors took during the 2020 pandemic within the applicable constitutional and legislative framework. The general goal is to identify what can be learnt about Mexico's federal system by analysing their behaviour; the argument made is that, in spite of a centralised federal system, states and municipalities played a significant role in combating Covid-19, thus reinvigorating that system.

The study covers the period from 18 March to 31 October 2020. During this period, in which the initial shock of the pandemic occurred, it was possible to observe key federal issues play out in regard to the distribution of powers and responsibilities and intergovernmental relations in the context of fighting the pandemic; in addition, demands and proposals were made for aspects of the federal system to be changed, chiefly ones relating to fiscal federalism.

12.2 The federal constitutional and legislative framework

12.2.1 Division of powers and functions

The principle by which powers and competences are allocated in Mexico's federal system is found in the residual clause of article 124 of the Mexican Constitution of 1917, according to which the powers not expressly attributed by the Constitution to the federal authorities are reserved to the states or Mexico City. There is a long list of such federal powers (Serna de la Garza 2013: 134–161). However, a number of policy areas are subject to a regime of concurrent powers, which entails that the Federal Congress can pass a statute distributing competences and responsibilities between the two (or among the three) levels of government – municipalities are recognised under article 115 of the Constitution as a third order of government.

Matters of 'general health' are subject to a regime of concurrent powers. The General Law on Health of 7 February 1984, passed by the federal Congress, distributes competences between the federal and state authorities in connection with different aspects of public health care. The federal government, through the Ministry of Health, has the power to issue general guidelines for the provision of public health services, powers of coordination of the National Health System,[1] and inspection powers to verify compliance with those guidelines. Moreover, the General Law on Health provides powers to the states in regard to the operation of public health services within their territories (González Block 2020).

The federal government provides health services and social security to two categories of insured people: private sector employees, through a federal entity called the Mexican Institute of Social Security (IMSS), and federal government employees, through the Institute for Social Security and Services for State Workers (ISSSTE). Some federal ministries or agencies have health services and social security schemes of their own for their employees. For their part, state governments likewise provide health services and social security for state employees. In addition, they have operative powers to provide public health services to the 'open' population, that is to say, to uninsured people.

Municipal governments do not have direct competence in the provision of health-care services, but do have constitutional powers that have an impact on public health, given that they are in charge of a variety of public functions and services. These include drinking water, drainage, and sanitation; street lighting; refuse removal; municipal markets and wholesale markets; cemeteries; slaughterhouses; streets, parks, and gardens; and public security, including preventative policing and traffic police (Graizbord 2009).

Public education is a subject matter that likewise falls under a regime of concurrent powers. In this regard, the General Law on Education of 30 September 2019 distributes competences and powers in this field among the different orders of government. Broadly speaking, the federal government, through the Ministry of Public Education, has the power to carry out global planning and programme direction of the national education system for the provision of public education, further to which it has powers of inspection over federal and state public schools as well as private education institutions; as for states, they are in charge of managing public state schools of the different levels of government.

12.2.2 Declaration of national disasters or states of emergency

Article 29 of Mexico's Constitution establishes a procedure for suspending or restricting rights by means of a declaration of a national disaster or state of emergency. In terms of this procedure, the President must obtain the approval of the Congress of the Union for such a declaration. The mechanism in article 29 has been activated only once, in the context of the Second World War, and was not to put to work during the Covid-19 crisis. Neither the states nor municipal governments have constitutional powers like these. States do not have the opportunity to participate in the procedure foreseen in article 29. This procedure is exclusively in the hands of federal entities, namely, the President of the Republic and the Congress of the Union.

In regard to disaster management, civil protection is a matter that falls under a normative regime of 'coordination', which is different from the regime of 'concurrency'. Under the latter, the federal Congress can pass a statute that distributes powers and competences among the different orders of government in a specific subject matter. Under 'coordination', the federal Congress does not distribute powers but creates mechanisms of coordination and collaboration among orders of government in a specific policy area (Serna de la Garza 2009). Accordingly, the General Law on Civil Protection of 6 June 2012, passed by the federal Congress, creates a system of coordination and collaboration between federal, state, and municipal authorities to react in cases of natural or man-made disasters. This system was, however, not put to use during the 2020 pandemic.

Article 73(XVI) of the Constitution defines two authorities that have the power to make decisions in a health crisis: the Ministry of Health and the Board of General Health. Both have the power to issue orders and provisions of mandatory compliance by the authorities of the three orders of government in the event 'of a serious epidemic or risk of invasion of exotic diseases'.

12.2.3 Health in the constitution and statute law

According to article 4(4), of the Constitution,

> [e]very person has the right to health protection. The law shall determine the bases and terms to access health services and shall establish the concurrence of the Federation and the States in regard to general health according to the item XVI in Article 73 of this Constitution.

In its development of this constitutional regime of concurrence, the normative scheme established by the General Law on Health in connection with fighting a pandemic can be summarised as follows: If a communicable disease threatens to become a serious danger in the territory of a state, the state authorities, in exercise of the reserved powers they enjoy in accordance with the logic of article 124 of the Constitution, can take such health measures as they are entitled to under the local legal order. Furthermore, this is particularly the case if, for some reason, the Federal Ministry of Health and the Board of General Health decide not to exercise their powers in the matter (e.g. if they regard the disease not as a threat to the general health of the republic, but as a problem limited to the territorial scope of a state). However, if the Ministry of Health and/or the Board of General Health decide/s to exercise their powers in this matter, then the state authorities must be subject to the general provisions, measures, and actions that these federal bodies dictate in addressing the health emergency.

12.3 Preparedness for a national disaster: The institutional framework

Normatively speaking, the Board of General Health has an intergovernmental dimension inasmuch as some state ministers of health form part of its structure and participate in its sessions, with voice though without vote. In theory, then, the Board should function as a forum for intergovernmental relations. However, in practice it does not function in a collegiate way, given that its decisions are taken by the Federal Ministry of Health. Prior to the 2020 pandemic, the last time the Board of General Health and the Ministry of Health issued general norms to control a pandemic was in 2009, in the context of the H1N1 influenza.

There is also a Federal Aid Plan for the Civilian Population in Disaster Cases known as the DN-III Plan, which is a military operational instrument that establishes general guidelines for the Mexican army and navy to carry out relief activities if the population is affected by disasters of natural or human origin. Its legal basis is in articles 21 and 73 of the General Law on Civil Protection and article 1 of the Organic Law of the Mexican Army and Air Force.

12.4 Rolling out measures to contain the pandemic

When the pandemic struck, party-political contestation was already much in the foreground, so governors and legislators duly responded to the crisis along party lines.[2] Supporters of the President, Andrés Manuel López Obrador, and his party, the Movement for National Regeneration, or *Movimiento de Regeneración Nacional* (MORENA), followed federal directives and guidelines with little criticism, although there were a few exceptions.[3] For their part, governors within the opposition established different groups (four in total) to form a common front in resisting particular federal directives.

These groups were organised along party and regional lines, with the most visible of them being the so-called Federalist Alliance. Made up of 10 governors, it drew together opposition parties on the left, centre, and right of Mexico's political spectrum. Its members were the governors of Aguascalientes (PAN), Coahuila (PRI), Guanajuato (PAN), Jalisco (MC), Colima (PRI), Michoacán (PRD), Nuevo León (no party affiliation), Tamaulipas (PAN), Chihuahua (PAN), and Durango (PRI). In September 2020, they decided to withdraw from the National Conference of Governors – which has represented all state governors since the early 2000s – on the grounds that it did not defend the sovereignty of the states, operate effectively, or serve as a forum for dialogue with the federal executive.[4]

The pandemic not only deepened political divisions but also further marginalised Mexico's indigenous peoples. Many such communities lack clinics, as a result of which some of them closed access to their towns or locales as the only way to avoid infection. Many of them had also not received information in their own languages on how to take care of themselves during the pandemic. For example, the leader of the Council of Community Government of Chilón, which represents about 600 communities of the Tzeltal ethnic group, accused health authorities of having done nothing to help them. Under circumstances like these, indigenous peoples resort to traditional medical practices but still claim for more assistance from health authorities. The Nich Ixim Midwife Movement of Chiapas, which advocates on behalf of indigenous midwives in the state of Chiapas, sought to guide community members on how to implement prevention measures in the absence of resources such as sanitisers and masks.

Such communities generally lack clinics, health services, and regular access to water and are challenged by linguistic barriers, inequality, exclusion, and historical neglect. During the pandemic, many were demanding that authorities at least provide mobile clinics, along with appropriate personnel and equipment (*Reforma*, 19 April 2020: 10). In the face of inaction by health authorities, some local authorities, such as the municipality of Ometepec (in the state of Guerrero), denied access to non-residents and imposed evening curfews, with sanctions of arrest of up to 36 hours for transgressors.

12.4.1 Taking the initiative

Some states, and even municipal authorities, were the first to take measures to combat the pandemic. On 13 March 2020, while the federal government was still denying the dangers of Covid-19, the governor of Jalisco, Enrique Alfaro, a member of the centrist opposition party *Movimiento Ciudadano* (MC), announced a number of response measures (*Reforma*, 18 March 2020: 1). First, he set up a panel of experts with advisory functions and, secondly, a coordination mechanism for engaging with municipal governments and academic institutions to reach consensus on what to do. On the same day, Alfaro announced the postponement of mass events including a film festival and pre-Olympic football tournament. On 15 March, he suspended in-person classes in state public schools and ordered the use of Covid-19 screening and sanitisation stations at state airports and bus stations.

Similarly, on 17 March 2020 both Alfaro and the governor of Nuevo Leon ordered the closure of public places such as bars, casinos, cinemas, and restaurants. At the local level, the municipal government of San Pedro Garza García (in the state of Nuevo León) also reacted rapidly. On 17 March 2020 it declared a 'state of emergency', ordering measures that included the temporary closure of bars, clubs, discos, breweries, gyms, and places of worship, as well as the cancellation of permits for all public and private events in public spaces (*Reforma*, 18 March 2020: 1).

Alfaro's precautionary measures drew criticism from the Federal Ministry of Health, which at that early, uncertain point in the pandemic deemed the state of Jalisco's actions as unnecessary. Federal-state tensions continued to rise, though, when the governor of Jalisco announced a programme of rapid tests for the coronavirus, thereby contradicting a federal policy stance that, then as later, gave little to no credence or importance to testing. Finally, on 16 April 2020, the Ministry of Health accused the government of Guadalajara (the capital city of Jalisco) of not complying with suspension of non-essential commercial activities as ordered by federal authorities (*Reforma*, 18 April 2020: 7).

In spite of the fact that the first infection in Mexico was reported on 27 February 2020, during the next 30 days the federal government continued allowing mass events and football games of the national league. Likewise, the President continued attending public meetings, shaking hands, and kissing people without him or other participants wearing face masks. On 22 March he was still inviting Mexicans to go out in the streets and dine at restaurants to strengthen the economy (*Reforma*, 13 May 2020: 12). The first action by the federal government came only on 30 March 2020, when the Board of General Health issued a decree by which a health emergency of *force majeure* was declared. One day later, the Ministry of Health issued a decree enumerating extraordinary actions to address this emergency. Among other things, the public, social, and private sectors had to implement measures that included the 'immediate suspension of non-essential activities'.

12.4.2 Federal action

12.4.2.1 Initial federal action

The Board of General Health's Declaration of Emergency was published on 30 March 2020. The main purpose of this Declaration was to open the door to the Extraordinary Measures taken by the Ministry of Health, which were published on 31 March. The latter ordered the immediate suspension of 'non-essential' activities for one month (the decree provided a list of activities considered 'essential'); set out rules on how to organise work in places where essential activities were allowed (concerning the number of people allowed in the workplace and the sanitary and control measures to be taken); and instructed people to stay at home. The decree also stated that the Ministry of Health, in conjunction with the Ministry for Economic Affairs and Ministry of Labour and Social Welfare, would issue guidelines for the country's orderly, phased, and regionalised return to work and social and economic activity (Ministry of Health 2020).

On 21 April 2020, another decree by the Ministry of Health extended the extraordinary measures for two months (until 31 May) and imposed a number of duties on state governments. Among other things, state governments were to keep a registry of patients in hospital with acute respiratory infections; implement prevention and control measures in line with the criteria issued by the Ministry of Health; establish mechanisms for restricting the municipal-level mobility of persons infected by or exposed to Covid-19; report to the Federal Ministry of Health on the implementation of these measures; and supervise changes to hospitals to guarantee the availability of beds for treating infected patients.

In addition, Aid Plan DN-III, mentioned earlier, was activated so as to make military hospitals available for patients with Covid-19; to make military personnel available to operate and protect hospitals; and to provide support in food distribution, transportation of supplies, repatriation of compatriots, and manufacture of medical supplies.

12.4.2.2 Federal-state conflict about reopening

In the same way as there were conflicts about the imposition of the lockdown, so there was conflict when it came to reopening schools and the economy. On 13 May 2020, the federal government announced its strategy for enabling the country to resume social and economic activity. This was to extend across three stages, each entailing a 'traffic-light' system of four phases (red, orange, yellow, and green), and to begin on 1 June.

GOAN, the association of nine governors from the opposition party PAN, reacted to the strategy on Twitter, saying in effect that its member states would heed their own counsel and decide for themselves when to reopen their states, taking into account local conditions and the advice of experts. The President replied that there would be no fight with the states in the event that their governors did not comply with the federal reopening plan:

> If there is a municipal or state authority that according to the characteristics of their own region or of each state, decides that they will not comply with the plan, there will be no controversy.… Though the plan was agreed in general, it also allows discrepancies, the right to think differently.
>
> (*Reforma*, 14 May 2020: 5)

Likewise, the Ministry of Health conceded that decisions on reopening according to the 'traffic-light' system would depend on the conditions in each state. States would be able to increase restrictive measures but not make them less restrictive or more flexible. Consensus, the Ministry said, had been reached on the issue (*Reforma*, 3 June 2020: 1).

The federal government and state governors also differed on the date on which to resume in-person classes in private and public schools. Initially, the Federal Minister of Education set 1 June 2020 as the date on which this would come to pass throughout Mexico. Numerous governors disagreed, arguing that in view of the differing conditions in the states, the decision to reopen schools should be taken by the authorities of each state. Ultimately, the Minister had to accede to this position (*Reforma*, 14 May 2020: 3).

12.4.2.3 Legal challenge by indigenous peoples

Flaws in the inclusivity and efficacy of Mexico's federal system, specifically when placed under the strain of pandemic crisis management, were highlighted in a number of legal challenges that communities of indigenous peoples mounted in reaction to alleged acts or omissions by the federal government in responding to Covid-19.

In one case, for example, the indigenous peoples of the Tsotsil, Tzeltal, Zoque, and Chol ethnic groups successfully filed a writ of *amparo*[5] demanding a guarantee of access to information about Covid-19 and its prevention in their respective home languages (*Reforma*, 8 April 2020: 1). In another, the Pueblo Maya Ch'ol (who reside in the municipalities of Palenque, Ocosingo, and Salto del Agua in the state of Chiapas) filed a writ of *amparo* against the continuation of a federal mega-project involving the construction of a railway line in the Southeast states. Here, the district judge ruled that the federal government had to desist from the project in the affected municipalities while the pandemic lasts, since continuation of work endangered the lives and health of the local population (*Reforma*, 23 June 2020: 1).

12.4.2.4 Accountability and the separation of powers

Mexico's pandemic response served to centralise power even further in the federal executive in the context of a system that, even before the health crisis, was focused on the President.

The two chambers of Congress stopped meeting from the end of March 2020, returning to work, albeit in a limited way, by mid-June. As a result, health measures and those related to mitigating the economic effects of the pandemic were adopted by the President and Ministry of Health with little deliberation. Especially controversial was the President's proposal, sent to Congress on 23 April 2020, which sought to empower him, in case of 'economic emergencies in the country', to 'redirect resources of the federal Budget, to allocate them to maintain the execution of the projects and priority actions of the Federal Public Administration and promote the country's economic activity, to face health emergencies and finance programs for the benefit of society' (Parliamentary Gazette 2020).

This proposal was not discussed in Congress – not only because of the difficulties of having meetings, but because the proposal was presented seven days before the end of the regular session of the Federal Congress, which each year begins on February 1 and ends on April 30. The proposal represented an attempt to take advantage of the crisis and absorb powers which are exclusive to the Federal Chamber of Deputies, such as the power to approve the federal budget. Furthermore, in the proposal, the power to declare when there is an 'economic emergency' was entirely at the discretion of the federal executive.

Apart from the case of the governor of Michoacán (mentioned below), there were cases in which federal courts were asked to clarify whether municipal governments have powers to establish harsh restrictions on the freedom of movement. The Courts determined that, according to the Constitution, municipal authorities are not allowed to suspend or restrict human rights.

12.4.3 State action

Some states asserted their autonomy with regard to their responsibilities and resisted being directed by the federal government. This is generally true for governors from opposition parties, as the examples below suggest.

12.4.3.1 Health measures

On 17 April 2020, the government of the state of Mexico, via its Ministry of Security, paroled 1,894 prisoners to avoid infections in state prisons. The releases were approved by the state Superior Court of Justice, which examined the proposal and allowed prisoners sentenced for 'non-serious' crimes (i.e., ones entailing

a prison sentence of less than 5 years) to be paroled subject to their wearing electronic bracelets. On the same day, the federal government announced that it was
considering paroling inmates in federal prisons and, to this end, utilising the
President's power of pardon.

On 25 June 2020 the government of Hidalgo established, in the state's capital city of Pachuca, the first of 30 health units to apply quick and free tests for
Covid-19 (this, contrary to federal policy that denied the usefulness of tests)
(*Reforma*, 26 June 2020: 6). Three days later, the same initiative was implemented
in the rest of the state. A similar policy was implemented in an important tourist
centre, namely Acapulco in the state of Guerrero.

12.4.3.2 Lockdown and mobility measures

The governor of Jalisco rejected the possibility of returning to in-person classes
on 1 June 2020, as ordered by the federal government. This contradicted what
the Federal Ministry of Education had declared regarding a possible return to
classes on 1 June or 17 July. Jalisco suspended classes on 17 March and resumed
them online on 17 April.

While the federal government was working out its plans and timelines for the
resumption of schooling, opposition governors announced unilateral decisions to
finish the then-current cycle and begin the next one. The governor of Jalisco said
that in spite of a decrease in infections in the state, there would not be a return
to in-person classes, as his government did not want to run any risks. Classes,
he said, would continue online or on television by way of programmes such as
Recrea Digital and *Learn at Home* (*Reforma*, 12 May 2020: 2).

Although federal policies entailed voluntary rather than mandatory confinement, some governors adopted more restrictive measures that indeed required
mandatory confinement, giving rise to lawsuits that claimed these measures were
unconstitutional. For example, on 20 April 2020, the governor of Michoacán
issued a decree declaring mandatory isolation and imposing strong restrictions on
people's mobility, along with sanctions for those who violated them. The decree
was challenged by a group of academics at the Faculty of Law of the Nicolaíta
University of Michoacán, who filed a writ of *amparo* against it. However, in the
end the collegiate circuit court that heard the case decided in favour of the governor, on the ground that the contested decree aimed to protect social well-being.[6]

Only a few states imposed border controls. For example, the government of
Tamaulipas did so on the state's border with Nuevo León to prevent the entry of
vehicles and persons deemed 'non-essential' (*Reforma*, 17 April 2020: 2).

12.4.3.3 Economic measures and reopening

In May 2020, Jalisco announced a plan for its economic recovery. Entitled *Plan de
Reactivación Económica*, its main thrust was to revise the state budget by taking austerity measures. The governor requested that the state executive, legislature, and

judiciary draft a plan to save money given that the pandemic had led to a major shortfall in a state budget of more than MXN 3 billion (*Reforma*, 2 May 2020: 3).

In the same month, the governors of Coahuila, Colima, Michoacán, Nuevo León, Tamaulipas, and Jalisco collectively determined their reopening plans. At a meeting on 15 May 2020, they agreed to work to a common agenda prioritising health, economic recovery, and assistance for the poor. An underlying premise of their collaboration was – as opposition governors argued on another occasion in a virtual meeting with federal authorities – that it is state governments, not the federal government, that have full knowledge of the conditions in their respective territories (*Reforma*, 16 May 2020: 1).

Even the governor of Puebla, a member of the same party as President López Obrador, announced that his state would have its own 'traffic-light' system for reopening. Although it would be similar to the federation's, he asserted that the 'new normality' in Puebla had to be defined by this state's own criteria. The governor said he did not want to be left waiting to take the lead from the federal government on the basis of assessments that were unrelated to circumstances in places where the real fight against the virus was being waged (*Reforma*, 23 May 2020: 3).

12.4.3.4 Cooperation among states

As has been suggested already, various states engaged in horizontal cooperation with each other along regional and political lines. For instance, in May 2020, the governors of Jalisco, Aguascalientes, Querétaro, and San Luis Potosí decided on a series of measures for addressing the pandemic in a coordinated manner, with such measures including reinforcing Covid-19 screening and sanitisation stations and devising ways to support the automobile and electrical industries. These states formed a regional alliance, the *Alianza Centro-Bajío-Occidente*, and agreed to assist one another with medical resources for their hospitals (*Reforma*, 1 May 2020: 8).

In addition, after initiating their own reopening plans, eight governors met in the state of Nuevo León to share their experiences on the matter and agree on simplified requirements for allowing businesses to reopen. According to the governor of Nuevo León, this involved using a system of 'economic intelligence' to monitor the impact of economic reactivation. He said the governors at the meeting agreed to support small enterprises through credit from public and private financial institutions and thus enable them to integrate themselves into the value chains of larger companies.

The governors present in the meeting were those of Tamaulipas, Coahuila, Jalisco, Michoacán, Durango, and Guanajuato. This bloc, located in the Northeast of the country and cutting across political parties, said it would seek a meeting with another regional alliance of governors, the *Alianza Bajío-Centro-Occidente*, to exchange information about what they had learnt from their experiences.

For their part, the nine opposition governors of GOAN proposed common areas of action in regard to economic reactivation. For example, they put forward a national strategy to address the economic crisis caused by the pandemic. It included creating an unemployment insurance scheme, implementing a programme of temporary employment, introducing tax incentives for new businesses, and providing soft loans for companies.

12.4.4 Local government action

The role of local authorities during the 2020 pandemic was mostly confined to implementing measures decided upon by the federal and state governments. There were exceptions to this, however. For example, in early March a number of municipalities took the initiative to shut down activities in public places; others yet, as mentioned, illegally closed their borders with other municipalities.

In this respect, the mayors of various municipalities disregarded the directives of the Federal Minister of the Interior, who told them not to limit freedom of movement in their goal of curbing infections. She explained to them that the federal government had authorised neither a curfew nor a suspension of rights; what it decreed was instead a health emergency in which Mexicans were requested to stay at home voluntarily. As such, municipalities could not close their 'borders', that is, their territorial limits, albeit that this is what happened in the states of Veracruz, Tamaulipas, Coahuila, and Nuevo León (*Reforma*, 25 April 2020: 7).

Another trend during the period was that mayors of the same party affiliation endeavoured to work together to leverage greater financial resources from the federation. For example, due to the fact that the income municipalities derived from municipal taxes decreased by 50 per cent as a result of the pandemic, mayors of the *Federación Nacional de Municipios de México* (FENAMM), linked to the Institutional Revolutionary Party, and of the *Asociación Nacional de Alcaldes* (ANAC), linked to the Party of National Action, asked the Federal Ministry of Finance to flexibilise the use of federal transfers and to authorise extraordinary transfers. The same was proposed by the *Asociación de Autoridades Locales de México* (AALMAC), which represents mayors from the ruling MORENA party at federal level (*Reforma*, 9 June 2020: 5).

Generally, the impression gained from media coverage of the pandemic is that there was a suspension of the usual modes by which executive mayors are held accountable, given that various municipal councils temporarily ceased operations. By the same token, many others decided to conduct their sessions online, while others yet resumed in-person sessions, with strict sanitary measures being observed. Nonetheless, the scope for public accountability diminished, particularly in those municipalities where there is the option of having public and open sessions of the municipal council.

12.4.5 Intergovernmental relations

Coordination among the different levels of government was patchy, if not dysfunctional. It is worth noting generally that Mexico lacks an institutional forum in which the federal executive can meet regularly with governors to reach consensus on public policies in matters related to health and education, among other things (see Hopkins 1990; Rodríguez 1998; Ward and Rodríguez 1999). Some governors had been requesting a meeting with the President since December 2019, without success. That meeting finally took place on 19 August 2020, by which point the country was nearing a total of 60,000 deaths from Covid-19.

In particular, there was a notable lack of communication between the Federal Health Ministry and state governments about 'general health', which is a concurrent responsibility of the federal and state governments. In the case of pandemics like Covid-19, the Ministry of Health may adopt 'extraordinary measures' in regard to health, with state governments then obliged to follow federal guidelines. However, what was witnessed throughout the crisis was a series of conflicts, disagreements, and failed encounters between federal and state authorities with regard to, inter alia, the point at which to declare a health emergency; the kinds of health-protection measures to adopt; and the timing and pace of reopening the national economy.

This was due in large part to the non-existence of an institutional mechanism to facilitate communication between the President and state governors and harmonise the development and implementation of public policy in the federation. Consequently, the lack of effective coordination and cooperation between the federal and state governments was evident from the outset of the 2020 pandemic – by mid-March 2020, state governments had taken the first measures to curb the spread of the virus, whereas the Federal Board on General Health did not meet until 19 March (and then only so as to make an evaluation of the situation).

An example of the disagreements between federal and state authorities occurred in mid-April when, after receiving federal aid in the form of materials to use in combating the pandemic, the governors of Michoacán, Aguascalientes, and Quintana Roo complained that the materials were of bad quality and returned them to the federal government as useless.

In another example, on 21 April 2020, the President threatened to expose those governors who did not comply with the measures stipulated by the federal government. He also said his government would not authorise the use of curfews, the police force, or monetary fines in the enforcement of those measures. On the next day, the spokesperson of the presidential office made public a list of municipalities that were not complying with the federal government's instructions to reduce the mobility of persons and have them stay at home. He said, however, that the vast majority – 97 per cent – were compliant. Some of the 'accused' municipalities responded to this by denying the charge and others, by adopting more effective measures for reducing mobility (*Reforma*, 23 April 2020: 3).

If the Covid-19 pandemic has taught us any lesson, it is the need to design better coordination and cooperation mechanisms between the three orders government of Mexico's federal system.

12.4.6 Intergovernmental fiscal relations

In economic affairs, the federal government has broad powers since it controls both monetary and fiscal policy, with the latter especially centralised given that 90 per cent of fiscal income comes from federal taxes, 8 per cent from state taxes, and 2 per cent from municipal taxes. States and municipalities are highly dependent on federal transfers to fund their activities in that they have only limited taxation powers. The transfers are the so-called *'participaciones'* (for discretionary use by state and municipal governments) and the *'aportaciones'* (restricted to the specific purpose defined by federal law). These federal transfers represent about 80 per cent of states' fiscal income.[7] Of the total federal transfers to the states, 42.9 per cent correspond to *'participaciones'* and 37.3 per cent to *'aportaciones'* (Centro de Estudios de las Finanzas Públicas 2019: 6)

By the end of April 2020, a group of opposition governors had begun to call into question the existing federal fiscal arrangement. The governors of Chihuahua (PAN), Nuevo León (no party affiliation), Tamaulipas (PAN), Jalisco (MC), and Coahuila (PRI) alleged that although their states contribute the most to the federal treasury, they receive the least in federal transfers. After proposing a national debate on this matter, they agreed to postpone it and instead work together in the next general election (2021) to win a majority in the Chamber of Deputies and use that majority to propose a change to the fiscal pact (*Reforma*, 20 April 2020: 1).

Opposition governors also started to demand more federal resources to fight the pandemic, arguing that 'extraordinary' federal resources were needed to address an extraordinary situation. However, the President's response was that they should reduce their spending and save money in order to procure those resources.

Finally, the governors of Nuevo León (no party affiliation), Tamaulipas (PAN), Coahuila (PRI), Durango (PRI), and Michoacán (PRD) – all with different political affiliations but sharing a regional interest – agreed to do a count of the expenses incurred to face the pandemic and claim reimbursement from the federation. They said that they had faced the crisis with their own ordinary resources and that these resources had to be reimbursed. In their view, it was not possible to face an extraordinary situation with ordinary resources.

The rather centralised arrangement of Mexico's fiscal federalism dates back to three national fiscal conventions that took place in 1925, 1933, and 1947. Today, and as a consequence of tensions derived from the pandemic, some opposition governors have proposed calling a new national fiscal convention, in order to review the rules and principles of the existing fiscal arrangement.

12.5 Findings and policy implications

Mexico has long had a highly centralised federal system, but it was during the 2020 pandemic that the shortcomings of centralisation in such a large and diverse country came fully to light. The federal government has broad legal powers in the fields of health and education, as well as in matters to do with reopening the economy. However, in spite of those powers, a good number of governors took the initiative to decide when to shut down their states' economies and schools, adopted public health measures contrary to federal guidelines (e.g., quick and large-scale testing for Covid-19), or decided for themselves when and how quickly economies should be reopened to suit the circumstances of their respective states.

The pandemic also revealed the displeasure numerous governors feel in connection with the fiscal arrangement in the country's federal system. This arrangement, which dates from the 1980s, is based on the premise that states have waived their powers to create state taxes by ceding them to the federal government in exchange for federal transfers. However, the arrangement has contributed to the subordination of the states to the federation, since the latter has an important margin of discretion in the distribution of federal transfers to the states. Moreover, states that contribute the most to the federal treasury contend that they are not adequately recompensed by what they get back in federal transfers.

Opposition governors of 12 states maintained that, due to a lack of a rational response to the pandemic and the lack of a plan for the economic reactivation of the federation, Mexico needs to move to a new federalism based on a new fiscal pact. This was declared by the governors who comprise the *Alianza Centro Bajío Occidente* and the *Alianza Federalista*. In a joint statement, they 'expressed the importance of advancing to a new cooperative and responsible federalism, that is, to a new model of decentralization articulated around powers, responsibilities and duties clearly defined that allow the strengthening of local capacities'. The statement continued:

> This new federalism will … take the maximum advantage [of] the USMCA,[8] [and] accelerate the country's economic recovery, the strengthening of public finances and the promotion of public and private investment in infrastructure and in public services.
>
> (*Reforma*, 4 July 2020: 11)

Whether this will happen or not will depend largely on the balance of power that emerges from the electoral processes of 2021, in which the 500 seats of the Chamber of Deputies and 15 governorships will be at stake. At the time of this writing, 14 of those governorships were controlled by opposition parties. If López Obrador's party wins these elections, the *Alianza Federalista* in favour of a 'new federalism', a 'new fiscal pact', and decentralisation will be severely weakened.

Notes

1 The national health system is made up of public administration agencies and entities at the federal, state, and local levels; individuals and organisations in the private sector and civil society that provide health services; and mechanisms for coordinating action. The system aims to fulfil the right to health protection (General Law on Health, article 5) and seeks to harmonise the programmes of the different public (federal and state) and private entities that provide health services in Mexico.

2 In March 2020, the political affiliations of Mexico's 31 governorships were as follows: *Partido Revolucionario Institutional* (PRI), 12; *Partido de Acción Nacional* (PAN), 9; MORENA, 7; *Partido de la Revolución Democrática* (PRD), 1; *Movimiento Ciudadano* (MC), 1; and one governor with no party affiliation. The percentage of seats in the Chamber of Deputies was MORENA, 50.4 per cent; PAN, 15.4 per cent; PRI, 9.6 per cent; Partido del Trabajo (PT), 9.2 per cent; MC, 5.4 per cent; *Partido Encuentro Social* (PES), 4.8 per cent; PRD, 2.4 per cent; and *Partido Verde Ecologista de México* (PVEM), 2.2 per cent; three deputies had no party affiliation. The split in the Senate was MORENA, 42.6 per cent; PAN, 19.5 per cent; PRI, 10.1 per cent; PT, 4.6 per cent; MC, 6.2 per cent; PES, 3.1 per cent; PRD, 2.3 per cent; and PVEM, 5.4 per cent; one senator had no party affiliation.

3 At the outset of the pandemic, the governing party MORENA and its allies (PT, PES, and PVEM) had a comfortable majority in both chambers of Congress, controlling 66.6 per cent of the seats in the Chamber of Deputies and 55.7 per cent of the seats in the Senate. The legislators of these parties have been always ready to cooperate with President López Obrador, and this support did not wither away as the pandemic continued.

4 The other three groups were the *Alianza Noreste-Pacífico*, comprising seven opposition governors (from Nuevo León (no party affiliation), Coahuila (PRI), Durango (PRI), Tamaulipas (PAN), Jalisco (MC), Colima (PRI) and Michoacán (PRD)); the *Alianza Centro-Bajío-Occidente*, comprising five opposition governors (from Aguascalientes (PAN), Guanajuato (PAN), Jalisco (MC), Querétaro (PAN) y San Luis Potosí (PRI)); and the *Asociación de Gobernadores de Acción Nacional* (GOAN), comprising the nine governors of the PAN.

5 A petition for a writ of *amparo*, or an *amparo* action, is, according to the Supreme Court of the Philippines (n.d.), 'a remedy available to any person whose right to life, liberty and security is violated or threatened with violation by an unlawful act or omission of a public official or employee, or of a private individual or entity'.

6 See *Amparo* 403/2020, filed by Jorge Alvarez Banderas against the decree of 20 April 2020 by the governor of Michoacán, which declared mandatory confinement as a measure to combat the pandemic.

7 See generally Cabrero Mendoza (2013) and Gershberg (1995); for a constitutional and comparative perspective, see Serna de la Garza (2000).

8 The United States-Mexico-Canada Agreement (USMCA) is a free-trade agreement in force since March 2020; it replaces the North American Free Trade Agreement (NAFTA).

References

Cabrero Mendoza, Enrique. 2013. 'Fiscal Federalism in Mexico: Distortions and Structural Traps', *Urban Public Economics Review*, 18: 12–36.

Centro de Estudios de las Finanzas Públicas. 2019. *Cuenta Pública 2018, Gasto Federalizado Ejercido en Entidades Federativas y Municipios*, Cámara de Diputados.

Gershberg, Alec Ian. 1995. 'Fiscal Decentralization and Intergovernmental Relations: An Analysis of Federal versus State Education Finance in Mexico', *Review of Urban and Regional Development Studies*, 7(2): 119–42.

González Block, Miguel, et al. 2020. *Mexico, Health System Review 2020*, 22(2). World Health Organization.

Graizbord, Boris. 2009. 'United Mexican States', in N. Steytler (ed.), *Local Government and Metropolitan Regions in Federal Systems*, pp. 200–33. Montreal and Kingston: McGill Queen's University Press.

Hopkins, Jack W. 1990. 'Intergovernmental Relations in Mexico and the United States: A Comparative Perspective', *International Review of Administrative Sciences*, 5: 403–20.

INEGI. 2010. *Volumen y Crecimiento. Población total según tamaño de la localidad para cada entidad federativa, México.*

Ministry of Health. 2020. *Acuerdo por el que se declara como emergencia sanitaria por causa de fuerza mayor, a la epidemia de enfermedad generada por el virus SARS-CoV-2 (COVID-19).* Official Gazette of the Federation, 30 March.

Parliamentary Gazette. 2020. '*Iniciativa con proyecto de decreto por el que se adicionan diversas disposiciones de la Ley Federal de Presupuesto y Responsabilidad Hacendaria, remitida por el titular del Ejecutivo federal*' (*Initiative with a draft decree that adds various provisions to the Federal Budget and Fiscal Responsibility Law, sent by the head of the federal Executive*), Parliamentary Gazette of the Chamber of Deputies, 23 April.

Reforma, Mexico City. 2020. News reports between 18 March 2020 and 31 October 2020.

Rodríguez, Victoria E. 1998. 'Recasting Federalism in Mexico', *Publius: The Journal of Federalism*, 28(1): 235–54.

Serna de la Garza, José Maria. 2000. 'Constitutional Federalism in Latin America', *California Western International Law Journal*, 30(2): 277–301.

Serna de la Garza, José Maria. 2009. 'Mechanisms of Cooperation in Mexico's Federal System', in B. de Villiers (ed.), *Crossing the Line: Dealing with Cross-Border Communities.* Johannesburg: Konrad Adenauer Stiftung.

Serna de la Garza, José Maria. 2013. *The Constitution of Mexico: A Contextual Analysis.* United Kingdom: Hart Publishing.

Supreme Court of the Philippines. n.d. 'The Rule on the Writ of *Amparo*', http://hrlibrary.umn.edu/research/Philippines/The%20Rule%20On%20The%20Writ%20Of%20Amparo.pdf (accessed on 1 December 2020).

Ward, Peter and Victoria Rodríguez. 1999. 'New Federalism, Intra-Governmental Relations and Co-Governance in Mexico', *Journal of Latin American Studies*, 3(3): 673–710.

PART III
South America

13

BRAZIL AND THE FIGHT AGAINST COVID-19

Strengthening state and municipal powers

Gilberto M. A. Rodrigues, Vanessa Elias de Oliveira, Marcelo Labanca Corrêa de Araújo and Sérgio Ferrari

13.1 Introduction

From the outset of the Covid-19 pandemic, a central feature of federalism in Brazil was the strong role played by state governors and the fact that this stood in contrast to the denialism of the President Jair Bolsonaro, who neglected his federal responsibilities. Whereas the President refused to support isolation measures and import medicines and supplies for curbing the pandemic, governors quickly performed these tasks. Subnational responsibility was confirmed by the Supreme Court, giving governors and mayors important political visibility and shaking up the entrenched structures of Brazil's centralised federalism.

This chapter discusses the dual nature of Brazilian federalism, as evidenced by the Covid-19 pandemic. On the one hand, the crisis highlighted the importance of the federal government in the institutional arrangement of Brazilian federalism, which is highly centralised; on the other hand, it has provided greater scope for action by state governments, whose political power has gradually diminished over the 30 years since the 1988 Constitution came into being.

The Federative Republic of Brazil is the largest country in South America and the fifth largest in the world. Its Constitution of 1988 makes it a significantly decentralised federation in terms of the distribution of political power and fiscal resources between the three levels of government – federal, state, and municipal – each of which consists of 'federative entities' (Souza 1997). Brazil is also highly socio-economically heterogeneous, a fact that presented considerable challenges in its efforts to confront the Covid-19 pandemic.

Politically, too, the country is fragmented, with 24 political parties represented in Congress, the federal parliament. The 10 with the largest congressional representation are the Brazilian Democratic Movement (MDB), Workers'

DOI: 10.4324/9781003166771-17

Party (PT), Brazilian Social Democratic Party (PSDB), Progressive Party (PP), Democratic Workers' Party (PDT), Brazilian Workers' Party (PTB), Democrats Party (DEM), Liberal Party (PL), Brazilian Socialist Party (PSB), and Republicans. However, governability in Congress depends as well on small parties without an ideological affiliation; in addition, a strong conservative multiparty caucus – the so-called beef, bullets, and bible lobby – supports the government in pursuit of specific interests, with the focus falling variously on agrarian matters ('beef'), law and order ('bullets'), and religion ('bible').

President Bolsonaro was elected by a small party, the Liberal Social Party (PSL), which espouses anti-political-system rhetoric. He left it in November 2019 but was unable to create a new one and thus remained without party affiliation during the 2020 pandemic. In the absence of a formal coalition, Bolsonaro relied on unstable support from conservative parties in Congress. In regard to state-level opposition politics, opposition governors are from a broad ideological spectrum ranging from the political left to the right.

The Brazilian population is relatively young: in 2019, 42.3 per cent of people in a population of about 210 million were less than 30 years of age (IBGE 2019a). Approximately 85 per cent of the population live in cities, but regional disparities are large: city dwellers make up 93 per cent of the population in the Southeast region of the country, but the proportion drops to 73 per cent in the Northeast. Although cities have a higher population density than peri-urban and rural areas and were disproportionately affected by the pandemic, health services are also concentrated in these areas, thanks to which treatment was readily accessible there.

Brazil has a mixed public and private health-care system, with the vast majority (75 per cent) of the population using the public National Health System (SUS) and only 25 per cent having private health insurance (Scheffer et al. 2015). Spending per capita is USD 1,282 when the public and private sectors are combined; however, it is much lower than this if one considers the public health service alone, which covers most of the population. Public health spending in this respect is USD 551 per capita per year (43 per cent of total spending in 2017, according to the Organisation for Economic Co-operation and Development (OECD 2019)). According to the World Bank, public spending on health in 2018 accounted for 3.9 per cent of gross domestic product (GDP) – this is lower than the average for Latin America and the Caribbean as a whole (4.1 per cent), and the average of 6.5 per cent presented by the OECD countries (OECD 2019).

It was in the big cities, especially São Paulo and Rio de Janeiro, that Brazil recorded its initial cases of Covid-19; the first to come to light was on 25 February 2020 and concerned a traveller returning from Italy (Department of Health 2020). Several days after a pandemic was declared by the World Health Organization (WHO) on 11 March, the states of São Paulo and Rio de Janeiro were the first in Brazil to introduce quarantine measures. On 20 March, the country's Ministry of Health confirmed the domestic spread of the virus.

Given that the federal government opposed isolation and quarantine, a policy of social distancing was not introduced uniformly across the country; even so, 15 of Brazil's 26 states, along with the Federal District, adopted these measures. The latter were important in reducing the initial transmissibility rate (i.e. the number of persons infected by one infected person), which was estimated at three – much higher than the average at the height of the pandemic in Europe, where the mean rate was 1.6. By 31 October 2020, Brazil had the third highest number of cases (about 5 million) and second highest number of deaths (more than 160,000) in the world, in this regard trailing behind only the United States. More than a third of the cases were concentrated in the Southeast region (Candido et al. 2020). On 14 November, the transmissibility rate had decreased to 0.94 (Imperial College 2020).

However, a series of problems indicated that the situation was more serious than the data suggested. Firstly, Brazil's rate of Covid-19 testing was very low; secondly, there would be a delay between the occurrence of a case and/or death and the official report of it; and, thirdly, in the middle of 2020, the Brazilian Ministry of Health changed the system for counting cases.

13.2 The federal constitutional and legislative framework

Brazil has a federal constitution that establishes three levels of government: the federation, the states, and the municipalities, each of which has its own administrative and legislative powers. States and municipalities enjoy political and constitutional autonomy (Ferrari 2015; Rodrigues 2018) whereby governments are chosen without the interference of the federal authorities, and legislative and administrative powers are held without the need to submit to any consultation, approval, or referendum at the federal level. Law-makers in the three spheres are elected in their respective constituencies, and, likewise, there is no interference on the part of any federal organ.

The division of powers adopted by the 1988 Constitution combines dual and cooperative models of federalism. Specific powers are reserved for the union (the federal government), with a residual clause pertaining to state governments (Constitution, article 25). This model is based on the United States' division of powers into those enumerated for the federal government and those reserved to the states, as provided for in the 10th Amendment. However, powers in a cooperative federation may also be shared or concurrent. In reference to the concurrent powers of cooperative federalism, the 1988 Constitution uses the expression 'in common' in article 23 to assign the administrative powers of entities, and the term 'concurrently' in article 24 to refer to legislative powers. The terms 'common' and 'concurrent' thus refer, in the system of shared powers of the 1988 Constitution, to the fields within which federal, state and municipal governments operate jointly in administrative or legislative matters (Rodrigues 2017).

Two features of Brazilian federalism tend to confer heightened status to cities. In the first, the political autonomy of municipalities is guaranteed in the

Constitution; in the second, municipalities are given extensive responsibility for social and urban policies. In regard to health care, they are responsible for the provision and management of primary health care ('basic care units') through municipal structures co-funded by the federal government. Municipalities are also responsible for urban transport, except for metropolitan bus services, while subways and urban railways are managed by the states. They (municipalities) are responsible too for establishing and running municipal schools for children between the ages of 6 and 15 years. In all such activities, mayors and city councils enjoy full jurisdiction.

One recurrent criticism of Brazilian federalism concerns the concentration of powers vested in the central government. Article 21 lays out 25 administrative matters over which the union has exclusive power, while article 22 lays out 29 further issues covered solely by laws of the union. The field of health is shared and, according to article 23, the promotion and protection of health is a concurrent power. The union has the power to draw up general legal frameworks in this field, leaving states and municipalities free to draft specific legislation. The actual provision of health services is the responsibility of all levels and should be accomplished in a decentralised manner (Constitution, articles 196 and 198(I)). Health legislation relating to Covid-19 passed by the National Congress thus fits into the category of a framework law, forming a kind of legislative condominium with state and municipal legislation.

With regard to disaster management-related legislation, four concepts in Brazilian law are to be distinguished from each other: a state of emergency, a state of disaster, a state of national defence, and a state of siege. The last two are provided for in the Constitution but have never been invoked (being for use when public order and the peace are threatened by extreme institutional instability, or in the case of war). Thus, in the Covid-19 crisis, Brazil declared, first, only a state of emergency and, then, a state of disaster. These two institutions are provided for by infra-constitutional frameworks without a specific constitutional foundation.

A state of emergency occurs when there are grounds to fear that the operation of the health system by public authorities may be overwhelmed and public safety jeopardised. It is declared to prevent harm. At the federal level, this issue is governed by Decree No. 7616 of 2011, which establishes the procedures to be followed when declaring a state of 'national health emergency' (ESPIN) in the case of epidemics, disasters, or lack of assistance to the population. Once an ESPIN has been declared, it is possible to adopt exceptional measures, such as the requisition of goods and services and the contracting of temporary staff. The federal government is required to act in conjunction with affected states and municipalities.

By contrast, a state of disaster occurs when the actions of public authorities and the health of the population have been compromised already in actuality (as opposed to when – as in a state of emergency – it is feared that this could happen). In case of disaster management, the federal government should play a coordinating role in which it works in concert with state and municipal plans to counter the effects of the disaster.

The Federal government has a National System of Security and Civil Defence (SINPEC) in which federal, state, and municipal authorities participate. Law 10954 of 2004 provides for emergency assistance to be given to the affected population, while Law 12340 of 2010 governs the transfer of funds from the union to state and municipal governments to support the emergency response and recovery of affected areas.

States and municipalities are not involved in the drafting of federal legislation other than, in the case of states, indirectly through the Federal Senate (which, in terms of article 48 of the Constitution, represents their interests); instead they implement and enforce national legislation, within the concurrent powers arrangement. Through their legislation, states and municipalities may also declare states of emergency or disaster (but not of defence or siege).

In principle, the federal government does not have the prevalence to declare a state of emergency and a state of disaster, since states and municipalities have equal powers to declare states of emergency or disaster within their respective remits. However, for states and municipalities to acquire funds from the federal government, they must submit to the legal criteria established by the federal legal framework.

Accordingly, Law 12608 of 2012 outlines national security and civil defence policy and stipulates the powers reserved to the union, in particular that of 'establishing the criteria and conditions for the declaration and recognition of situations of emergency and a state of public disaster' (article 6(10)). Thus, despite the autonomy of the states and municipalities in authorising the declaration of a state of emergency or disaster, its recognition by the federal government may operate as a form of control. Law 12608 contains a section that defines the powers of each unit of the federation – the union (article 6), the states (article 7), the municipalities (article 8) – and, finally, all three (article 9).

The situation in Brazil during the 2020 pandemic was unparalleled in recent history. States of emergency and disaster had been declared before, especially in the event of natural disasters, but not on the same scale as in the response to Covid-19. In such events, the federal government produces central records recognising states of emergency and disaster (many of which relate to droughts, floods, and landslides) and monitors the situation by means of an integrated disaster information management system indicating the locations on the map where the crisis is in force.

13.3 Preparedness for a national disaster: The institutional framework

Despite the existence of the SINPEDC national security and civil defence system, Brazil has no agency specifically responsible for responding to disasters. Disaster management is provided as the situation demands and organised in a decentralised way. Civil defence is coordinated at the state and municipal levels.

The organisation best equipped to deal with disasters is the Fire Service, which is a state-level entity organised as a military fire service. In cases of accidents or environmental disasters, such as the bursting of dams built by mining companies, the civil defence force and the Fire Service (both of which are state organisations) work together with the civil defence forces of the municipalities concerned. In such cases, federal agencies conduct investigations, initiate administrative procedures, and impose administrative fines and punishments. In extreme cases, the (federal) armed forces may be used, but this must be at the request of the governors.

In regard to public health, the prevention and management of disasters depend on agencies and organisational systems specific to this field. Under normal political circumstances, public health crises of national proportions are addressed primarily by the Ministry of Health and the National Health Council.

The federal government has at its disposal an autonomous agency – the Brazilian National Health Regulator (ANVISA) – which has administrative policing power to intervene in the national territory in cases of epidemics and pandemics. Its scope of action is broad and affects various aspects of public health. Under normal circumstances, it provides health surveillance in border regions, ports, and airports; approves medication for use; and oversees health conditions at industrial, commercial, and service establishments in cities and rural areas. ANVISA is an agency that enjoys widespread public confidence. At the federal level, it has a well-trained professional technical staff that follows the recommendations of the WHO and the Pan-American Health Organisation.

The Brazilian National Health System (SUS) has a federated structure and depends on cooperation between the three levels of government. It has some institutional instruments for coordination, such as the Two-Party Inter-Administration Commission (which brings together municipal and state managers) and the Three-Party Inter-Administration Commission (involving all three levels of government). These management structures promote dialogue between governments within each state and in the federation as a whole.

A number of previous health crises, such as the Zika and H1N1 virus epidemics, have posed a significant challenge to the Brazilian public health system, but nothing has been comparable to the challenges posed by Covid-19. For example, the low rate of testing by the three levels of government adversely affected Brazil's efforts in dealing with the pandemic (Magno et al. 2020). Eight months after the first case in Brazil, the federal and state governments were still unable to solve the problem of insufficient testing, as a result of which the number of infected individuals continued to be underestimated. In April 2020, the number of tests per thousand inhabitants in Brazil was 0.63, which was far lower than the rate in other Latin American countries (Our World in Data 2020). The only persons who were tested were frontline health workers, those who had been hospitalised, and, in some states, those suspected of having died as a result of Covid-19. Consequently, as França et al. (2020: 1) noted, 'the two major challenges are that of estimating the scale of underreporting Covid-19 deaths and that of determining what the exact figure should be'.

In addition, richer states conducted more testing than poorer ones, both because these states could afford to do so and because of the huge presence within them of the private health system. Richer states also paid for patients' tests.

13.4 Rolling out measures to contain the pandemic

Since President Bolsonaro took office, the political situation in Brazil has been anomalous due to his ideologically polarising rhetoric and adoption of an agenda that denies science. Under the circumstances, the federal executive did not, as it should have, respond effectively to the outbreak of the pandemic by heeding practical administrative and technical expertise in this field. There was, from the outset, thus no coherent political approach to the pandemic, which worsened as time went on. The fact that opposition parties governed the major states and cities exacerbated the lack of unity of purpose.

One of the tragic aspects of federal mismanagement of the pandemic was the negligence shown towards indigenous populations. Brazil has a diversity of indigenous ethnic groups, who inhabit territories that are scattered across the country and which comprise 13 per cent of the national territory (Castro and Rodrigues 2010). The indigenous population is estimated to number 1 million people (IBGE 2019b). Although their immunological status puts them at a high risk of infection and fatality, the federal government refused to adopt protective measures suited to their needs. The Covid-19 pandemic worsened the plight of indigenous peoples, who were already burdened by the Bolsonaro government's regressive environmental and human rights policies. They have been threatened with forced assimilation, the suspension and revision of their land rights, and the re-demarcation of their territories. Allegations of genocide against indigenous peoples by President Bolsonaro were referred not only to the United Nations Human Rights Council but the International Criminal Court (ICC), whose Rome Statute Brazil has ratified and whose decisions it is thus legally bound to accept (Connectas Human Rights 2020).

In reaction to the President's Covid-19 denialism, the Federal Supreme Court supported states and municipalities, thereby strengthening their role in the federation during the pandemic. It held in particular that the federal government was neglecting its coordinating role and, worse yet, flouting the recommendations of the WHO. The Court maintained that this jeopardised the security of the Brazilian population and necessitated decentralised government action in line with the recommendations. The ruling would appear to reflect a political position on the value of health and human life rather than a change in the Court's interpretation of the Brazilian federal system (Araújo and Liziero 2020).

13.4.1 Taking the initiative

The first political reactions, both from the President and the governors, revealed the leaders' differences in viewpoint on the pandemic. While President Bolsonaro minimised it, describing Covid-19 as a 'small flu', governors quickly sought to tackle it by setting up teams of political leaders and medical experts. Despite the President's stance, the federal health minister acted promptly; their divergent perspectives on viral transmission led to conflict, however, and culminated in the health minister's resignation a month after the health crisis began.

On 3 February 2020, the Brazilian Ministry of Health published Ordinance No. 188, marking the start of the state of emergency relating to Covid-19. Law No. 13979 of 6 February 2020 likewise established the basis for adopting a series of measures for confronting the Covid-19 emergency, such as isolation and quarantine, compulsory medical examinations, and restriction of movement within and into the country. Moreover, a state of disaster was declared in Brazil by Legislative Decree No. 6 of 20 March 2020.

Directly after the first federal initiatives, state governors began to react. The Federal District of Brasilia was the first subnational entity to adopt restrictive measures, doing so on 11 March when it suspended classes in all educational institutions. In the most populous state in the country, São Paulo, restrictive measures were taken on 13 March with the suspension of commemorative events. Then, still in March, all shops, restaurants, and schools were closed. Other states followed suit and took similar measures, such as Rio de Janeiro on 19 March. The states adopted measures based on their monitoring of infection rates and the occupancy rates of hospital beds (Agência Brasil 2020).

A key feature of Brazil's management of the pandemic was the conflict between the federal and subnational governments regarding social isolation. As noted, President Bolsonaro reacted to the first cases of Covid-19 by denying the gravity of the situation and the need for social isolation. Despite clear scientific proof of the importance of isolation in containing transmission, the President continued to argue that the policy of social isolation adopted by state and municipal governments was damaging to the economy and should therefore be discontinued.

Under such circumstances of inaction and misrepresentation by the federal government, various state governors used the power they share with the union in managing public health crises to introduce measures, rejected by the President, regarding social isolation and the obligatory use of masks in public places. The suspension of operations at schools, businesses, services, and locations open to the public was decreed by state governments as an emergency measure to contain the pandemic.

The President made several verbal attacks on isolation measures and governors and mayors who adopted them – through social media, he continued all the while to incite his supporters to flout these measures. For their part, states began to implement various public health measures. State opposition to the federal government on these issues had no direct relationship to party politics; indeed, at the time, the President had no party. The opposition by states was instead due to his denialist attitude towards science.

13.4.2 Federal action

Numerous federal laws were enacted in response to Covid-19. Among others, Provisional Measure 927 of 22 March 2020 concerns labour law during the pandemic; Law No. 14010 of 10 June 2020 established an emergency legal framework for legal relations in private law; and Law No. 14021 of 7 July 2020 set out measures to protect indigenous and *quilombola* (African-Brazilian) communities from the pandemic. The measures were intended to protect jobs and also to adapt contracts signed between private actors in a way to fit them into the new panorama of the pandemic. In relation to indigenous peoples and *quilombolas*, the measures were intended to protect them and their cultural heritage through the provision of an emergency plan that included quick tests and construction of field hospitals near their villages. Various laws were also passed to mitigate the economic consequences of the pandemic and assist the most vulnerable sectors of the population. The congressional legislature was not suspended during the pandemic but continued operations by way of virtual sessions.

This legislative industriousness gives little indication, though, of the tensions that underlay the federal government's pandemic response, in particular the controversies surrounding its Ministry of Health. Brazil had three health ministers during the 2020 pandemic. After clashing with the initial Minister of Health, Luiz Henrique Mandetta – events that culminated in the latter's resignation on 16 April 2020 – the President appointed the renowned doctor, Nelson Teich, in Mandetta's stead; he, however, did not accept the President's anti-scientific stance, either, and spent only a month in office. Thereafter the President decided to militarise the Ministry. Eduardo Pazzuelo, a general specialising in logistics and with no prior experience in public health, was made Minister of Health in September 2020 after having held the position on an interim basis for around four months.

Arguably, President Bolsonaro impaired a crucial office and misused resources of specialist expertise that could have helped the executive branch manage the pandemic at federal level. As mentioned, he underplayed the risk of contagion and its grave consequences for the health of the population, and questioned the WHO's recommendations regarding the use of masks and social isolation. He also urged the population to remain at work and lead normal lives, thereby giving priority to the economy to the detriment of public health. The resignation of two health ministers sent a clear message that the President had decided not to accept WHO protocols; instead he elected to adopt obscure, non-transparent criteria to manage the pandemic, to publish incomplete accounts of case numbers and fatalities, and to support Covid-19 treatments not endorsed by the WHO, such as hydroxychloroquine.

Given the President's stance, Brazil was soon to face a conflict over jurisdiction in emergency measures. Law No. 13979 of 6 February 2020 drew up a list of drastic measures that could be adopted, including isolation, quarantining, restriction of activities, compulsory medical examinations, restrictions on entering and leaving the country, and requisitioning goods and services. Although subnational administrations are empowered to take measures to counter pandemics, Provisional Measure 926 of 20 March amended the federal legal framework to determine that the President would have the competence to list the essential services that could not stop, as well as to establish the need for previous authorisation from the regulatory agencies so that the restriction measures could be adopted by governors and mayors.

This requirement was challenged before the Supreme Court, which in two decisions came down firmly in favour of the states. In the first case (*Unconstitutionality Direct Action* 6341/DF), the Democratic Workers' Party sought to ensure that the measures provided for in the federal law would not exclude the possibility of state action and would not depend on authorisation from the federal government. The Court decided on 15 April, confirming an earlier injunction of 24 March, that the possible measures adopted by the federal government did not exclude the possibility of normative and administrative measures by the states, the federal district, and municipalities.

In the second case (*Non-compliance of Basic Principles* 672/DF), the Brazilian Bar Association asked the Court, on April 1st, to order the President to abstain from committing acts contrary to the social isolation policies adopted by the states and municipalities. The Court responded quickly, on April 9th, reinforcing subnational governments for issuing decrees, free of federal government supervision, legally provisioned restrictive measures, such as social distancing and isolation, suspension of activities at schools and universities, and restrictions on commercial and cultural activities and the free movement of people.

The Court thus adopted a position affirming decentralisation and recognising the action of states and municipalities in introducing measures to control the pandemic. Justice Ricardo Lewandowski expressly said in a conference at an academic congress (organised by the Brazilian Bar Association) that the Federal Supreme Court had reassessed federalism during the pandemic and that the ruling did not reflect the Court's traditional position (Notícias STF, 2020). Indeed, the literature shows that Brazilian federalism is usually centralised and that the Supreme Federal Court has tended either to reinforce this (Lorencini et al. 2017) or to ignore the debate on federal powers, with the Court in various cases having sided with the federal government and overruled state governments (Araújo 2009).

Apart from the dispute between federal entities about social isolation, another controversial measure by the federal government was its promotion of hydroxychloroquine as an effective treatment for Covid-19. The day after Eduardo Pazuello took office as interim Minister of Health, he signed an ordinance authorising the use of this medication in the public and private health-care system, doing so without prior authorisation by the country's health regulator, ANVISA, which is responsible for approving medications for clinical use. As an emergency measure, the Brazilian Army Pharmaceutical Laboratory (LQFEx) then started to produce hydroxychloroquine, for which it had acquired BRL 1.5 million worth of hydroxychloroquine powder without putting the acquisition out to competitive tender. In June 2020, the Federal Court of Accounts (TCU 2020) launched an investigation into the purchase, which was suspected to have involved overbilling.

The medication thus produced, amounting to three million pills, did not go unused, though. The President's vocal support of it led to a frenzied rush to acquire it, especially by the mayors of rural towns, who, as part of their campaigns for re-election in November 2020, distributed it as a way of associating themselves with the President and demonstrating they were in control of the disease. By mid-August, Minister Pazzuelo announced that there was a shortage of hydroxychloroquine; however, the army had not resumed production (CNN Brasil 2020).

Despite the federal government's disastrous performance, autonomous federal institutions made significant contributions to the effective management of the pandemic. Public federal universities (of which there are 68 in the country) undertook important studies on diagnostic tests, vaccines, and improved treatment of Covid-19. Another key federal institution is the Oswaldo Cruz Foundation, which conducted diagnostic tests and research (Fiocruz 2020).

13.4.3 State action

State governments played an outstanding role in curbing the pandemic. They did so primarily by responding promptly to the first cases of Covid-19 and adopting quarantine and other social isolation measures, such as the closure of schools and public parks and suspension of non-essential commerce and services. Moreover, the failure of the federal government to provide technical and financial assistance to the states, which are responsible for a large number of public hospitals, prompted some governors to pursue alternative routes, such as importing medical equipment (masks, tests, ventilators, and the like) directly from foreign countries without the intervention of the federal government. São Paulo, Rio de Janeiro, and Maranhão (all governed by President Bolsonaro's opponents) were among the states to take steps of this kind.

In particular, the need to purchase large numbers of ventilators and expand intensive care units (ICUs) posed a significant challenge to the health-care system in Brazil. The federal response in this regard was slow, resulting in shortages of beds and equipment. Several states hired private facilities to enable the public health system to meet demand, with some seeking alternatives on the international market, such as the purchase of breathing ventilators and PPE. The fact that they often did so without logistical assistance from the Ministry of Health meant that they encountered great difficulty in managing these imports, making the latter a further point of tension between the federal and state governments.

The commendable performance that states delivered at the start of the pandemic was, however, not always sustained. For example, economic and political pressures from the private sector, mainly from service associations wishing to reopen, led to various state governors relaxing restrictions sooner than recommended, with the result that the numbers of new cases and fatalities remained unchanged or even increased. Opinion polls suggest that governors hence saw a decline in their popularity ratings (Uol 2020a).

One crucial measure that states undertook was to set up field hospitals to increase the availability of ICUs. Prior to this, the number of ICU beds available differed substantially from state to state. It thus became necessary to provide beds urgently, especially in states with lower capacity. Ministry of Health data provided a clear picture of the inequality between states, showing that, on average, the SUS was meeting the WHO recommendations of one public bed per 1,000 inhabitants. However, 17 of the 26 states and the Federal District had not met this quota, while others (mostly in the Sand Southeast regions) greatly exceeded it (Albuquerque et al. 2017).

The urgent need to provide ICU beds gave rise to questionable administrative practices, with corruption scandals emerging in connection with the acquisition of materials and equipment as well as the contracting of service providers to establish and run Covid-19 field hospitals, in the process raising doubts about the probity of government officials. For instance, the governor of the state of Rio de Janeiro was temporarily removed from office by the courts due to suspicion of involvement in pandemic-related fraud (Superior Court of Justice, 2020).

What also became apparent was that inequalities in facilities translated into huge disparities between states in case numbers and fatalities. São Paulo, Bahia, Rio de Janeiro, and Ceará saw the largest numbers of cases and, by the same token, placed greater restrictions on people's movement than elsewhere; nevertheless, the federal government did nothing to address the situation, leaving states to their own devices and consequently aggravating the inequalities between the richest and the poorest. As an illustration, a judge from the state of Maranhão in the Northeast region ordered a full lockdown in its capital, São Luis, and three cities of the metropolitan region due to the lack of beds and high level of infections and deaths – the decision led to a 10-day lockdown and arose from a lawsuit filed by the office of the state public attorney (Carta Capital 2020). The governor, Flavio Dino, of Brazil's Communist Party and strongly opposed to Bolsonaro, received insufficient support from the union to combat Covid-19.

13.4.4 Local government action

Municipalities are recognised in the Constitution as federative entities with the autonomy to legislate and manage action on the basis of their local interests (Ribeiro and Pinto 2009). State capitals and large cities are the main actors in the local government scene. During the 2020 pandemic, many city councils stayed in operation by virtual means. For example, the city councils of Rio de Janeiro and São Paulo passed laws concerning the pandemic during virtual sessions. Some mayors, especially those of state capitals and large cities, introduced stricter measures than those adopted by state governments. These included making it mandatory to wear face masks and suspending or curtailing the provision of goods and services.

Municipalities too were subject to economic pressure from the sectors of the population that wished to reopen activities and see the adoption of more flexible modes of social isolation. Reopening has thus not always been in response to a reduced number of cases. State capitals such as Porto Alegre and São Paulo, which adopted responsible measures at the beginning of the pandemic, gave in to pressure and reopened, causing a drastic increase in the numbers of new cases and deaths. The pressure was not only economic but also political, given that, by virtue of a decision of the Superior Electoral Court, municipal elections took place throughout the country in November 2020; moreover, local politicians were reluctant to impose drastic social isolation measures for fear of paying the political cost in lost votes.

Another issue that merits attention is the capacity of local authorities to deal with the pandemic, including their technical capacity to provide adequate health care for patients with Covid-19. As noted, there were enormous disparities in the number of beds available from state to state and even within the same state. Many municipalities did not have ICUs and had to send patients to larger nearby municipalities; given that some states had very low capacity, citizens in towns often had to travel long distances to receive adequate care, losing precious treatment time as a result. In the state of Amazonas, for example, some localities were 12 hours' drive away from the nearest ICU, which they could sometimes access only by riverboat.

The pandemic has revealed Brazil's shortage of primary health-care resources and the failure on the part of the authorities to provide support for frontline health workers. Lotta et al. (2020) found that community health workers (CHWs) had not received enough training and safety equipment to be able to attend to patients or identify cases requiring hospitalisation. In July 2020, only 9 per cent of CHWs reported having received proper instruction in how to deal with patients (Lotta et al. 2020). In some cities, CHWs with chronic health issues were asked to confine themselves to administrative duties and work remotely, while in others, such workers were obliged to continue providing direct care. This fact highlights that the wide-ranging autonomy the Constitution grants municipalities can lead to inequalities in the provision of public services to citizens.

Another situation that illustrates the extensiveness of local autonomy and the problems arising from it is the absence of regional coordination in metropolitan areas. A bizarre but representative case was that of a shopping mall in the state of São Paulo that straddles the boundary between the municipalities of Sorocaba and Votorantim. As no more ICU beds were available in the public sector in Sorocaba, the municipal authorities decided to reintroduce the policy of suspending commercial activities. Votorantim, however, kept the mall open for four hours a day, as mandated by the state government for municipalities in Phase 2 of the state's lockdown plan. As a result, the section of the mall located in the municipality of Votorantim reopened stores, while, in the section falling under the municipality of Sorocaba, stores remained closed. The mall thus remained partially open, and partially closed, as a result of a lack of regional coordination (Uol 2020b).

Although this is an extreme example, it shows the negative effects of the extensive local autonomy that is permitted in Brazil's federal system notwithstanding the absence of institutional mechanisms for horizontal intergovernmental coordination in cases of disaster management. This affects not only the opening of stores but also strategies to counter the pandemic itself, as the virus makes no distinction between the commerce of one municipality and that of a neighbouring one within an urban conurbation.

It was only in a few locations, such as the ABC region in the metropolitan area of São Paulo (with 20 million inhabitants), that municipalities engaged in horizontal intergovernmental cooperation with a view to addressing the pandemic in a coordinated way (Rodrigues and Oliveira 2020). This was especially important due to the large flow of people between these cities, mainly for work reasons.

13.4.5 Intergovernmental relations

Although its elements are envisaged as functioning cooperatively, the federal system in Brazil has not – except for single issues such as fiscal policy – developed or constitutionalised structures and mechanisms to enable vertical intergovernmental relations between the union and the states, despite the country's long history of shortcomings in the area of policy coordination (Arretche 2015; Souza 1997).

Intergovernmental coordination in Brazil varies not only in function of the institutional framework (polity), but also in regard to the specific design of the public policies. As such, because it stems from policies rather than being systemically embedded, the problem is that it is an unstable practice, one easily modified by changes in ordinary laws by the government of the day. A dramatic case in point is that the Bolsonaro government has been dismantling important structures for coordinating public policies, both in health and other socioeconomic such as social assistance. This was the case, for instance, with federal programmes, such as the *Bolsa Família*, that could be used to render emergency assistance for the low-income population. It was discarded by the federal government in preference for providing federal resources to citizens through the *Caixa Econômica Federal*, a bank run by the federal government. With more than 60 million beneficiaries entitled to emergency benefits in Brazil, the bank was finding it difficult to distribute these benefits due to its capacity constraints (Stuchi et al. 2020).

In a crisis such as the Covid-19 pandemic, people tend to look for guidance to the President because of his or her ability to bring the nation together around a consensus or majority position regarding the implementation of policy, a power which in most cases is accompanied by the transfer of federal resources to states for emergency action. This did not happen during the Covid-19 crisis.

To turn from vertical to horizontal intergovernmental relations, some states cooperated horizontally with each other during the 2020 pandemic. The states of the Northeast mobilised a regional consortium, one created in March 2019, and established the Scientific Committee to Control Coronavirus to advise governors on the political and administrative decision-making process regarding prevention and control of the pandemic (IREE 2020). As mentioned, instances of horizontal intergovernmental relations between municipalities were few and far between, even in situations where – as in the case of the bi-municipal shopping mall in São Paulo – their absence resulted in measures glaringly at cross-purposes with each other.

13.4.6 Intergovernmental fiscal relations

The pandemic had a major impact on the economic welfare of Brazil. Its gross domestic product (GDP) declined by 7.05 per cent from March to June 2020 (compared to June 2019), making this arguably the worst recession the country has witnessed in the past 120 years. The impact was especially detrimental for the states since their main revenue derives from their collection of value-added tax, or *imposto sobre valor acrescentado* (IVA), the amount of which was seriously affected by social isolation measures.

Although they have fiscal autonomy, states also receive federal transfers. In view of the pandemic, they were consequently more dependent on these transfers, as well as on public and private debts. By constitutional provision (article 158, IV Federal Constitution), local governments must receive 25 per cent of the IVA revenue collected by the states, in proportion to the economic activity in each one. Therefore, local government finances were also in peril, also because, especially in urban municipalities, the service tax (ISS) is one of the main sources of revenue, strongly impacted by the suppression or reduction of activities.

Public spending is also regulated by the Fiscal Responsibility Act of 2000, which establishes several limits and permanent procedures to avoid financial imbalance. Some of its main provisions are the limitation of spending on public employees and the prohibition on borrowing in the last year of the term. The declaration of a state of disaster via the Legislative Decree of 6 March 2020 enabled governments to dispense with some of the fiscal obligations imposed by the law. However, Constitutional Amendment 95 of 2016 established a 'ceiling' on federal government spending for 20 years, starting in 2017, to contain the growth in public debt. This ceiling was neither suspended nor relaxed during the pandemic.

Furthermore, Complementary Law 173 of 27 May 2020 established the Federal Covid-19 Control Programme, with measures such as suspension of payment of state debts to the union, restructuring of financial credit operations, and the transfer of financial assistance from the union to the states. It also stipulated that the federal government has to provide financial aid to the states, the federal districts, and the municipalities to the sum of BRL 60 billion. The funds were to be distributed according to a number of criteria, including on the basis of demographic data and the incidence rate of Covid-19.

One of the great debates in Congress and among the financial sector was about the extent to which Brazil would be able to respect its debt ceiling or, failing that, the extent to which it was at risk of having to increase its domestic and international debt to unsustainable levels.

13.5 Findings and policy implications

Eight months after the first Covid-19 case in Brazil, the federal government was still berating subnational governments with the claim that governors and mayors were responsible for more than 160,000 deaths nationwide. Although the federal system has traditionally been centralised, management of the pandemic revealed the potential for decentralisation and for strengthening the scope of action of states and municipalities, which received support from the Supreme Court in their appeal for legitimisation of their measures to combat the virus.

Brazil saw a shift in the play of federative forces, with states and municipalities taking the lead in fighting the pandemic; conversely, the federal government, which usually has a coordinating role, saw two ministers of health leave the post amid a pandemic and wound up playing a secondary role in which it followed the actions of subnational entities – that is, when it was not intent on sabotaging them without proposing viable alternatives.

It may be argued therefore that the intergovernmental relations generated by the very nature of federalism were indispensable in enabling Brazil to address the pandemic and so prevent worse outcomes in terms of public health. Relations between states and municipal governments were fundamental in the struggle to contain the 2020 pandemic – although on occasion the country functioned as a unitary entity with a single central command structure directing public health measures, the present government alone would certainly not have been capable of providing effective responses to protect the health of the population, given that the President's denialist policy led him to act in opposition to WHO recommendations.

It is thus fair to say that federalism in Brazil fulfilled its core purpose of decentralising power and thereby protecting fundamental rights by instituting checks and balances on a wayward president. Ultimately, the role of the states was strengthened by the pandemic and their governments conducted themselves in a manner that warrants public trust. Local governments at city level nevertheless showed wide variation in their responses, which suggests that coordination with states was insufficient and should be improved.

Yet it is uncertain if the expanded autonomy of states and municipalities during the pandemic, due the Supreme Court decision, will lead to a more decentralised federation in the middle and long terms. Nevertheless, this precedent may produce an impact on the perception that decentralisation is not only good, but sometimes necessary, to protect lives against a centralist, non-rational rule.

References

Agência Brasil. 2020. https://agenciabrasil.ebc.com.br/saude/noticia/2020-03/veja-medidas-que-cada-estado-esta-adotando-para-combater-covid-19 (accessed on 31 October 2020).

Albuquerque, Mariana Vercesi de, et al. 2017. 'Regional Health Inequalities: Changes Observed in Brazil from 2000–2016', *Ciência & Saúde Coletiva*, 22(4): 1055–1064.

Araújo, Marcelo Labanca Corrêa de. 2009. *Jurisdição Constitucional e Federação: o princípio da simetria na jurisprudência do STF*. Rio de Janeiro: Elsevier.

Araújo, Marcelo Labanca Corrêa de and Leonam Liziero. 2020. *'Reposicionando o debate federalista no Brasil em razão da pandemia COVID-19: há mesmo uma tendência à descentralização?'*, in João Paulo A.Teixeira (ed.), *Pensar a Pandemia*, pp. 380–391. Curitiba:Tirant Lo Blanch Brasil.

Arretche, Marta. 2015. 'Intergovernmental Relations in Brazil: An Unequal Federation with Symmetrical Arrangements', in J. Poirier, C. Saunders and J. Kincaid J (eds), *Intergovernmental Relations in Federal Systems: Comparative Structures and Dynamics*, pp. 108–134. Oxford: Oxford University Press.

Candido, D. S. et al. 2020. 'Evolution and the Pandemic Spread of Sars-CoV-2 in Brazil', *Science*, https://science.sciencemag.org/content/369/6508/1255 (accessed on 1 November 2020).

Carta Capital. 2020. https://www.cartacapital.com.br/sociedade/justica-ordena-lockdown-em-sao-luis-no-maranhao/ (accessed on 1 November 2020).

Castro, Marcus F. and Gilberto M. A. Rodrigues. 2010. 'Brazil', in C. Colino and L. Moreno (eds), *Diversity and Unity in Federal Countries*, pp. 76–108. Montreal: McGill-Queens University Press.

CNN Brasil. 2020. https://www.cnnbrasil.com.br/nacional/2020/11/16/sem-demanda-nos-estados-400-mil-comprimidos-de-cloroquina-encalham-no-exercito (accessed on 15 November 2020).

Connectas Human Rights. 2020. 'Why Bolsonaro could be Denounced at the International Criminal Court', https://www.conectas.org/en/news/why-bolsonaro-could-be-denounced-at-the-international-criminal-court (accessed on 15 November 2020).

Department of Health. 2020. 'Coronavirus (Covid-19)', https://coronavirus.saude.gov.br/linha-do-tempo (accessed on 31 October 2020).

Ferrari, Sergio. 2015. 'Local Government in Brazil and Switzerland: A Comparative Study on Merger an Inter-Municipal Cooperation', pp. 36–43, Institute of Federalism, University of Fribourg, https://www3.unifr.ch/federalism/en/assets/public/files/Workingpercent20Paperpercent20online/06_Sergiopercent20Ferrari.pdf (accessed on 31 October 2020).

Fiocruz. 2020. https://portal.fiocruz.br/pesquisas-notas-tecnicas-e-relatorios (accessed on 28 November 2020).

França, Elisabeth Barboza et al. 2020. 'Deaths Due to COVID-19 in Brazil: How Many Are There and Which Are Being Identified?', *Revista Brasileira de Epidemiologia, Rio de Janeiro*, 23, e200053.

IBGE (Instituto Brasileiro de Geografia e Estatística). 2019a. 'Pirâmide Etária', https://educa.ibge.gov.br/jovens/conheca-o-brasil/populacao/18318-piramide-etaria.html (accessed on 31 October 2020).

IBGE (Instituto Brasileiro de Geografia e Estatística). 2019b. 'Data base on Indigenous Peoples and Quilombolas', https://www.ibge.gov.br/en/geosciences/territorial-organization/territorial-typologies/27488-base-de-informacoes-sobre-os-povos-indigenas-e-quilombolas-2.html?=&t=o-que-e (accessed on 31 October 2020).

Imperial College. 2020. https://mrc-ide.github.io/global-lmic-reports/BRA (accessed on 31 October 2020).

Instituto para Reforma das Relações entre Estado e Empresa (IREE). 2020. https://iree.org.br/consorcio-nordeste-entenda-o-que-e-a-iniciativa/ (accessed on 30 October 2020).

Lorencini, Marco A. G. L, Gilberto M. A. Rodrigues, and A. Zimmermann. 2017. 'The Supreme Federal Court of Brazil: Protecting Democracy and Centralized Power', in N. Aroney and J. Kincaid (eds), *Courts in Federal Countries: Federalists or Unitarists*, pp. 103–134. Toronto: University of Toronto Press.

Lotta, G. et al. 2020. 'Community Health Workers Reveal COVID-19 Disaster in Brazil', *The Lancet*, 396: 365–66.

Magno, L. et al. 2020. 'Challenges and Proposals for Scaling up COVID-19 Test and Diagnosis in Brazil', *Ciência & Saúde Coletiva*, 25(9): 3355–64.

Notícias STF, 2020. http://www.stf.jus.br/portal/cms/verNoticiaDetalhe.asp?idConteudo=448639 (accessed on 21 January 2021).

OECD. 2019. 'Health at a Glance 2019: OECD Indicators', OECD Publishing, https://www.oecd-ilibrary.org/social-issues-migration-health/health-at-a-glance-2019_4dd50c09-en (accessed on 31 October 2020).

Our World in Data. 2020. 'Table (line 9488, column AB)'. https://ourworldindata.org/coronavirus-testing (accessed on 31 October 2020).

Ribeiro, L. C. de Queiroz Ribeiro and Sol Garson B. Pinto. 2009. 'Brazil', in N. Steytler (ed.), *Local Government and Metropolitan Regions in Federal Systems*, pp. 75–105. Montreal: McGill-Queen's University Press.

Rodrigues, Gilberto M.A. 2017. 'Concurrent Power and Local Interest in Brazil's Federalism', in N. Steytler (ed.), *Concurrent Powers in Federal Systems: Meaning, Making, and Managing*, pp. 206–221. Leiden, Boston: Brill Nijhoff.

Rodrigues, Gilberto M. A. 2018. 'Are Cities Constituent Units in Brazil's Federalism?', *50 Shades of Federalism*, http://50shadesoffederalism.com/case-studies/cities-constituent-units-brazils-federalism/ (accessed on 31 October 2020).

Rodrigues, Gilberto. M. A. and Vanessa E. Oliveira. 2020. 'Brazil and Covid-19: the President against the Federation', *UACES Territorial Politics*, https://uacesterrpol.wordpress.com/2020/06/05/brazil-and-covid-19-the-president-against-the-federation/ (accessed on 31 October 2020).

Scheffer, Mário, et al. 2015. *Brazilian Medical Demographics (Demografia médica no Brasil)*. São Paulo: Departamento de Medicina Preventiva da Faculdade de Medicina da USP; Conselho Regional de Medicina do Estado de São Paulo; Conselho Federal de Medicina.

Souza, Celina. 1997. *Constitutional Engineering in Brazil: The Politics of Federalism and Decentralization*. London: Palgrave Macmillan.

Stuchi, Carolina G., Vanessa E. Oliveira and Gilberto M. A Rodrigues. 2020. 'Covid-19 and Emergency Grant: Brazil's Populist Policy?', *UACES Territorial Politics*, https://

uacesterrpol.wordpress.com/2020/09/24/covid-19-and-emergency-grant-a-brazils-populist-policy/ (accessed on 31 October 2020).

Superior Court of Justice. 2020. https://www.stj.jus.br/sites/portalp/Paginas/Comunicacao/Noticias/28082020-STJ-afasta-o-governador-Witzel-do-cargo-e-prende-seis-investigados-por-irregularidades-na-Saude-do-Rio.aspx (accessed on 30 October 2020).

Tribunal de Contas da União (TCU). 2020. https://portal.tcu.gov.br/english/inside-tcu/the-court/ (accessed on 4 September 2020).

Uol. 2020a. http://media.folha.uol.com.br/datafolha/2020/06/26/66ed4921092c48022554df364b7a3464gvnts.pdf (accessed on 4 September 2020).

Uol. 2020b. https://noticias.uol.com.br/cotidiano/ultimas-noticias/2020/06/24/votorantim-promotor-diz-que-shopping-dividido-e-absurdo-e-pede-explicacoes.htm (accessed on 28 August 2020).

14

FEDERALISM AND COVID-19 IN ARGENTINA

Centralisation and hyper-presidentialism

Antonio María Hernández and Cristian Altavilla

14.1 Introduction

Argentina has a federal system comprising 23 states, known as provinces, and the Autonomous City of Buenos Aires, or *Ciudad Autónoma de Buenos Aires* (CABA), which is the seat of the national capital.[1] There is substantial asymmetry between the CABA and the provinces[2] in terms of wealth, territory and population size. Within this federal arrangement, the country has a republican and presidential form of government, with powers separated between the executive, legislative, and judicial branches and direct election of the federal president and provincial governors. The bicameral legislature, called the National Congress, consists of the Senate and Chamber of Deputies. It is elected independently of the executive branch for fixed terms – four years in the case of deputies, and six in the case of senators.

In the elections of October 2019, the *Frente de Todos* ('Everybody's Front') coalition won 48.1 per cent of the presidential vote, with Alberto Fernández and Cristina Fernández de Kirchner becoming president and vice president, respectively. *Frente de Todos* is a centre-left coalition of political parties largely Justicialist-Peronist in orientation. It defeated *Juntos por el Cambio* ('Together for Change'), a centre-right coalition composed mainly of the Republican Proposal and Radical Civic Union parties. The latter coalition had been in power since 2015 under then President Mauricio Macri, who sought re-election.

To turn to the results in the federal legislature, the governing coalition won 43 of the 72 seats in the Senate (59.7 per cent of the total) and *Juntos por el Cambio*, 29 (40.3 per cent). The outcome in the Chamber of Deputies was far more evenly matched: of the 257 deputies, 119 (46.3 per cent) were of *Frente de Todos* and 116 (45.1 per cent) were of *Juntos por el Cambio*. At the provincial level, *Frente de Todos* governed in 20 provinces at the time of the Covid-19 outbreak, while

DOI: 10.4324/9781003166771-18

the opposition *Juntos por el Cambio* was confined to the provinces of Mendoza, Corrientes and Jujuy and, at city level, the CABA.

As for health care in Argentina, the Pan American Health Organization describes the country's health system as 'one of the most fragmented and segmented' in Latin America (PAHO 2017). Likewise, Isuani (2020) asserts that it is characterised, inter alia, by fragmentation, variation in quality, and irrationality. Inequality of access to health benefits and services is compounded by geographical disparities, given the extreme socio-economic differences that are evident from region to region. Such fragmentation is due to the country's federal organisation, which enables each of the 24 jurisdictions to run its own health system, as well as to a historically uneven pattern of development and a lack of national coordination.

Health matters are a concurrent competence among the four orders of government, namely the federal, provincial, municipal, and federal district (i.e. governance pertaining to the CABA).[3] Health care is provided by a varying combination of employer- and labour-union-sponsored plans, government insurance plans, public hospitals and clinics, and private health insurance. More than 300 health-care cooperatives (200 of which are related to labour unions) provide care for half the population. The Federal Health Council, presided over by the national Minister of Health, is responsible for intergovernmental coordination in health matters and is composed of the highest health authorities of the nation, provinces, and CABA.

It is in this overall context that Argentina's first case of Covid-19 was recorded on 3 March 2020 and its first death on 7 March. Early cases were concentrated in the CABA and its metropolitan area. On 11 March, the government announced a mandatory 14-day-quarantine of returnees to Argentina from highly affected countries such as China, South Korea, Japan, Iran, and the United States. The first domestic restrictions were imposed on 19 March when the federal government ordered a lockdown of the whole country by way of the Decree of Necessity and Urgency (DNU) No. 297.

Adopted at a point when there were still fewer than a dozen cases in the country, the measure had the support of federal legislators, the leaders of all political parties, and the governors of all provinces. It was generally considered the correct step to take in order to buy time in which to strengthen a health system unprepared for the pandemic. Borders were duly closed, all air and land transport was halted, only essential work and movement were allowed, and the population was confined to its homes; on 14 April, a further restriction was introduced that made it obligatory for everyone using public transport or otherwise out in public to wear face masks. Although the initial lockdown was for two weeks, it was extended incrementally until 10 May, at which time certain restrictions were lifted in areas beyond Greater Buenos Aires.

On 23 March, Ministry of Health officials reported that the coronavirus was spreading via community transmission in the CABA and its surroundings, as well as in cities in the provinces of Chaco, Córdoba, and Tierra del Fuego; by the end of March, there were 1,054 confirmed cases of Covid-19 and 27 deaths. Then, as later, the major location of infections and fatalities was the province of Buenos Aires, in particular the 40 municipalities that make up the Buenos Aires Metropolitan Area – with a population of more than 12 million people, this is the part of the country where its greatest problems of poverty and social exclusion are found; a related area of concern was the CABA and its 3 million inhabitants, which also forms part of the metropolitan area. Other high-infection locations were the provinces of Santa Fe, Córdoba, Jujuy, Río Negro, Neuquén, and Chaco.

By 3 July, cases of Covid-19 had been found in every province of the country, but it was thought that the pandemic was abating: July concluded with 191,289 confirmed cases, 3,543 deaths, and 83,767 recoveries. However, on 31 July, President Fernández announced that the lockdown restrictions would continue until 16 August, as there had been a record number of cases and deaths in the previous days.

On 9 August, the Ministry of Health confirmed a total of 61,867 new recoveries on that day. This big jump was due to a change in the definition of recovery, which now included (along with discharges from hospitals) mild cases that the Covid-19 monitoring system would discharge automatically 10 days after the onset of symptoms. The recovery rate thus rose to 70 per cent of confirmed cases until that date. President Fernández on 28 August authorised meetings throughout the country of up to 10 people in the open air, providing they used face masks and practised social distancing, and announced that the eased lockdown would be extended again until 20 September. Shortly before then, on 10 August some 10,000 students in San Juan became the first to return to face-to-face classes. Most other provinces either did not attempt this or faced strong resistance from teachers' unions.

The lockdown was extended for three more weeks on 18 September. After reaching a maximum level of infection of 7.591 cases per day in late August, the infection rate started to decrease in Greater Buenos Aires at the beginning of September and was officially said to be 'stabilising'. At the same time, however, the virus increased in spread in the country at large. In the first 15 days of September, the provinces of Córdoba, Jujuy, La Rioja, Mendoza, Neuquén, Río Negro, Salta, Santa Cruz, Santa Fe, Tierra del Fuego, and Tucumán registered exponential increases in case numbers, with most of their health-care systems facing high levels of strain. The lockdown was again extended, now by another two weeks until 25 October.

On 20 October, Argentina, with a population of 45 million, confirmed more than 1 million positive cases, becoming the fifth country in the world and the second in South America to pass this landmark. Three days later, it was announced that the lockdown would continue for another two weeks in provinces with a high daily number of confirmed cases. By 29 October, official figures set the accumulated national total at 30,071 deaths, 1.1 million cases, and nearly 3 million tests (or 64,257 per million inhabitants).

At the time of writing, the pandemic was ongoing and Argentina's anticipated phase of social and economic recovery had not begun – one consequence of the country's protracted lockdown. Poverty increased from 35.5 per cent at the end of 2019 to 40.9 per cent in the first half of 2020, while inflation had risen over the past 12 months to 35 per cent in November 2020. Similarly, the unemployment rate rose to 13.1 per cent in the second quarter of 2020, compared to 10.6 per cent in the same period in 2019 and 10.4 per cent in 2018, making the increase a 15-year record (Infobae 2020). Economic activity rose by 1.1 per cent in August 2020, but this was still 11.6 per cent lower than in August 2019.

These economic stressors came in addition to the huge fiscal deficit, tax pressures, and enormous external debt with which Argentina was encumbered even before the pandemic broke out.

14.2 The federal constitutional and legislative framework

14.2.1 Division of powers and functions

Article 1 of the Constitution of 1853 declares Argentina a federal country. The provinces and CABA have their own constitutions and are empowered to create institutions and be governed by them. Although they have to comply with the Constitution, provinces enjoy significant autonomy in the legislative, administrative, and juridical domains. Their governments have three branches (executive, legislative, and judicial). The executive branch is led by a governor, while the legislative branch may be unicameral (as is true of 15 provinces and the CABA) or bicameral (as is the case with eight provinces).

The Constitution divides power and functions between the federal and provincial levels. In this regard, there are three main types of competence: exclusive, shared, and concurrent.

The federal government's exclusive competences pertain to, inter alia, international relations, the armed forces, citizenship, currency, air and aerospace navigation, telecommunications services, and federal intervention, while those of the provinces relate to, for instance, primary education, electoral systems, creating own institutions and establishing local government structures. By contrast, shared competences apply in matters requiring joint decisions, such as the creation of new provinces, the establishment of the capital city, and the enactment of the so-called co-participation regimen – a special tax-sharing arrangement between federal and provincial levels.

As for concurrent competences, they can be decided and implemented independently by any level (Bidart Campos 1998). Both the federal and provincial levels are endowed with powers and functions related to social policies and general welfare: health care, education, science and culture, employment and labour, environmental affairs, and housing are all concurrent competences. The main principle informing the distribution of power is contained in article 121, which states that provinces reserve to themselves all the powers not delegated to the federal government. As such, federal powers are limited and enumerated, whereas provincial powers are numerous and indeterminate.

In practice, though, the federal level plays the role of developing and coordinating policies and establishing general guidelines, while the provinces are in charge of implementing and administering these policies. This arrangement is especially apparent in the areas of health care, education, and housing. The federal government plays a key – almost exclusive – role in the areas of social assistance and social security, two competences which have been re-centralised in recent decades.

14.2.2 Declaration of states of emergency

In terms of the Constitution, a state of emergency may be declared if there are exceptional social, political, economic, or natural situations that could affect the constitutional order. The power to declare an emergency lies with the National Congress, which can create various emergency powers that are subject to the Constitution. The Congress has to decide whether there is a true state of need, formally declare the emergency, establish its duration, and set out the main measures to be taken. In general, while those measures increase the powers of the state – particularly of the executive – and correlatively limit the rights of individuals, they may not in any way suspend or limit the republican and federal system.

The Emergency powers foreseen by the 1853 constitutional text are federal intervention (article 6) and a state of siege (article 23); those contemplated by amendments to the Constitution in 1994 are decrees of necessity and urgency (DNUs) (article 99(3)) and legislative delegation to the executive (article 76) (Hernández 2012a; Midón 2001).

A state of siege ('*estado de sitio*' in Spanish), or what is more commonly known as a state of emergency, is provided for in the 1853 Constitution in the event of the emergencies of war ('external attack') and domestic disorder ('internal commotion'). These situations have to meet the requirements, first, of endangering both the Constitution and the authorities created by it, and, secondly, presenting a disturbance of order. Since 1853 there have been 53 states of siege, and in 60 per cent of them the executive acted by decree; exorbitant powers were given to the President; congressional functions saw evident decline; and notable harm was done to individual rights and guarantees (Hernández 2020a, 2012b).

With regard to DNUs, the President is not allowed under any circumstances to issue provisions of a legislative nature, which would be entirely null and void; however, in exceptional circumstances where the ordinary constitutional procedures for the enactment of laws are impossible to follow, he or she may issue decrees on the grounds of necessity and urgency. Even then, the President cannot issue decrees on criminal matters or issues of taxation and electoral or political-party systems. As regards formal requirements, the Constitution stipulates that this kind of decree has to be decided together with all the ministers and the Chief of Cabinet and be submitted to the consideration of a joint standing committee of Congress composed of representatives of both houses.

Finally, legislative delegation is a mechanism whereby Congress can delegate the power to regulate certain issues concerning administration and public emergency to the executive arm of government. The legislature empowers the executive to create norms (which, from a purely material point of view, are laws) that determine the content and timing of the decision previously taken and owned, so to speak, by the legislature (Quiroga Lavié 2009: 1172).

14.3 Preparedness for a national disaster: The institutional framework

As noted, the national constitution does not specifically provide for institutions to respond to a disaster such as Covid-19. In the case of a health crisis, the Federal Health Council, comprising the federal and provincial ministries of health, could be used, but at the time of this writing it had not convened during the pandemic.

Argentina recorded its first case of Covid-19 on 3 March 2020. At that point, it was in the midst of a severe economic, social, and health crisis that had been formally declared as a public emergency by the National Congress in December 2019. This declaration put in place most of the legal framework within which national and local authorities acted during the 2020 pandemic.

The background to it is that in late December 2019, the National Congress, at the request of the new government, enacted Law No. 27541 which declared a public emergency in nine areas, including economic, financial, fiscal, administrative, pension, tariff, energy, health and social matters, and, under article 76 of the Constitution, expressly authorised the delegation of powers to the President, although in broad terms.

Consequently, when the pandemic reached Argentina in March 2020, a public emergency had already been declared, with the President enjoying legislative delegations and in no need of a further declaration by Congress. The latter commenced its ordinary session on 1 March, but adjourned in the course of the month and did not meet again until mid-May.

14.4 Rolling out measures to contain the pandemic

With the coronavirus spreading across the world and its arrival in Argentina imminent, the country's three levels of government began to take measures. Provincial governors were the first to do so, followed rapidly by the federal government; numerous municipalities were also quick to respond to the looming health crisis. Once the federal government had taken the lead, however, the other levels acted within its framework.

14.4.1 Taking the initiative

As stated above, the three levels of governments reacted automatically to the first cases of Covid-19. Indeed, the three levels acted first independently and within their own respective constitutional competencies – although, many local and provincial decisions where considered unconstitutional by local literature. The federal government announced a lockdown throughout the country on 19 March 2020, following which provincial and municipal governments accepted the decision and acted accordingly. Making use of a certain margin of discretion within the federal legal framework, subnational governments added restrictions of their own, with provinces closing borders between each other and many municipalities doing the same with their neighbours.

These actions reflected a lack or failure of coordination in multilevel governance. From the outset, questions emerged about which level of government has constitutional competence to deal with emergencies and which has emergency police powers. The country's literature is unanimous in recognising that health care is a concurrent competence both in times of normality as well as emergency; what was in question was the extent to which each level could limit fundamental rights in exercising its emergency powers.

14.4.2 Federal action

In the face of an imminent viral outbreak, President Fernandez on 12 March 2020 issued Decree No. 260, in terms of which the health emergency declared by Congress previously in December was extended for one year 'in accordance with the pandemic declared by the World Health Organisation (WHO) in relation to the coronavirus Covid-19'. The measure was criticised as unconstitutional, on the grounds that no emergency can be established by means of DNUs and that the President is not authorised to extend an emergency already declared by a law of Congress, especially when Congress is still in session – as the Supreme Court of Justice found in *San Luis Province v. Estado Nacional* [J.A.] (2003-I-188).

One week later, on 19 March, a compulsory lockdown was imposed on the entire country by way of DNU No. 297. This was initially successful, since it had the support of all political parties as well as provincial, CABA, and municipal governments (Porto and Di Gresia 2020; Tortolero Cervantes 2020). There was widespread agreement that mandatory social distancing was the primary way to curb the pandemic, regardless of the constitutional rights it affected.

The first renewals of the lockdown were announced jointly on 26 April by the President, and the governor of the province of Buenos Aires, who belonged to the governing party, and the head of government of the CABA, who was of the opposition party. Later, though, when the President continued issuing decrees in violation of the republican and federal form of state, resistance, accompanied by public protests, grew throughout the country.

The justification consistently offered for the lockdown was that the health of the population was more important than the economy. Accordingly, the Ministry of Health established an Emergency Operations Centre, or *Centro de Operaciones de Emergencia* (COE), comprised of epidemiologists and public health experts whose function was to advise the government. Before each renewal of the lockdown, the COE met with the President and national Minister of Health – arguably, the President was seeking thereby to be absolved of responsibility for the social and economic consequences of his actions, as he could claim that, in the name of rationality, he had to follow scientific advice for the good of population health.

From the outset of the pandemic, the federal government implemented a series of socio-economic measures to mitigate the impacts of quarantining. In the first place, it formed an 'economic cabinet' or cabinet committee, albeit without provincial representatives.[4] This cabinet sought to speed up assistance to small and medium enterprises, vulnerable sectors, and taxpayers financially affected by the lockdown.

As part of these initiatives, the federal government introduced two special financial support packages: the Emergency Family Income package, which provided AMD 10,000 (less than USD 100) to each of more than 8 million people, and the Emergency Assistance Program for Work and Production, aimed at providing economic support to affected businesses and workers for the duration of the pandemic.

It also regulated aspects of business activity that have key socio-economic impacts. Among other things, it froze the price of housing rentals, fixed the maximum prices of basic products, introduced tax exemptions, and prohibited layoffs in the private sector. The President adopted these measures unilaterally by executive decree – although Congress validated most of them, they ought to have come about by means of laws of Congress.

The federal government continued to govern by means of decrees and resolutions as the year wore on. By the end of October 2020, the President had issued 38 DNUs and 12 Delegated Decrees (Cavallini Viale and Ferreyra 2020), facing increasing resistance from the opposition due to Congress's irregular functioning.

Indeed, Congress was bypassed by the DNUs issued by the President, in part because it was closed from the beginning of the lockdown until it began to meet virtually on 13 May. The situation was not helped by the fact that the Senate was presided over by the Vice President, Cristina Kirchner, who steadfastly resisted calls to debate the pandemic response; her son, meanwhile, was the head of the governing-party legislative bloc in the Chamber of Deputies. The opposition was also hindered from taking recourse to judicial measures because both the federal and provincial judiciaries decreed an extraordinary recess for the first months of the pandemic (from March until July), as a result of which – barring a few isolated cases – they all but ceased to operate.

Moreover, when Congress began to meet virtually on May 13 and thereafter, it gave only brief attention to presidential DNUs – some 20 of these were approved in the Senate meeting of that day. Before the online sessions became operative, both houses had spent considerable time deliberating such a possibility informally and in the media before deciding to proceed with remote sessions paired with the physical presence of a minimum of legislators (restricted to parliamentary office-holders and leaders of legislative blocs). In the Senate, this mixed mode of operation was extended by decree of the Senate leader, yet without the two-thirds votes required to amend the relevant laws pursuant to article 227 of the Senate's Rules of Procedure;[5] the same occurred in the Chamber of Deputies, where the government extended the remote sessions without the required consensus.[6]

It is evident that the federal government's only strategy in response to the 2020 pandemic was the nationwide lockdown. The national lockdown was the longest in the world and caused a multitude of social and economic, as well as educational and psychological, problems in all sectors of the population, including notably the poor, children and youth, and the elderly. The lockdown was mandatory and sanctions were imposed for non-compliance, all of which resulted in violations of fundamental rights that were not sufficiently reviewed by the judiciary.

The situation was well illustrated by the Single Certificate for Circulation, issuable only by the Ministry of Interior. In terms of Resolution 48/2020 of the Ministry of Interior dated 28 March 2020, permission for any individual to travel outside his or her place of residence depended on the national authority. Thus, all authorisation of movement, and hence of circulation of the population and the resumption of social, economic, and educational activity, rested with the federal government, irrespective of the prevalence – or, in some provinces, or in many areas within different provinces, the virtual non-existence – of the pandemic. By the logic of the Resolution, no one anywhere in the Argentine federation could at any time make a move without the say-so of the centre.

14.4.3 Provincial action

All 23 provinces and the CABA formally declared public health emergencies in their respective jurisdictions and according to their own constitutions and laws, thereby enabling their authorities to exercise emergency powers. In many cases, these declarations were effected by executive decrees rather than laws, as required by provincial constitutions. The provinces adopted, and complied with, federal decrees and resolutions, in addition to which they added their own restrictions. In fact, Tierra del Fuego was put under lockdown on 16 March 2020, three days before the rest of the country, while the provinces of Chaco, Misiones, Salta, Jujuy, and Mendoza closed their borders to other countries on 18 March.

The federation as a system of federal and provincial governments was important in health-care provision. As noted, public health services are under the administration of provinces, the CABA, and municipalities, with more complex institutions falling under provincial governments or the private sector via private health insurance. Provinces thus had to respond to the emergency as well, which many did by repurposing facilities as Covid-19 treatment centres, building new hospitals, or setting up tent and mobile hospitals. Accordingly, provincial COEs were established, with these composed of provincial health ministers and specialists in different fields (e.g. physicians, epidemiologists, and lawyers). COEs decided on measures to combat the pandemic, which in effect subordinated municipal governments to provincial ones, since the former had no say in decisions made by the latter.

Operating within a thin margin of autonomy, provinces were allowed to reduce or expand the activities permitted during the lockdown. In some cases, provinces took measures that went beyond the restrictions of the federal government, such as preventing interprovincial transit and imposing curfews, thus affecting the fundamental rights and federal principles contained in the Constitution. For example, numerous provinces closed the roads leading into them, often by digging up road to make them impassable or leaving trucks parked across them; such actions led to legal challenges.

In general, though, the provinces' role in the quarantine was merely to implement federal decisions, especially regarding DNU 297 and its successive extensions. This is so because any measures implemented by a province were carried out within the national legal framework. The DNU 297 measures were highly restrictive and imposed a rigid framework within which local authorities were also required to act.

Like their federal counterpart, the provinces were prone to a state-level version of hyper-presidentialism. Provincial legislatures and municipal councils were not fully operational, though there were exceptions. Some provincial legislatures held meetings that were attended in person, in which they adhered to hygiene and safety protocols (as is the case in Neuquén, San Juan, Catamarca, Tucumán, and Jujuy, among others) while in other provinces, legislatures proceeded with remote sessions (as in Córdoba, Santa Cruz, Misiones, or La Rioja, for example) or a mixture of online participation and a minimum physical presence of legislators (as in San Luis and Formosa). Although provincial legislatures were operational in one way or another, the general trend was for government by gubernatorial decree, or even by resolutions or administrative decisions issued by lower-level officials such as provincial COEs, which are not legislative bodies (Hernández 2020a).

The role of provincial government was far from insignificant. Provinces are in charge of police forces, which were drawn on extensively to enforce pandemic control measures. Crucially, too, provinces are responsible for the administration of the health-care system and all it entails, ranging from hospitals and health centres to personnel, resources, and infrastructure.

14.4.4 Local government action

Municipal governments also had an important role to play in the 2020 pandemic, primarily because their broad competences in health matters are concurrent with those of the provincial and federal levels. Of the 25,751 facilities that make up Argentina's health system, a total of 4,056 (15.75 per cent) depend directly on municipal governments, which all developed prevention, containment, and support activities in the fight against Covid-19. Their role – specifically the role played by primary health-care centres – was especially critical given their close, direct relationship with the most vulnerable sectors of the population, which are present in small towns as well as intermediate cities and large metropolitan areas.

This immediacy led some local governments to take preventive measures ahead of the federal or respective provincial government. For example, Bahía Blanca in the province of Buenos Aires issued Decree 317/2020 on 12 March 2020 prohibiting large-scale public events and activities; a few days later, other municipalities followed suit, among them La Plata, Tandil, Olavarría, Pilar, Avellaneda, Mar del Plata, and Brandsen (Malavolta and Pulvirenti 2020).

Some local government orders were controversial, such as blockades of inter-provincial or municipal boundaries or the imposition of curfews. A notable case was the local government of Puerto Iguazú, which announced the closure of the Tancredo Neves Bridge linking Brazil and Argentina but which was prevented by a warning from the Federal Judge of El Dorado (Azarkevich 2020).

14.4.5 Intergovernmental relations

Cooperative and coordinated federalism are fundamental to the constitutional reform of 1994 (Hernández 2009), but the intergovernmental relations (IGR) they entail were not given full effect to during the pandemic or, for that matter, before it. The federal government's hyper-presidentialism and attendant centralised approach meant that Congress, provinces, the CABA and local governments were marginalised (Hernández 2020a, 2020c) – arguably, a serious error to make in the management of Covid-19 in what is, after all, the eighth-largest country in the world.

This occurred notwithstanding that certain DNUs refer explicitly to multilevel coordination in implementing control measures. Article 3 of DNU No. 355/2020 stipulates that federal authorities, 'in coordination with their peers from the provincial jurisdictions, from the CABA and from the municipal authorities, each one in the scope of their competences, will arrange the measures …'. However, article 2 of the same decree in effect subordinates subnational governments and curbs their leeway for movement, since only the Chief of Cabinet of the federal government is authorised to make exceptions to the orderly exit from lockdown, exceptions which have to be requested by provincial governments. Similarly, DNU No. 408/2020 permits provinces to determine their respective activities and protocols, only to constrict them tightly again by reaffirming that it is the Federal Ministry of Health and Chief of Cabinet that have the final say on these matters.

At an institutional level, a variety of spaces exist for deliberating on and implementing joint, consensual intergovernmental decisions, in particular federal councils such as the previously mentioned Federal Health Council, along with the Federal Education Council and Investment Education Council. However, the latter were inactive and unutilised in the 2020 pandemic response, an act of omission that amounted to a missed opportunity for fostering IGR generally and so, among other things, averting or mitigating the conflicts that would inevitably arise in a nationwide effort of this kind. For instance, the decision of the federal government to centralise the purchase of respirators prevented the provinces of Mendoza, Jujuy, Chubut, and Corrientes from buying their own even though they had already placed orders with the company concerned (Mozetic 2020) and as a consequence of that decision, these provinces were unable to buy those respirators.

To turn from vertical to horizontal IGR, inter-state cooperation was rare. In Patagonia, for instance, an enormous region encompassing the provinces of La Pampa, Neuquén, Río Negro, Chubut, Santa Cruz, and Tierra del Fuego, all but two interprovincial initiatives were carried out: the creation of the Interprovincial Commission for Monitoring the Epidemiological Situation (Covid-19), set up by the governors of Neuquén and Río Negro on 19 April 2020; and a meeting of the Patagonian Forum of the Superior Courts of Justice to prevent and minimise the pandemic's effects on the administration of justice.

Far more common was inter-state conflict. A case in point was that between the neighbouring provinces of Corrientes and Chaco. Separated by a river and joined by a bridge, the one province, Chaco, had a high level of Covid-19 infection, while the other, Corrientes, had none; their dispute turned around two contradictory court rulings to do with medical personnel living in the province of Corrientes but working in Resistencia, the capital of Chaco.

When the government of Corrientes prohibited them from crossing the bridge between the two provinces, the federal judge of Resistencia ordered the opposite; in turn, the province of Corrientes resorted to the federal judge of Corrientes (the city of the same name), who ruled that this resolution was unenforceable in the province of Corrientes's jurisdiction. Once again, the federal judge of Resistencia ordered Corrientes not to prevent the medical personnel from performing their duties in accordance with the federal government's emergency decree. This precautionary measure was ratified by the federal judicial chamber of Resistencia in a resolution, dated 20 April 2020, that allowed medical personnel from Corrientes entry to Chaco (Pulvirenti 2020).

A similar issue arose between the federal court of Rio Cuarto (province of Córdoba) and the province of San Luis. In response to a precautionary measure issued by the former, which ordered the lifting of the blockade imposed by the province of San Luis on national and provincial routes connecting both jurisdictions, the federal judge of San Luis issued a counter-measure requested by the provincial government itself. In the meantime, an *amparo* action was filed before the federal judge of Río Cuarto by four entities – representing thousands of citizens of the south of the province of Córdoba – in regard to the fundamental rights violated by the blockade ordered by the provincial government of San Luis.

In view of the conflict of jurisdiction, the federal judge of Río Cuarto referred the case to the Supreme Court of Justice of the Nation, which has competence in such matters under article 117 of the Constitution. Its ruling was awaited at the time of writing, and it was anticipated that it would clarify the position not only as regards Córdoba and San Luis but also the several other provinces and municipalities which had declared similar prohibitions of interprovincial or inter-municipal transit. The Supreme Court had requested that the provinces of San Luis, Córdoba, Corrientes, Salta, and Formosa submit reports detailing citizens' complaints about the prohibitions. In one such instance, it ordered the province of Corrientes to allow a person to enter the provincial jurisdiction so as to assist his mother, who was ill with cancer (*Maggi, Mariano v. Provincia de Corrientes*, 10 September 2020).

14.4.6 Intergovernmental fiscal relations

The pandemic had a highly adverse impact on the economy, all the more so given that Argentina was already in the midst of a major economic crisis when Covid-19 broke out. Unemployment rose to 13.1 per cent in the second quarter of 2020, while between March and November, poverty rates increased and inflation climbed to 35 per cent. Due to the slump in economic activity, tax collection decreased, thus hampering federal transfers to provinces. Fiscal federalism is highly centralised in Argentina, where it is the federal government that collects the lion's share – nearly 82 per cent – of tax revenue generated by the country. Federal taxes represent 32 per cent of the tax burden as a percentage of gross domestic product (GDP), while provincial taxes represent only 5.6 per cent (Altavilla 2019).

Under normal circumstances, the federal government provides provinces with resources by way of various transfers. Chief among these is the co-participation regime, or *Régimen de Coparticipación Federal de Impuestos* (RCFI), which accounts for a little more than 50 per cent of all federal transfers. Provincial finances are heavily dependent on these transfers. Most provinces rely on them for more than 50 per cent of their revenue, and in some extreme cases, for nearly all of it: in Formosa, federal transfers cover as much as 94.5 per cent of its budget, in La Rioja, 92.5 per cent, in Catamarca, 90.2 per cent, in Santiago del Estero, 89 per cent, and in Chaco, 88.1 per cent (Altavilla 2019).

As mentioned, from the outset, the federal government adopted measures to mitigate the lockdown's socio-economic impacts. Between March and October 2020, it transferred AMD 1.55 trillion to the provinces by means of discretionary federal funds, such as food programme funds or the fund, Contributions from the National Treasury, or *Aportes del Tesoro National* (ATN). As these are discretionary funds, the federal government was free to distribute them to any province according to its own criteria.

Furthermore, in April 2020, it created the Provincial Financial Emergency Programme, or *Programa para la Emergencia Financiera Provincial* (PEFP), capitalised to a total amount of AMD 170 billion (made up of AMD 60 billion from the ATN fund and ADM 110 billion from the Provincial Development Trust Fund (FFDP)). Predetermined federal transfers continued to be assigned to provinces. However, since transfers are composed of federal taxes, their amount depends on tax collection; during the pandemic, tax collection declined, as did the amounts directed to provinces. As such, transfers via the FFDP compensated for the decrease in RCFI amounts.

Critical problems in intergovernmental fiscal relations surfaced, nonetheless. For one, at the time of writing, the federal government had not yet distributed all the FFDP's budgeted amounts (to date, only AMD 46 billion of AMD 60 billion had been transferred from the ATN fund). For another, some reports show that the distribution of resources to provinces has been linked less to their degree of Covid-19 infection than to whether they are governed by the national ruling party (Aerarium 2020). Looking at federal transfers as a whole, only five provinces received more resources in 2020 than in the previous year (Buenos Aires, La Rioja, Neuquén, Santa Cruz, and the CABA); the other 19 provinces received less than before.

Certain decisions by the President caused major intergovernmental conflict. In a sudden, unilateral decision, he issued decree No. 735 on 9 September on tax relations which provided for a 1.18 per cent reduction of the co-participation regime of the CABA (in opposition hands) to be granted to Buenos Aires province, ostensibly to help tackle the pandemic, and immediately sent a bill to Congress to reduce the tax share due to the CABA. The bill, approved by the Senate, was in relation to the 2016 Security Transfer Agreement. In that year, federal and city governments agreed to transfer more than 20,000 federal police to the CABA since the latter were providing services in the city but were funded by the national budget. For this reason, the CABA's tax share was set at 3.50 per cent. Decree 735 reduced this to 2.32 per cent, while the bill passed in the Senate reduced the percentage further to 1.4 per cent. The CABA rejected the federal government's policy as unconstitutional and approached the Supreme Court, whose decision was pending at the time of this writing.

Other serious infringements of federalism also occurred, such as the fact that the process of transferring companies providing water and electric power services under the federal jurisdiction to the province of Buenos Aires and to the CABA were stopped. Also, in the proposed federal budget most of the transport subsidies are targeted at the Buenos Aires Metropolitan Area at the expense of other jurisdictions, which has led to claims by the mayors of the metropolitan areas of Córdoba, Rosario, Salta, and Bariloche, among others.[7]

In short, the main economic measures were taken at the centre, while the intergovernmental fiscal structure was not adapted in response to the pandemic. The pandemic and lockdown worsened the country's economic situation, both generally and specifically in the provinces. Federal transfers depend on tax collection, and because tax collection declined, federal amounts paid to the provinces were reduced – at the same time, there were no compensatory measures to mitigate the provincial financial crisis.

14.5 Findings and policy implications

Emergency powers should conform to the principles and rules of Argentina's constitutional, democratic, liberal, and republican order. The standards set by the jurisprudence of the Supreme Court of Justice and of the Inter-American Court of Human Rights should be applied, based on reasonable and proportional limitations to fundamental rights. In contrast, what occurred in practice is that most of the decisions made and measures taken in response to the pandemic were adopted through presidential decrees with a centralist bias and in violation of the concurrent powers of subnational entities and the formal division of power. There was a de facto subordination of provinces, the CABA and local governments to the federal government, rather than coordinated federalism based on adequate IGR.

Although the country's executive authorities are endowed with the highest of powers for dealing with exceptional situations, this does not mean that Congress and other legislative bodies should cease to play their oversight role with regard to emergency measures – the same is true as well at the subnational level. In responding to emergencies, the country's measures need to balance effectiveness, on the one hand, with democratic legitimacy and constitutionality, on the other. This is not easy to do, but if the mistakes of the past are to be avoided, it is a challenge that has to be taken up (Hernández 2020d).

Argentina has returned to hyper-presidentialism in which power is concentrated in the hands of the President beyond what is prescribed in the Constitution, a situation that stands to the detriment of the division of powers in multilevel government and the principles of constitutional democracy (Hernández 2012b; Hernández et al. 2016; Nino 1992a, 1992b). The country has often suffered from circumstances such as these, which point to low institutional capacity, a weak culture of legality, and a strong culture of corporatism and centralism (O'Donnell 1992). The executive branch also reverted to its old habit of using emergency powers for personal or political advantage.

In view of the complexity of the pandemic, deliberation by legislative bodies should not have been dispensed with. The national union (mentioned in the preamble of the Constitution as one of the objectives of the nation) that needs to be defended in times of threat should be imagined as a plural, open society and sustained by democratic consensus rather than centralist thinking. The pandemic and the consequences of its governance have now been added to Argentina's many other national problems.

In conclusion, the pandemic has brought out new issues and has revitalised some old problems that have affected the Argentine Federation for a long time. Centralised decision-making without consulting the provinces and municipalities has damaged the already weakened intergovernmental relation network. While at the beginning of the pandemic, the process of decision-making seemed to follow some intergovernmental logic (previous reunion between the president and governors), however, soon thereafter the practice of decision-making turned to be centralist (Hernández 2020b). No institutional channel was used (such as the existing federal councils) not even a new one was established (for instance, some federal emergency committee).

Undoubtedly, federal institutions were helpful and useful in addressing the pandemic because of the effectiveness of the preventive measures that were implemented, and the swiftness with which they were implemented. However, a great opportunity to improve intergovernmental relations was lost, and Argentine federalism failed, in some way, to address this emergency situation from a federal perspective, using all the institutional resources provided by the Constitution. Yet, the pandemic is still ongoing – and while it is not yet feasible to reach a definitive conclusion – it can be said that a window of opportunities for improving intergovernmental relations is still open.

Notes

1 Greater Buenos Aires, also known as the Buenos Aires Metropolitan Area, is an agglomeration consisting of the CABA and 40 adjacent districts within the province of Buenos Aires.
2 The 23 provinces are Buenos Aires, Catamarca, Chaco, Chubut, Córdoba, Corrientes, Entre Ríos, Formosa, Jujuy, La Pampa, La Rioja, Mendoza, Misiones, Neuquén, Río Negro, Salta, San Juan, San Luis, Santa Cruz, Santa Fe, Santiago del Estero, Tierra del Fuego, and Tucumán.
3 See Hernández (2003, 2009); on concurrent municipal powers, see Marchiaro (2020a, 2020b).
4 This cabinet was composed of, among others, the Chief of Cabinet; the federal Economy Minister, Minister of Productive Development, and Minister of Labor, Employment and Social Security; the president of the Central Bank; the president of the AFIP (Federal Administration of Public Revenues); and the Secretary of the Treasury. All of these office-holders were federal public servants.
5 For this reason, an *amparo* action (special proceedings for urgent protection of constitutional rights) was filed before the Supreme Court on 22 September by the *Interbloque de Juntos por el Cambio* of the National Senate, which brings together the opposition parties Republican Proposal and Radical Civic Union parties, with Antonio María Hernández and Ricardo Gil Lavedra as lawyers for the plaintiff.
6 An *amparo* action was also filed on 8 September by the *Interbloque de Juntos por el Cambio* of the Chamber of Deputies, with Antonio María Hernández and Juan Vicente Sola as lawyers for the plaintiff.
7 Practically 90 per cent of the subsidies are provided to the Buenos Aires Metropolitan Area, with the balance going to the main cities of the country.

References

Aerarium. 2020. *Transferencias federales a provincias. Automáticas y discrecionales: ¿quiénes ganan y quiénes pierden?*, https://434938b4-9b8e-4a95-9c6f-bd5ed403809f.filesusr.com/ugd/2f2254_5db2cd19bae04127b7819a2a3c2547cc.pdf (accessed on 11 December 2020).

Altavilla, Cristiàn. 2019. *Decentralization, Intergovernmental Relations and Regional Inequality in Argentina*. Conference at Harvard Law School, 18 April.

Azarkevich, Ernesto. 2020. 'Coronavirus in Argentina: Finally Puerto Iguazú Did Not Close Its Border with Brazil', *Clarín*, 25 March.

Bidart Campos, Germán. 1998. *Manual de la Constitución Reformada. Vol. I.* Buenos Aires: Ediar.

Cavallini Viale, Delfina and Leandro Ferreyra. 2020. '*Cincuenta Decretos de Fernández*', *Palabras del Derecho*, 19 May.

Hernández, Antonio María. 2003. *Derecho Municipal*. Mexico: UNAM.

Hernández, Antonio María. 2009. *Federalismo y Constitucionalismo Provincial*. Buenos Aires: Abeledo Perrot.

Hernández, Antonio María. 2012a. 'El Poder Ejecutivo', in Hernández, Antonio María (ed.) *Derecho Constitucional*. Buenos Aires: La Ley.

Hernández, Antonio María. 2012b. *Fortalezas y debilidades constitucionales. Una lectura crítica en el Bicentenario*. Buenos Aires: Abeledo Perrotáá.

Hernández, Antonio María. 2020a. *Emergencias, Orden Constitucional y COVID-19 en Argentina*. Buenos Aires: Rubinzal Culzoni Editores.

Hernández, Antonio María. 2020b. '*El Retorno Al Peor Pasado Centralista*', *La Nación*, February 27.

Hernández, Antonio María. 2020c. '*Federalismo y Covid-19*', *Clarín*, 24 April.

Hernández, Antonio María. 2020d. '*Las Emergencias y el Orden Constitucional*', *Clarin*, 23 March.

Hernández, Antonio María, Daniel Zovatto and Eduardo Fidanza. 2016. *Segunda Encuesta de Cultura Constitucional. Argentina, una Sociedad Anómica*. Buenos Aires: Eudeba.

Infobae. 23 September 2020. '*Tasa de Desempleo de Argentina Trepa a 13,1% en Segundo Trimestre: Oficial*', https://www.infobae.com/america/agencias/2020/09/23/tasa-de-desempleo-de-argentina-trepa-a-131-en-segundo-trimestre-oficial-3/ (accessed on 29 November 2020).

Isuani, Aldo. 2020. '*Frente a la Pandemia: ¿tenemos un Sistema de Salud?*', *Clarín*, 1 October.

Malavolta, Víctor and Orlando Pulvirenti. 2020. '*El Federalismo y el Municipalismo en Tiempos de Pandemia*', 28 April, http://www.saij.gob.ar/victor-malavolta-federalismo-municipalismo-tiempos-pandemia-dacf200078-2020-04-28/123456789-0abc-defg8700-02fcanirt-cod?& (accessed on 11 December 2020).

Marchiaro, Enrique. 2020a. 'Cierres Municipales y Pandemia', *DPI, Diario Administrativo*, 273, 7 April.

Marchiaro, Enrique. 2020b. 'Son Válidos Los Cierres Municipales de Circulación y Actividad General en Tanto No Impidan Los Servicios Esenciales', in Cristiàn Altavilla and Candela Villegas (eds), *Los Desafíos del Derecho Frente a la Pandemia COVID-19. Mirada del Derecho Argentino con Aportes del Derecho Comparado*, pp. 133–36. Buenos Aires: Universidad Siglo 21 – IJ Editores.

Midón, Mario. 2001. *Decretos de Necesidad y Urgencia*. Buenos Aires: La Ley.

Mozetic, Daniela. 2020. 'Cruce Entre Ginés y Gobernadores por la Compra de Respiradores', *Perfil*, 28 March.

Nino, Carlos Santiago. 1992a. *Fundamentos de Derecho Constitucional*. Buenos Aires: Astrea.

Nino, Carlos Santiago. 1992b. *Un país al margen de la ley.* Buenos Aires: Emecé.

O'Donnell, Guillermo. 1992. 'Delegative Democracy'. Kellogg Institute working paper no. 172.

Pan American Health Organization (PAHO). 2017. 'Health in the Americas: Argentina', https://www.paho.org/salud-en-las-americas-2017/?p=2706 (accessed on 11 December 2020).

Porto, Alberto and Luciano Di Gresia. 2020. *El Rol de los Gobiernos Subnacionales (Provinciales y Municipales) en la Pandemia Covid-19*, 13 April. Universidad Nacional de La Plata.

Pulvirenti, Orlando. 2020. *Tres Fallos y el Federalismo en la Pandemia*, Microjuris.com, MJ/DOC/15283/AR, 14 April.

Quiroga Lavié, Humberto. 2009. *Derecho Constitucional Argentino. Vol. II.* Santa Fe: Rubinzal-Culzoni.

Tortolero Cervantes, Francisco. 2020. 'La Pandemia como Oportunidad para Relanzar el Rol de las Entidades Subnacionales Latinoamericanas', in Nuria González Martín and Diego Valadés (eds), *Emergencia Sanitaria por COVID-19-Federalismo.* México: Instituto de Investigaciones Jurídicas de la UNAM.

PART IV
Asia and Australia

15
PANDEMIC GOVERNANCE IN INDIA

The ongoing shift to 'national federalism'

Ajay Kumar Singh

15.1 Introduction

Covid-19 broke out in India in January 2020, soon placing a federation already embattled by authoritarian centralism under strain, yet without successfully containing the spread of the pandemic in what, after China, is the second-most populous country in the world. The pandemic further pushed the polity towards national federalism, emphasising national executive governance of public policies and state subjects.

With a population density of 382 per km², India's population, according to the 2011 census, stood at 1.21 billion in 2011 (Union Ministry of Information and Broadcasting 2020: 7), while estimates by the United Nations in 2019 put the figure as high as 1.37 billion (United Nations, Department of Economic and Social Affairs, Population Division 2019: 12). Roughly 29.5 per cent of people are in the age group 0–14 years, 62.5 per cent in the age group 14–59 years, and 8 per cent 60 years and older (Office of the Registrar General and Census Commissioner of India 2011). About 31.2 per cent of the population reside in urban areas that range from towns to cities and metropolises. Hindus comprise approximately 79.8 per cent of the population, followed by Muslims (14.2 per cent), Christians (2.3 per cent), Sikhs (1.7 per cent), Buddhists (0.7 per cent), and Jain (0.3 per cent).

Politically and administratively, India is a federation consisting of 28 states and nine union (or federal) territories, 734 districts, 4,470 urban bodies, and 255,544 village *panchayats* (grass-roots councils). Over the past decade, especially since 2014, parliamentary democracy has been overshadowed by what many regard as an authoritarian regime in the form of the Bharatiya Janata Party (BJP), a right-wing Hindu formation which rules at the centre and in most of the states

DOI: 10.4324/9781003166771-20

demonstrates little respect for constitutional principles. Secularism and multi-culturalism have been under attack in the face of the BJP's efforts to establish a Hindu-ised socio-political order, with anti-minority sentiment and exclusionary politics becoming the norm (Diamond 2020: 1–7; Gandhi 2020: 1–4; Mukherji 2020: 91–105; Patnaik 2019: 6–9; Picketty 2020: 944–948).

Notably, in August 2019, the special autonomy status of Jammu and Kashmir regions was revoked (Basu 2020: 287–294), while in December, amendments under the Citizenship (Amendment) Act 47 of 2019 granted citizenship to members of non-Muslim religious communities from Afghanistan, Bangladesh or Pakistan who had entered India by 31 December 2014 (Tharoor 2020: 258–277; Union Ministry of Law and Justice 2019). This led to violent protests, with fears being voiced that the Act is discriminatory to Muslims and intended to make indigenous peoples minorities in their homelands.

Other aspects of India's democracy are also in danger. Freedom of expression is suppressed by state organs such as police, investigative agencies, surveillance systems, and tax authorities (Yadav 2020: 351). Parliamentary processes are subverted in the making and amendment of laws; parliamentary accountability is at its lowest ebb; and the autonomy of independent institutions, including the judiciary, Election Commission, Central Information Commission, and other regulatory bodies, is under constant threat (Ramakrishnan 2020). The pandemic has further incentivised illiberal repressive measures by Prime Minister Narendra Modi's government (Diamond 2020: 1–7; Mukherji 2020: 91).

Economically, at the beginning of 2020 India found itself in the midst of a growth crisis, one that worsened as the pandemic unfolded. Gross domestic product (GDP) has been in decline since 2016, when it recorded growth of 8.2 per cent. By 2019, GDP decreased by 3 per cent (World Bank 2020), after which it saw negative growth of 23.9 per cent in the first quarter (April–June) and 8.6 per cent in the second quarter (July–September) of the 2020–2021 fiscal year (Reserve Bank of India 2020). Unemployment, always a cause of concern, was aggravated by the pandemic, with salaried jobs decreasing from 86 million in 2019–2020 to 65 million in August 2020 (Vyas 2020).

On the medical front, India has a three-tier system consisting of primary health care (provided at sub-district level), secondary health care (provided at district level), and specialised services at the tertiary level. Public health expenditure has, however, never exceeded 1.6 per cent of GDP (PRS Legislative Research 2020a: 1), resulting in a significant misalignment in India between population size and health infrastructure; likewise, the doctor-population ratio is low at 1:1,343. The country has about a thousand district hospitals, 5,335 community health centres, 24,855 primary health centres, and 157,411 sub-centres in outlying areas. More tellingly, Jaffrelot and Shah (2020), referring to a study by the Centre for Disease Dynamics, Economics and Policy (India) and Princeton University, noted that 'public hospitals have only 713,986 beds, including 35,699 in intensive care units and 17,850 ventilators'.

It was in this context that India reported its first case of Covid-19 on 30 January 2020, with the infection coming to light in the state of Kerala; the first Covid-19 death occurred on 12 March. The authorities continued with their wait-and-see policy until 14 March, at which point the pandemic was declared a national health emergency. Prior to this, the official response was virtually non-existent. Health screening at airports and international borders was not up to the standards set in World Health Organization (WHO) advisories, and almost no cases were reported in the intervening month of February.

When the first national lockdown was announced on 24 March 2020, India had only 519 recorded cases. Between then and 31 October, it conducted 108.8 million tests, with the total number of cases amounting to 8.1 million; during this period, 121,000 people died of Covid-19. In terms of territorial distribution, nearly all states and union territories were affected. However, about 75 per cent of cases were reported in ten states, namely, Andhra Pradesh, Chhattisgarh, Delhi, Karnataka, Kerala, Maharashtra, Tamil Nadu, Rajasthan, Uttar Pradesh, and West Bengal (Union Ministry of Health and Family Welfare 2020a). About 130 districts were hotspots, while the worst affected cities included Mumbai, Chennai, Delhi, and Ahmadabad. In a cumulative analysis, 97.72 per cent of the cases were reported during the period of phased reopening from 1 June to 31 October, which supports the thesis that India imposed a national lockdown too early and hastily.

This chapter argues that, under the helm of Prime Minister Narendra Modi, India's response to the pandemic resulted in the suspension of federalism in favour of highly centralised, unitary executive governance, and, concomitantly, severe curtailment of state autonomy. Elsewhere, I have argued that Indian federalism since 2014 (the year the BJP rose to power) is best described as undergoing a phase of national federalism marked by a shift of sovereignty from states to the centre and from the centre to the Office of the Prime Minister (Singh 2019). Pandemic governance is no exception to this trend. It is also argued that centralisation has not yielded the desired result of containing and managing Covid-19, which instead has placed further strain on centre-state relations, particularly when it comes to fiscal issues.

15.2 The federal constitutional and legislative framework

India's union model of federalism is a curious blend of the characteristics of dual, cooperative-collaborative, and organic-interdependent federalism (Singh 2009). Under the Constitution of India of 1950, the distribution of powers between the different levels of government tilts the balance in favour of a strong centre, with centralisation rationalised as a measure to secure national unity and interests, promote general public welfare, and advance national economic integration (Jain 2019: 739).

Schedule 7 of the Constitution grants the centre residual powers and exclusive authority over 97 subjects including the deployment of the central armed forces;

major industrial operations; national highways and transport (including inter-state movements of goods, services, and people); regulation of higher education; inter-state migration and quarantine; and offences against union laws.

In comparison, important competences of states pertaining to Covid-19 are public order and safety; policing; public health and sanitation; hospitals and dispensaries; local and intra-state transport and communications; agriculture and allied activities; local industry and manufacturing; market operations; theatres, amusement parks, and the like; civil works and construction; and school and university education. In many of these subjects, states have only qualified and conditional competence. For example, in public health matters, the central government regulates clinical trials, treatment protocols, drug use, and medical standards, in addition to disease-specific measures (Singh 2015: 139–142).

States and the centre have shared competencies in matters such as civil and criminal law and procedure, social and economic planning, labour, education, social security, and employment. Nevertheless, central laws and regulations override state laws.

The Constitution provides for only two kinds of national emergency – the first due to war, external aggression or armed rebellion, and the second a financial emergency in which India's fiscal stability is under threat. In the event of a breakdown of governance in a state, presidential rule from the centre is imposed on the state. The declaration of an emergency is subject to parliamentary approval within a specified period (Basu 2019: 15061–233). In the absence of constitutional provisions specifically dealing with a pandemic emergency, the central government invoked three legislative enactments to declare a national pandemic emergency on 15 March 2020: the Epidemic Diseases Act (EDA) of 1897, the Disaster Management Act (DMA) of 2005 and Criminal Procedure Code (CPC) 1973 (Parliament of India, Rajya Sabha 2020a). The EDA was used to declare Covid-19 a national pandemic and the DMA to declare it as a 'notified disaster' and a 'national health emergency'. The CPC 1973 enabled police and other authorities engaged in pandemic management to take preventive and punitive action on any breach of the government's order on Covid-19 and to impose punishment for offences.

The EDA has four significant features: it allows the centre to declare a dangerous epidemic a national pandemic; it empowers state authorities to initiate corrective, preventative and regulatory control measures which are otherwise not feasible under the ordinary laws; it allows the government to inspect passenger traffic on air, land, or water and detain any person; and it protects health-care providers from any act of violence committed by any individual or group (PRS Legislative Research 2020b). The EDA was invoked previously during outbreaks of malaria, cholera, dengue, and swine flu (Nomani and Parveen 2020: 156).

The DMA 2005 was invoked, for the first time, to declare Covid-19 a national health emergency. The central government assumed all powers from the local to the national level related to pandemic care, control, and management. The DMA also empowers the central government to issue directives and orders on pandemic management and related matters. The orders made by the centre are binding (although barely accountable to Parliament); conversely, states and local authorities cannot take any measures contrary to central directives. For instance, during the phased reopening after India's lockdown, states wished to regulate inter- and intra-state movement of people but could not contradict an order of the central authority forbidding this.

15.3 Preparedness for a national disaster: The institutional framework

After enacting the DMA in 2005, India established a three-layered hierarchy for managing disasters, with the National Disaster Management Authority (NDMA; hereafter 'National Authority') at the central or national level, the State Disaster Management Authority (SDMA) at the state level, and the District Disaster Management Authority (DDMA) at the local level.

The National Authority is led by the Prime Minister: in the event of emergency, he or she can 'exercise all or any of the powers of the National Authority' (DMA 2005, section 3), which are ratified *ex post facto* by the NDMA. The latter comprises not more than nine members, each of whom is nominated by the Prime Minister; currently, it has five expert members. The NDMA is vested with the authority of planning and policy formulation. It approves the disaster management plans prepared by ministries, as well as coordinating and enforcing the policies and guidelines it prepares or approves; accordingly, it also has the authority to direct central ministries, departments, and state and district authorities in compliance with its orders and guidelines. It ensures funding and other measures of support necessary for disaster management. The National Authority can sanction concessional loans to persons and establishments affected by disaster of a severe magnitude, in addition to providing for basic necessities such as food, shelter, and health care. In other words, ensuring social and economic welfare is a principal responsibility of the National Authority.

The National Authority is assisted by the National Executive Committee (NEC). Headed by the union home secretary, it is a committee of secretaries in charge of ministries or departments involved in disaster-management work. As a 'coordinating and monitoring body for disaster management', the NEC is responsible for the preparation of a national plan to be approved by the National Authority, which lays down guidelines and their administration by departments of the central government as well as state authorities and ministries. It monitors and evaluates progress in disaster mitigation and management.

The SDMA in turn is headed by the chief minister of the state concerned. In case of a localised state disaster, the state authority has powers and functions similar to those of the National Authority. However, in the event of a declaration of a national disaster, its authority has no autonomous domain. Like the National Authority, the state authority is assisted by the State Executive

Committee (SEC), which is chaired by the state chief secretary – the latter is the executive officer responsible for implementing disaster mitigation plans and guidelines issued by the state authority.

The district authority is in charge of district-level planning and led by the district magistrate, collector or deputy commissioner, who appoints executive magistrates as 'incident commanders' responsible for the implementation of disaster mitigation measures in their respective local jurisdictions. All other line department officials work under the instruction of the chair of the DDMA, which means in practice that *panchayats* and municipal authorities serve under his or her authority.

In declaring Covid-19 an epidemic, the National Authority (read: the Prime Minister) on 24 March 2020 invoked its power under the DMA 2005 to 'direct ministries/departments of government of India, state governments and state authorities' to take nationally consistent and uniform measures for the prevention of the spread of disease (section 6(2)(i)). It further authorised the NEC to issue necessary guidelines.

In this context, three sections of the DMA 2005 must be highlighted. Section 35 allows the central government unilaterally to control, command, and coordinate disaster measures across India, while section 62 endows it with extraordinary authority to issue directives to statutory authorities, officers, and employees at any level of government. In other words, the pandemic is to be governed through a unified system of command and compliance. Furthermore, section 65 grants the leviathan of the state the 'power of requisition of resources, provisions, vehicles, etc.' from any public authority or person.

In summary, in the event of disasters of a national scale, the DMA 2005 provides for a pyramidal structure of governance with the Prime Minister at the top and incident commanders at the bottom. Authority begins and ends with the Prime Minister. It is from here that the overall national power structure, its political composition, ideologies, and leadership have a determining impact on disaster management.

15.4 Rolling out measures to contain the pandemic

When the pandemic struck, the BJP – either on its own or as part of the National Democratic Alliance (NDA) – was firmly in control at the centre and in 21 states, which approximates to about 70 per cent of India's population. The Indian National Congress (INC) party is in power in but five states, the Communist Party of India in one, and other regional or local parties preside over three states (Maps of India 2020). Of the 545 seats in the Lok Sabha ('House of the People'), the lower chamber of India's bicameral parliament, the BJP has 302 and the INC only 51; of the 250 seats in the upper house of parliament, the BJP has 92 and the INC, 37. The picture which emerges is that India has a nationally weak opposition, and hence one that cannot ensure the accountability of a nationally dominant ruling party.

Against the backdrop of this imbalance, India in recent years witnessed an escalation in communal polarisation directed at Muslims, a trend that continued into the Covid-19 period. When infections began rising in the national capital and other cities, members of the Tablighi Jamaat sect were targeted by Hindu fundamentalists as 'super-spreaders' of the coronavirus (Salam 2020: 59–60). The Bombay High Court, in clearing Muslims of this pejorative label, was moved to remark that 'a political government tries to find the scapegoat when there is [a] pandemic or calamity' (Aurangabad Bench, Criminal Writ Petition No. 548 of 2020, 21 August 2020: para 27). Despite incidents like these, people in India generally responded supportively to government health measures, with community-driven food-relief initiatives for the needy coming into operation almost everywhere during the national lockdown.

15.4.1 Taking the initiative

In early January 2020, the government issued advisories to states to improve preparedness and health infrastructure in the event of a pandemic. On 18 January, thermal screening of passengers from China and Hong Kong was introduced at entry-points. A committee of five union ministers – those of health, aviation, shipping, home affairs, and foreign affairs – was formed to monitor the pandemic. On 11 March, the NEC, acting in terms of the DMA 2005, delegated powers to the union health secretary to boost preparedness and containment. Once a national disaster is in force, union ministries do not enjoy equal status but exercise their authority only with the consent and approval of the NDMA and NEC.

Point-of-entry surveillance was introduced by the end of January, and on 4 March, thermal screening was made mandatory for all international passengers. Travel bans, visa cancellation, and quarantining were effected from 13 March, and on 14 March, Covid-19 was (as noted) declared a national health emergency, which enabled states to withdraw monies from the State Disaster Response Fund (SDRF) (Parliament of India, Rajya Sabha 2020b: 6). States were instructed to ensure strict implementation of union advisories and guidelines. In terms of advisories issued by the Union Ministry of Health and Family Welfare, education facilities, cinemas, malls, and gyms were closed, and social and cultural gatherings were restricted. On 22 March, all international flights to India were suspended, as were mass transport services such as railways and buses. Domestic flights were suspended on 24 March.

On that same day, Prime Minister Modi, in a televised address at 20:00, announced a 21-day national lockdown, effective from midnight. The public had barely four hours' notice to gather essential items, nor for that matter had states or political parties been given much or any forewarning of the announcement (Mukherji 2020: 93); indeed, it was only later that night that chief secretaries of states were briefed about the lockdown (PIB 2020). Once the lockdown had been announced, states and political parties extended their support to the central government. For instance, the INC president, Sonia Gandhi, welcomed the decision in a public letter to the Prime Minister on 26 March, although also raising concerns among the medical fraternity about their safety and among workers about financial aid (The Print 2020a).

On 29 March 2020, the Union Home Secretary, as chair of the NEC, set up 11 specially empowered groups of officials to plan and manage the implementation of various aspects of pandemic response such as medical-emergency planning, disease surveillance, critical-care infrastructure, the supply of food and essential goods, and economic and welfare measures. Furthermore, working under the direction of the NEC, the Union Ministry of Health and Family Welfare coordinated health-care preparedness across states, issuing SOPs (standard operating procedures) and guidelines in this regard. The union agency, the Indian Council of Medical Research (ICMR), appointed technical experts to attend to the clinical aspects of health management, which included identifying laboratories in the states to conduct testing, and approve modes of treatment, drug prescriptions, and medical interventions.

Looking briefly at the initial state-level response, Kerala, led by the Communist Party, was the first to respond substantively to Covid-19. Even before the national lockdown, a stringent local lockdown was in effect, with schools having been closed and social gatherings banned; in fact, Kerala had issued coronavirus guidelines setting out case definitions and procedures for screening, quarantine, isolation, and treatment four days before India's first case of Covid-19 was reported on 30 January (NDMA 2020a). Rajasthan was also quick to respond to a possible emergency by taking measures in regard to quarantining and containment, with a state-wide curfew imposed on 18 March some days before the national lockdown. Likewise, Punjab adopted similar measures between January and early March. Prior to the lockdown, every state had a protocol of its own for contact tracing, isolation, and treatment.

Once Covid-19 had been declared a national pandemic on 14 March, states no longer had autonomy in their response measures and were obligated to follow national directives – if they wished to depart from them, they had to obtain permission in advance from the central government. Moreover, what was missing from the outset was the dimension of inter-state coordination – hardly any formal or informal inter-governmental mechanism was utilised.

15.4.2 Federal government action

In India, central government action in response to Covid-19 had four aspects to it. A first set of interventions were non-pharmaceutical and non-clinical and involved containing viral spread through closures, including lockdown and other modes of suspension and regulation of activity. A key outcome was that nationwide lockdown gave the central government time to ramp up health infrastructure. In the second place, there were pharmaceutical-clinical interventions carried out in terms of the regulatory guidelines of the ICMR and other central-level medical agencies. This involved centrally monitored hospital management and treatment of Covid-19 cases on a uniform national basis – to which one should hasten to add that it intruded significantly on state autonomy and jurisdictional authority over public health, given that states could not initiate medical measures contrary to central guidelines.

A third kind of action entailed providing information to the public about dietary and other means for building immunity, including through the use of Ayurvedic (alternative) medicine, while a fourth involved welfarist interventions geared towards the socio-economically vulnerable groups. This included supplying food relief over six months to two-thirds of the population (in the form of free rations consisting of 5 kg of rice and wheat and 1 kg of pulse foodstuffs such as beans and lentils) and paying INR 500 per month for an initial three months to about 200 million women holding accounts under the Pradhan Mantri Jan Dhan Yojana (PMJDY) financial inclusion programme; in addition, free gas cylinders were provided for three months to some 83 million families living below the poverty line (NDMA 2020b: 33).

The lockdown was effected through a series of orders issued by the Ministry of Home Affairs. The first 21-day national lockdown started on 25 March (Order No. 40-3/2020-DM-I/(A)). Except for the partial relaxation of the opening of states' administrative offices, and agricultural operations, the second lockdown order (MHA Order No. 40-3/2020-DM-I/(A), 15 April 2020) kept the stringency of the first and did not return states' powers. The third lockdown order (MHA Order No. 40-3/2020-DM-I/(A), 1 May 2020) brought some easing of trade restrictions allowing standalone shops in urban residential localities, and all shops in rural areas to operate. During the fourth lockdown (MHA Order No. 40-3/2020-DM-I/(A), 17 May 2020), states were allowed to start market operations with staggered opening times and Covid-19 preventive measures. States by mutual agreement were allowed to start interstate movement of vehicles. For better focused pandemic measures at the local level, the centre conceded the request of states to delineate red, green, and buffer zones in accordance with parameters laid down by the Union Ministry of Health and Family Welfare.

With the economic slump in sight, India started to unlock on a monthly basis from 1 June when hospitality services, markets, shopping malls, and limited religious worship in temples were allowed. During August the night curfew was removed and inter- and intra-state travel and transportation were permitted. In September, socio-religious, political, and academic gatherings could be held, while states were allowed to open schools and colleges and other educational institutions from 15 October.

Overall, pandemic governance under the institution of the NDMA consisted principally in executive governance little impeded by accountability to Parliament. As one contributor to the magazine *Frontline* observed, the pandemic seemed to have given the central government the opportunity to engage in 'muting parliament' (Ramakrishnan 2020: 21–23).

Despite resistance from opposition parties, major instruments of parliamentary accountability were suspended during the legislature's 2020 monsoon session, namely, private members' bills, question hour (except for questions requiring written answers), and 'zero hour' (a procedural innovation allowing members to raise issues on matters of national concern without prior notice). Notably, too, the government did not accede to a demand for a debate on Covid-19, as this would have put it in the embarrassing position of explaining its handling of the pandemic and the effect it had on the economy.

The well-known parliamentarian Shashi Tharoor said the Modi government was attempting to reduce Parliament to 'a notice-board' and was '[using] its crushing majority as a rubber stamp for whatever it wants to pass' (cited in Ramakrishnan 2020: 21–22). This was especially true of labour laws passed during the monsoon session, and three controversial farm bills that were introduced and passed on the same day, thereby short-circuiting amendment procedures and truncating opportunity for debate in spite of stiff resistance from farmers, non-BJP-ruled states, and several regional political parties.

Together, the three bills – the Farmers' Produce Trade and Commerce (Promotion and Facilitation) Bill, the Farmers (Empowerment and Protection) Agreement on Price Assurance and Farm Services Bill, and the Essential Commodities (Amendment) Bill – leave India's farmers without security of pricing and the minimum guarantee of assured income and assistance they enjoyed hitherto. The effect of the three new legislative enactments is to privatise farming and bring agriculture within the ambit of inter-state trade, with the centre having exclusive jurisdiction – a move in keeping with the Modi government's wider efforts to use the pandemic as an occasion to promote privatisation and policy centralisation under the much-vaunted doctrine of *Aatma Nirbhar Bharat* ('self-reliant India').

This extends beyond agriculture. Although education is a concurrent subject, a new education policy (Union Ministry of Human Resource Development 2020) adopted in 2020 shifts the constitutional scales in favour of the centre rather than seeking to secure a fine federal balance between states and centre. Apart from promoting privatisation, the policy introduces structural changes in education governance by creating a single regulator for higher education as well as regulating the school curriculum, a matter that otherwise falls within the competence of states. In a similar vein, the Banking Regulation (Amendment) Bill of 2020 removes cooperative banking from the regulatory control of states and assigns it to the Reserve Bank of India.

15.4.3 State government action

As noted, prior to the declaration of a national disaster, states introduced measures of their own, given that they could issue orders under their state disaster management acts or state legislation on epidemics and public health. However, once central directions were issued, states had to comply with them.

Kerala, for instance, allowed short-distance city bus travel and the reopening of local barber shops and restaurants. The centre considered it a violation of national lockdown measures, and the union home secretary instructed Kerala to adhere to them 'without any dilution and to ensure strict compliance [with] lockdown measures' (D.O. 40-3/2020-DM-I(A), 19 April 2020). The state was left with no choice but to rescind its order.

Nevertheless, states were allowed to introduce stricter containment measures if necessary. In addition, in later phases of the lockdown (1 June–31 October), they were permitted a partial degree of autonomy, but again only in accordance with central guidelines and SOPs.

The leeway available for individuality and locally responsive agency and innovation in state-level responses to the pandemic was thus highly constrained, a situation compounded by wide variation in resource capacities from one state to the next and hence in what each would be capable of doing anyway even if given a free hand. States largely performed similar functions such as border screening and control and enforcement of quarantining and isolation, although some states were innovative, as illustrated below:

- Kerala, with a highly decentralised and well-equipped public health system, followed a community-based approach in successfully containing two waves of Covid-19. It developed a network of neighbourhood surveillance systems for contact tracing. Its response further included effective provision of medicines, community kitchens, food relief, and social assistance worth INR 1,000 to families not receiving welfare grants (Kerala Chief Minister 2020).
- Karnataka optimised information technology and conducted a health-risk survey of about 15 million households that enhanced its management of Covid-19. It was also the first state to invoke provisions of the Epidemic Diseases Act, in addition to which it capped the cost of testing and hospitalisation in private hospitals (NDMA 2020c).
- Andhra Pradesh introduced innovations in ward surveillance and in managing multiple lockdowns, which were accompanied by highly regulated reopening.
- Tamil Nadu, apart from rigorously implementing lockdown measures, provided social assistance of INR 1,000 to all ration-card holders and INR 1,500 per month to persons with disabilities. (Most states provided free rations and cash transfers to the needy in the initial few months of lockdown.)
- Apart from implementing a community-based surveillance system, Madhya Pradesh introduced 'fever clinics' serving as '[first] points of contact for suspected Covid patients' (NDMA 2020d).
- Rajasthan's success story lies in decentralised public health and rigorous containment measures, while Punjab and Delhi were the first few states to introduce plasma therapy for Covid-19 treatment.

State high courts – notably in Delhi and Maharashtra, among others – intervened, either on their own initiative or on the basis of public appeals, in matters relating to migrant workers, disease testing, the disposal of dead bodies, the condition of facilities in quarantine centres, and capping fees charged by private laboratories. During the August and September 2020 phased re-opening, state legislative assemblies began to convene; however, there are no inspiring tales of legislatures securing executive accountability in Covid-19 management.

The commanding authority of the central government was further upheld in two rulings by the Supreme Court of India. In *Alakh Alok Srivastava v. Union of India*, it pronounced that 'state governments, public authorities and citizens of this country will faithfully comply with the directives, advisories, and orders issued by the union of India in letter and spirit in the interests of public safety' (Supreme Court 2020, WP(C) No. 469). Then, in *Praneeth K and Ors v. University Grants Commission (UGC) and Ors*, it quashed the decisions of the SDMAs of Maharashtra and West Bengal to promote students to the following semester or year without holding year-end or term-end exams.

Stating that this was contrary to the guidelines of the University Grant Commission of India (UGC), the Court ruled that an SDMA was not authorised to take such a decision while the NDMA is in force. It also upheld the federal authority of the central government to regulate the examination and promotion of students in colleges and universities; conversely, SDMAs and other state authorities have no such jurisdiction (Supreme Court 2020, WP (C) No. 724).

15.4.4 Local government action

Although the 73rd and 74th Amendments to the Constitution in 1992 put *panchayati raj* institutions and municipal bodies on a sound constitutional footing, the devolution of functions, funds, and functionaries to them was left to the discretion of states (Basu 2020: 304). Some states, such as Kerala, Karnataka, and Rajasthan, have devolved considerable powers and authority to local bodies, while others, such as Bihar and Uttar Pradesh, are yet to do so. From the perspective of pandemic control, then, local government has been implemented unevenly and, in constitutional terms, is asymmetrically positioned in relation to state government.

Moreover, in terms of the DMA 2005, local bodies have to work under the control and direction of SDMAs. Their role ranges from raising public awareness about health issues and disposing of dead bodies to distributing welfare goods, providing sanitation and conducting community surveillance. In Kerala, for instance, panchayats were engaged, inter alia, in quarantine-centre work, door-to-door surveys, and keeping lists of migrants (Dutta and Fischer 2020). In Karnataka, they played a proactive role in delivering goods under government schemes in rural areas. In urban areas, municipal bodies were mainly responsible for the surveillance of hotspots and containment zones, over and above providing sanitation services.

In India, local bodies do not have the fiscal authority to defer or waive service charges, defer housing-loan payments, or grant concessions in property taxes, all of which are done either by states or the centre. For example, soon after the imposition of the first national lockdown, the central government announced that housing-loan repayments would be deferred for three months, later extending this by yet another three months; this measure did not affect local authority income, however.

15.4.5 Intergovernmental relations

Intergovernmental relations (IGR) are conducted both formally and informally (see Singh and Saxena 2015). The Constitution establishes the Inter-State Council to promote cooperation and coordination between the centre and states and among states on crucial issues of IGR and on matters of national importance. Its composition – consisting of all chief ministers, heads of union territories, the Prime Minister and six cabinet ministers of the union government – makes it a truly federal forum. However, in the three decades since it was constituted in 1990, it has met only 11 times, with the last meeting to date having been held in July 2016; on the matter of the global pandemic, it had not met once.

As for the DMA 2005, it does not provide any structured mechanism for IGR to facilitate policy consensus and coordination of measures among different levels of government. Instead, as noted, it institutes an executive, unilateral model of pandemic governance in which orders and commands flow top-down and permit only one-way traffic.

Informal mechanisms of intergovernmental relations include chief ministers' conferences and governors' conferences. Although not required to do so under the DMA 2005, Prime Minister Modi convened eight virtual meetings with state chief ministers and addressed the heads of local bodies once, and at the bureaucratic level, union home and health secretaries held several briefings and preparedness meetings with their state counterparts.

An overall assessment is that IGR has been at a low ebb in recent years and notably so in the Covid-19 period, with Prime Minister Modi showing scant regard for federal IGR institutions. At state level, instances of inter-state cooperation in pandemic management have been few and far between and, where they arose, limited to sharing cadres of health professionals, as happened between Kerala and Maharashtra.

In the grand scheme of pandemic governance, cooperative or competitive inter-state relations have little substantive role to play. For example, states have acted on their own rather than in concert in capping the prices of Covid-19 testing kits and treatment; at the same time, given that the centre monitors the prices of essentials, the resultant ceiling has prevented price wars or resource competition among the states.

15.4.6 Intergovernmental fiscal relations

The states raise about 52.5 per cent of their revenue, of which state GST constitutes about half of that (Reserve Bank of India 2019: 28–36), with central transfers constituting the remaining 47.5 per cent, following the recommenda-tions of the Finance Commission of India. The decline in tax collection by the centre during the pandemic also caused a drop in the states' share of central taxes (Union Ministry of Finance 2020a).

The pandemic had a colossal impact on goods and service taxes (GST), which usually make up about 42 per cent of states' own tax revenue. Overall state GST collection in April–May 2020, India's two months of complete lockdown, declined by more than 44 per cent year-on-year, and in April–August, by more than 30 per cent; states' revenue deficit was estimated to be over INR 3,000,000 million (The Indian Express 2020a). Except Nagaland, which recorded a growth of 12 per cent, almost all states recorded a decline in the collection of state GST during April–August 2020 (Union Ministry of Finance 2020b).

Any shortfall in GST has an adverse impact on capital expenditure by states. Given that states ceded tax sovereignty in favour of a one-nation-one-tax model, a key issue is whether or to what extent the central government is under an obligation to compensate them for their GST shortfalls. It presented options for borrowing money from the Reserve Bank of India or from the open market, but non-BJP ruled states, such as Kerala, West Bengal, Punjab, and Delhi, demanded compensation to avoid the debt trap (The Indian Express 2020b).

As far as disaster funding is concerned, Bhaskar and Kelkar point out that, unlike the Government of India, 'state governments do not levy taxes/cesses to directly fund disaster relief' (Bhaskar and Kelkar 2019: 41). Annual expenditure in this regard is generally managed in four ways: by spending funds earmarked for relief expenditure such as 'gratuitous relief', food supplies, and the like; by tapping into funds allocated for capital works; by taking out loans for restoration work, such as 'repair of damaged houses and loans for purchase of agricultural inputs'; and by using money released from the SDRF (ibid). With a few excep-tions, health infrastructure in India's states is poor; faced with the critical need to improve it yet also lacking adequate fiscal resources to meet expenditure on hos-pital facilities, quarantine centres, testing kits and similar necessities, states had to rely on the SDRF, other central assistance towards Covid-19 preparedness, and borrowing from the market.

Within the existing fiscal arrangements, disaster financing is shared between the centre and states in the ratio of 75:25 for general-category states and in the ratio of 90:10 for north-eastern and Himalayan states such as Uttarakhand and Himachal Pradesh. The Fifteenth Finance Commission, by way of grant-in-aid, allocates funds to the SDRF: for 2020–2021, the allocation was INR 289,830 million. SDRF funds are shared among states on the basis of criteria such as the state's size, population, disaster risk profile, and expenditure responsibility in regard to disaster management (Fifteenth Finance Commission 2019: 55–60). Unless permitted by the central government, states on their own may not with-draw from the SDRF (Union Ministry of Home Affairs 2020a).

As at 20 September 2020, releases from the SDRF totalled INR 115,659.25 million. The central government also released INR 16,246.3 million from the National Disaster Response Fund (NDRF) to give Manipur, Meghalaya, Odisha, Rajasthan, Tripura, and West Bengal additional support in their fight against Covid-19 (Union Ministry of Home Affairs 2020b). Assistance under the SDRF and NDRF was geared mainly towards meeting expenditure on quarantine measures and the procurement of essential equipment.

Moreover, states were provided with once-off central assistance of INR 42,567.9 million from the India Covid-19 Emergency Response and Health System Preparedness Package to set up dedicated hospitals and procure diagnostic and protection kits as well as other essentials for managing Covid-19. With a corpus fund of INR 150,000 million, the Package was created in April 2020 for strengthening national and state health systems and promoting pandemic research. Allocations to states were generally made on a combination of criteria such as case numbers and health infrastructure indexes (Union Ministry of Health and Family Welfare 2020a). To meet growing expenditure on health, states were also granted an additional borrowing limit of up to 2 per cent of gross state domestic product (GSDP) and permitted borrowing of 0.50 per cent of their respective GSDP from the market in the 2020–2021 financial year (Union Ministry of Finance 2020a).

In spite of these various measures by the central government, states have faced a severe cash-flow crisis. During April–June 2020, their fiscal deficit swelled to 36.5 per cent (The Print 2020b), adversely affecting expenditure on salaries and pensions as well as infrastructure, while their market borrowing in 2020–2021 soared to INR 3 trillion rupees – a figure estimated to be 52 per cent higher than borrowing in the previous year.

15.5 Findings and policy options

As this analysis shows, federalism in India was for all practical intents and purposes suspended during the Covid-19 pandemic in favour of highly centralised and personalised executive governance. The Indian polity accordingly tilted strongly towards unitary government: the power structure came to resemble a pyramid, with the Prime Minister placed at its apex and wielding extraordinary authority in commanding his subordinates at the state and local levels.

One explanation for this may be that the Constitution does not lay down a federal framework of pandemic governance. It is, indeed, a constitutional paradox that public health is a state matter, yet states are not allowed to govern it during a declared national disaster. The DMA 2005 entails a deeply unitary system of governance with little conformity to federal principles – as was evident in the practice it enabled, shaped, and sanctioned.

States were not part of central decision-making on the pandemic: a federal political culture of negotiated cooperation was missing, and neither states nor opposition parties were taken on board in any decision of the centre. Powers were concentrated in the centre; the normal functioning of centre-state relations was suspended. The centre exploited the pandemic to encroach upon important state-level fields such as agriculture, school and tertiary education, local economic, industrial and market operations, local transport, and intra-state movement of people and goods. The pandemic, in sum, did not retard or interrupt the general trend towards centralisation: it accelerated it.

Despite all the centre's measures, the pandemic continued to spread and intensify in its multiplying impacts. The lockdown failed to achieve its stated objective of breaking the chain of viral transmission; instead, the sudden declaration of a national lockdown caused the virus to spread from urban to rural areas due to massive labour migration. In the midst of all this, the federal government continued to control reporting on Covid-19 data, with the media and other independent agencies prevented from reporting any alternative information. The public had little option but to trust, or accept, central data on the pandemic.

By way of policy suggestions, there is, first, a need to review the DMA 2005, which was originally intended to respond to disasters on an emergency basis: it allows for short-duration centralisation and executive governance, but was never architected with a long-duration national pandemic emergency in mind. Thus, to cater for biological emergencies of an extended duration, it is necessary either to create a separate law or institution conforming to the principles of federalism and parliamentary accountability, or to amend the DMA 2005.

Secondly, the pandemic exposed the cracks in the system in India's primary and secondary levels of health care: even district hospitals, never mind grassroots facilities, lacked facilities adequate to the task of responding to a biological emergency. Given that the problem is due mainly to poor investment in health care, it needs to be re-emphasised, as has been done time and again, that the country should invest 2.5 per cent of its GDP in the health sector. The current budgetary allocation is insufficient to respond to biological emergencies such as Covid-19, while states are unable to meet rising health expenditure from their own pockets. There is hence a manifest need to revisit centre-state financial allocations.

References

Basu, Durga Das. 2019. 'Commentary on the Constitution of India' *Articles 311 to 368*, 9th ed. Vol. 14. Gurgaon: LexisNexis.

Basu, Durga Das. 2020. *Introduction to the Constitution of India*, 24th ed. Gurgaon: LexisNexis.

Bhaskar, V. and Vijay Kelkar. 2019. 'Financing Disaster Management: Options for the GST Council and the Fifteenth Finance Commission', *Economic & Political Weekly*, 54(25): 39–47.

Diamond, L. 2020. 'Democracy versus the Pandemic', *Foreign Affairs*, June 13, https://www.foreignaffairs.com/articles/world/2020-06-13/democracy-versus-pandemic (accessed on 13 February 2020).

Dutta, Anwesha and Harry W. Fischer. 2020. 'The Local Governance of Covid-19: Disease Prevention and Social Security in Rural India', *World Development*, 138: 105234.

Fifteenth Finance Commission. 2019. *Report for the year 2020–21*. New Delhi: PRS.

Gandhi, Supriya. 2020. 'When Toppling Monuments Serves Authoritarian Ends: India's Hindu Nationalists Erects an Imagined Past on Modern Ruins,' *Foreign Affairs* 13 July. https://www.foreignaffairs.com/articles/india/2020-07-13/when-toppling-monuments-serves-authoritarian-ends (accessed on 28 July 2020).

Jaffrelot, Christophe and Utsav Shah. 2020. 'The Health Care Gap', *The Indian Express*, 9 June.

Jain, M. P. 2019. *Indian Constitutional Law*, 7th ed. Vol. 1. Gurgaon: LexisNexis.

Kerala Chief Minister. 2020. 'Kerala's Fight against Covid-19', *Official Website of Chief Minister of Kerala Pinarayi Vijayan*, https://www.keralacm.gov.in/kerala-fight-against-covid-19/ (accessed on 24 September 2020).

Maps of India. 2020. 'Ruling Parties in Different States of India.' https://www.mapsofindia.com/maps/india/states-political-parties.html (accessed on 3 December 2020).

Office of the Registrar General and Census Commissioner of India, 2011. '2011 Census Data', https://censusindia.gov.in/2011-common/censusdata2011.html (accessed on 13 February 2020).

Mukherji, Rahul. 2020. 'Covid vs. Democracy: India's Illiberal Remedy', *Journal of Democracy*, 31(4): 91–105.

National Disaster Management Authority (NDMA). 2020a. 'Response to Covid-19: Kerala', https://ndma.gov.in/sites/default/files/PDF/covid/response-to-covid19-by-kerala.pdf (accessed on 20 October 2020).

National Disaster Management Authority (NDMA). 2020b. COVID-19 Impacts and Responses: The Indian Experience, January–May 2020. India: NDMA, https://ndma.gov.in/sites/default/files/PDF/covid/COVID-19-Indian-Experience.pdf (accessed on 20 October 2020).

National Disaster Management Authority (NDMA). 2020c. 'Response to COVID-19: Karnataka', https://www.ndma.gov.in/sites/default/files/PDF/covid/response-to-covid19-by-karnataka.pdf (accessed on 20 October 2020).

National Disaster Management Authority (NDMA). 2020d 'Response to COVID-19: Madhya Pradesh', https://ndma.gov.in/sites/default/files/PDF/covid/MP_English.pdf (accessed on 20 October 2020).

Nomani, Zafar Mahfooz and Rehana Parveen. 2020. 'Contextualising Epidemic Diseases (Amendment) Ordinance, 2020 in Epidemic-Pandemic Syndrome of Covid-19 in India', *Systematic Reviews in Pharmacy*, 11(8): 156–160.

Parliament of India, Rajya Sabha. 2020a. '229 Report on the "Management of Covid-19 Pandemic and Related Issues" of the Departmentally Related Standing Committee on Ministry of Home Affairs'. Report presented on 21 December.

Parliament of India, Rajya Sabha. 2020b. '123 Report on "the Outbreak of Pandemic Covid-19 and its Management" of the Departmentally Related Standing Committee on Ministry of Health and Family Welfare'. Report presented on 17 November.

Patnaik, Prabhat. 'Shadow of Fascism.' 2020. Frontline, April 12, https://frontline.thehindu.com/cover-story/article26641337.ece (accessed on 13 February 2020).

Picketty, Thomas. 2020. *Capital and Ideology*. Cambridge MA: The Belknap Press of Harvard University Press.

Press Information Bureau (PIB). 2020. 'States Briefed on Lockdown Measures and Guidelines', Release ID: 1608012, 24 March, https://pib.gov.in/Pressreleaseshare.aspx?PRID=1608012 (accessed on 24 March 2020).

PRS Legislative Research. 2020a. 'Demand for Grants 2020–21 Analysis: Health and Family Welfare', https://www.prsindia.org/parliamenttrack/budgets/demand-grants-2020-21-analysis-health-and-family-welfare (accessed on 18 May 2020).

PRS Legislative Research. 2020b. 'The Epidemic Diseases (Amendment) Bill, 2020', http://www.prsindia.org/billtrack/epidemic-diseases-amendment-ordinance-2020 (accessed on 3 December 2020).

Ramakrishnan, Venkitesh. 2020. 'Muting Parliament', *Frontline*, 37(19), 21–23.

Reserve Bank of India (RBI). 2019. *State Finances: A Study of Budgets of 2019–20.* Mumbai: RBI.

Reserve Bank of India (RBI). 2020. Press Release: 2020–2021/623, 11 November, https://www.rbi.org.in/Scripts/BS_PressReleaseDisplay.aspx?prid=50650 (accessed on 13 November 2020).

Salam, Ziya Us. 2020. 'Tablighi Jamaat: Vindicated, Finally', *Frontline*, 37(19). September 25, https://frontline.thehindu.com/the-nation/vindicated-finally/article32516103.ece (accessed on 13 February 2020).

Singh, Ajay Kumar. 2009. *Union Model of Indian Federalism.* New Delhi: Manak Publications.

Singh, Ajay Kumar. 2015. 'Constitutional Semantics and Autonomy within Indian Federalism', in Fransceco Palermo and Elisabeth Alber (eds), *Federalism and Decision Making: Changes in Structures, Procedures and Policies*, pp. 120–47, Leiden: Brill Nijhoff.

Singh, Ajay Kumar. 2019. 'An Emerging National Federalism.' *Seminar*, 717: 68–71.

Singh, M. P. and R. Saxena. 2015. 'Intergovernmental Relations in India: From Centralisation to Decentralisation', in Johanne Poirier, Cheryl Saunders, and John Kincaid (eds), *Intergovernmental Relations in Federal Systems: Comparative Structures and Dynamics*, pp. 239–271, Don Mills: Oxford University Press.

Tharoor, Shashi. 2020. *The Battle of Belonging: On Nationalism, Patriotism and what it means to be Indian.* New Delhi: Aleph Book Company.

The Indian Express. 2020a. *Issues in GST Compensation*, p. 13, August 29.

The Indian Express. 2020b. *GST Revenue Deficit: 20 States Get Nod to Borrow Rupees 68,825 Cr*, p. 15, October 14.

The Print. 2020a. 'In a Letter to PM Modi, Sonia Gandhi Says 21-Day Coronavirus Lockdown a "Welcome Step"', 26 March, https://theprint.in/india/in-letter-to-pm-modi-sonia-gandhi-says-21-day-coronavirus-lockdown-a-welcome-step/388697/ (accessed on 14 September 2020).

The Print. 2020b. '52% Higher Borrowing: Big Drop in Revenue – Why States Are Despairing about Their Finances', http://theprint.in/india/governance/52-higher-borrowing-big-drop-in-revenue-why-states-are-desparing-about-their-finances/501948/ (accessed on 19 October 2020).

Union Ministry of Finance. 2020a. 'Monthly Review of Accounts of Union Government of India Up to the Month of September, 2020 for the Financial Year 2020–21', https://pib.gov.in/PressReleasePage.aspx?PRID=1668448 (accessed on 29 October 2021).

Union Ministry of Finance. 2020b. Reply to Rajya Sabha Unstarred Question No 206, 15 September 2020.

Union Ministry of Health and Family Welfare. 2020a. PIB release ID 1669006. 31 October, http://pib.gov.in (accessed on 31 October 2020).'

Union Ministry of Home Affairs. 2020a. Reply to Lok Sabha Unstarred Question No. 1541. 20 September 2020.

Union Ministry of Home Affairs. 2020b. 'Press Release: Stimulus Package for COVID-19', 15 September, https://pib.gov.in/PressReleasePage.aspx?PRID=1654599 (accessed on 15 September 2020).

Union Ministry of Human Resource Development. 2020. *National Education Policy 2020.* https://www.education.gov.in/sites/upload_files/mhrd/files/NEP_Final_English_0.pdf (accessed on 20 October 2020).

Union Ministry of Information and Broadcasting. 2020. *India 2020.* New Delhi: Principal Director General, Publication Division.

Union Ministry of Law and Justice. 2019. The Citizenship (Amendment) Act, 2019. http://egazette.nic.in/WriteReadData/2019/214646.pdf (accessed on 15 October 2020).

United Nations, Department of Economic and Social Affairs, Population Division. 2019. *World Population Prospects 2019: Highlights*. New York: United Nations.

Vyas, Mahesh. 2020. '21 Million Salaried Jobs Lost', Centre for Monitoring Indian Economy (CMIE), 5 September, https://www.cmie.com/kommon/bin/sr.php?kall=warticle&dt=2020-09-07%2017:57:52&msec=996 (accessed on 20 Sept 2020).

World Bank. 2020. *GDP Growth (Annual %) – India*, https://data.worldbank.org/indicator/NY.GDP.MKTP.KD.ZG?locations=IN (accessed on 20 October 2020).

Yadav, Yogendra. 2020. *Making Sense of Indian Democracy*. Ranikher: Permanent Black.

16

THE AUSTRALIAN FEDERAL RESPONSE TO THE COVID-19 CRISIS

Momentary success or enduring reform?

Nicholas Aroney and Michael Boyce

16.1 Introduction

The Commonwealth of Australia is a federation of six constituent states and two self-governing territories. With an area of almost 7.7 million km², it is the world's sixth largest country and the only nation-state occupying an entire continent. With a total population of just over 25 million, Australia is one of the most sparsely populated countries in the world; however, it is also one of the most urbanised, with more than half of its population living in five urban centres of more than 1 million persons. The Australian states and territories differ vastly in land area and population. The largest state, Western Australia, is more than 2.2 million km², while the smallest, Tasmania, is less than 70,000 km²; the most populous state, New South Wales (NSW), has more than 7.7 million people, while the least populous, Tasmania, has a little over 520,000. Australia has a highly developed economy, with one of the largest gross domestic products (GDPs) per person in the world and with Australians enjoying an average life expectancy of more than 83 years – also among the highest in the world.

In 2020, Australia experienced two waves of Covid-19 cases, the first in March–April and the second in July–August. At the time of writing (November 2020), a total of more than 9 million Covid-19 tests had been administered, 27,668 cases confirmed, and 907 deaths recorded, 819 of which were in the State of Victoria. More than 93 per cent of Covid-19-related deaths were among persons older than 70, with 685 of these associated with aged-care facilities and 655 occurring in Victoria (Department of Health 2020c; Pagone and Briggs 2020: 2, 15). Cases and deaths were concentrated in densely populated urban centres; by contrast, there were many regional and remote communities that experienced very few or no cases.

DOI: 10.4324/9781003166771-21

The Australian policy response was coordinated between the Commonwealth, states, territories, and local government through a newly formed 'National Cabinet' consisting of the Prime Minister, the Premiers of the states and the First Ministers of the territories, supported by an array of health officers and expert advisers. This response was built on legislative frameworks and policy plans that were already in place to deal with national emergencies, including pandemics. Collectively, the implemented measures were remarkably successful in containing the virus despite occasional but serious administrative failures.

The main tension points concerned differences in policy goals (containment versus eradication) and the appropriate policy settings to achieve these goals (e.g., strict lockdowns and state border closures), with differences in political ideology as well as variations in local conditions driving disagreements between right-of-centre Liberal-National Party coalition governments at a Commonwealth level and in NSW, South Australia and Tasmania, and left-of-centre Labour Party governments in Victoria, Queensland, Western Australia, and the two territories. Despite these tensions, the federal system has worked relatively well overall, enabling a nationally coordinated approach with localised variations in governmental response, at least at a state and territory level, though not always in a manner well adjusted to the needs and circumstances of smaller local communities, especially in remote regions.

16.2 The federal constitutional and legislative framework

Under the Australian Constitution, the states continue to exercise the general legislative, executive, and judicial powers they possessed prior to federation, while the Commonwealth is vested with overriding legislative powers over a range of specific topics. These powers enable the Commonwealth to control Australia's national borders, such as by restricting entry of persons into the country and imposing quarantine requirements. In most other respects, governmental responses to the Covid-19 pandemic were implemented by the states and territories, including management of hospitals and intensive care facilities, restrictions on personal movement and interaction, and imposition of social distancing and lockdown requirements. The powers of both the Commonwealth and the states are subject, however, to a constitutional requirement that 'trade, commerce and intercourse' among the states be 'absolutely free', potentially restricting their ability to control personal movement across state borders.

The Commonwealth, states, and territories each have their own democratically elected legislatures and executive governments responsible to those legislatures. They also have independent taxing and spending powers, except that the Commonwealth has a constitutional monopoly over taxes on goods and has in effect monopolised taxes on individual and corporate income. Consequently, the states are dependent on the Commonwealth for approximately half of their revenues and the Commonwealth has the capacity to make conditional grants to the states that require them to pursue particular policies and meet operational benchmarks. The Commonwealth also has much greater capacity to provide general financial support and welfare benefits by way of income supplementation and economic stimulus.

Local governments, on the other hand, are creatures of the states and have had relatively limited capacity to develop policies responsive to the pandemic. Nonetheless, they initiated measures to support local communities and businesses, such as through relief from council rates, fees and other taxes, and engaged with state and territory governments in developing and implementing coordinated government responses.

The constitutional settings of the Australian federal system enable three principal modes of governmental response: (1) *independent* policy-making by the Commonwealth, states, and territories, each exercising autonomous powers of governance within its particular jurisdiction; (2) *coordinated* policy-making based on agreement among the Commonwealth, state, and territory governments, each exercising its constitutional powers as mutually agreed; and (3) *coercive* policy-making by the Commonwealth using its overriding legislative powers and financial capacities to determine or shape the policies to be implemented by the states and territories. The extent to which each of these approaches is adopted in response to any emergent issue or problem has significant implications for the efficiency and effectiveness of the policy response. As Alan Fenna (2020: 1) has put it:

> Federalism might have hindered an effective response to the crisis by creating obstacles to action or discoordination. On the other hand, it might have encouraged a proportional and appropriate response by opening the way to regionally varied measures and by mustering the greater wisdom of a more collective decision-making process.

16.3 Preparedness for a national disaster: The institutional framework

Prior to the emergence of the pandemic, the Commonwealth, states, and territories had enacted legislation authorising the use of emergency powers to respond to bio-security threats, such as by imposing quarantine requirements, restricting movement, controlling commerce, and prohibiting gatherings. These included the National Health Security Act of 2007, which establishes a national system of public health surveillance, and the Biosecurity Act of 2015, which facilitates management of biosecurity risks and emergencies. The Biosecurity Act gives the federal Health Minister expansive powers to issue directions and impose requirements to combat human biosecurity emergencies. Each state and territory also has its own disaster response and public health laws which authorise officials to declare a state of emergency and issue orders and directions to deal with natural disasters and public health emergencies.

The Commonwealth had also developed the Australian Health Management Plan for Pandemic Influenza (AHMPPI), which was used to guide Australia's response to the H1N1 pandemic in 2009 and was revised in 2014 and again in late 2019 (Department of Health 2019). More broadly, in 2011 the Council of Australian Governments (COAG) adopted a National Strategy for Disaster Resilience to support the development of coordinated policies at all levels of government for preventing, preparing for, responding to, and recovering from disasters of all kinds (Council of Australian Governments, 2011). Following Australia's adoption of the United Nations Sendai Framework for Disaster Risk Reduction 2015–2030, the country's policies also focused on preventing the emergence of new disaster risks and reducing existing ones. This is reflected in the National Disaster Risk Reduction Framework (2018), which was co-designed by all three levels of government with input from the private sector.

16.3.1 *Commonwealth*

The Biosecurity Act was enacted to manage biosecurity risks caused by diseases and pests entering, establishing or spreading in any part of Australian territory and thereby causing harm to human, animal or plant health, to the environment or, as a consequence, to the economy. To enact the statute, the Commonwealth relied on an array of legislative powers. Recognising that the Act presses these powers to their outer constitutional limits, and quite possibly beyond them, a 'severance' clause was included which provides that the Act is to have the effect it would have if its operation were limited to its constitutionally valid operation under any one of these alternative heads of power. To date there have been no court cases testing the constitutionality of the Act, even though its constitutionality is in some respects questionable (Aroney 2020: 14).

The Act empowers the Commonwealth Chief Medical Officer (CMO) to issue 'biosecurity control orders' in respect of persons exposed to 'listed' diseases. Recognising the federal context, the CMO must first consult with the state and territory chief health officers (CHOs) before doing so. Biosecurity control orders can require a person to provide contact information, report signs or symptoms, remain confined to his or her place of residence, wear particular clothing or equipment, undergo decontamination, undergo examination, provide body samples, or receive vaccination, treatment or medication.

The Biosecurity Act has been described as 'shift[ing] the constitutional boundaries between the Commonwealth and States with respect to civil emergencies' (Lee 2018: 170) and as 'an unprecedented expansion of power by the federal executive' (Brenker 2020), particularly because it encroaches on areas of regulation which would usually be within the states' domain and because Parliament has delegated to the executive branch the power to legislate and override pre-existing legislation. Possibly for these reasons, the powers available under the Biosecurity Act have been exercised sparingly and only in relation to matters generally outside of the states' areas of primary responsibility or control (see Section 4.2).

16.3.2 States and territories

The states and territories have passed general emergency management laws that confer an array of extraordinary powers on public officials following the declaration of a state of emergency. Of special relevance to the Covid-19 crisis is that Public Health Acts in each jurisdiction allow for the declaration of a state of public health emergency, triggering specific emergency powers that can be exercised following such a declaration. In some jurisdictions (Queensland, Victoria prior to August 2020, and the two territories), these powers have been exercised exclusively by their respective CHOs. In the largest jurisdiction, NSW, it is the responsible minister who issues public health orders directly, while in three other states (Western Australia, Tasmania, and South Australia), the responsibility to exercise emergency powers is shared between the public health authorities and the general emergency authorities, giving rise to risks of administrative overlap.

The powers exercisable by the CHOs are extensive. They include powers to detain or restrict the movement of persons; restrict contact between persons; prevent entry into the jurisdiction; close any premises; enter any premises without a warrant; search for and seize anything; subject persons and places to decontamination procedures; direct persons to undergo medical observations, examinations or treatments; direct the destruction of any substance or thing; and issue any other directions considered reasonably necessary to protect public health.

16.4 Rolling out measures to contain the pandemic

Having conferred most of the necessary powers by legislation, the Australian parliaments played a largely passive role during the Covid-19 crisis. The bulk of the decision-making was undertaken by the executive and administrative branches of government, particularly by public health officials. Most intergovernmental coordination was executive-led, principally through the conversion of the preexisting COAG into the newly minted National Cabinet, which met frequently throughout the crisis. The National Cabinet generally exhibited a notable degree of unity when compared with the often fractious intergovernmental relationships that tended to characterise COAG. The Prime Minister exercised leadership but appeared most often to have sought to develop policy responses by consensus on the basis of shared expert advice. This allowed each jurisdiction to tailor its particular measures to its specific conditions, including in addressing some residual disagreement over policy goals and means. Through these mechanisms, the Prime Minister brokered what may prove to be an enduring change to the system of intergovernmental relations in Australia, even if the underlying political and fiscal tensions will remain and could become more apparent as time goes by.

16.4.1 Taking the initiative

On 21 January 2020, after undertaking the required consultations with his state and territory counterparts, the then CMO, Dr Brendan Murphy, determined that the 'human coronavirus with pandemic potential' was a listed human disease due to its communicable nature and its potential to cause significant harm to human health. This determination activated an array of powers under the Biosecurity Act. Two days later, Australian federal biosecurity officials began screening arrivals on flights from Wuhan, China, seven days before Covid-19 was declared a pandemic by the World Health Organisation. Another two days later, Australia recorded its first case.

On 1 February 2020, the Commonwealth government required returning citizens who had been in mainland China to self-quarantine for 14 days, and closed the border to all foreign nationals arriving from that country. The same rules were soon applied to persons who had been in Iran, South Korea, and Italy. During this time, the Australian states and territories initiated testing and contact-tracing regimes, while hospital, intensive care, and ventilator capacities were ramped up across the country. From 16 March, all travellers arriving in Australia from any destination were required to self-isolate for 14 days, and on 20 March the national border was entirely closed to non-residents and non-citizens. These measures were supplemented by a declaration by the Governor-General on 18 March that a human biosecurity emergency existed with respect to Covid-19, triggering additional powers under the Biosecurity Act. On the same day, the federal Minister for Health used these additional powers to prevent international cruise ships from entering Australian ports except in specific circumstances.

These and other measures limited the initial spread of the disease, such that of the 300 cases identified by mid-March 2020, most were returning travellers. However, towards the end of that month, as instances of community transmission increased and national case numbers doubled every three to four days, the Commonwealth, states, and territories agreed to a nationally coordinated lockdown in which indoor and outdoor gatherings were restricted to two persons, with only limited exceptions. Several states and territories also introduced hard border closures and restrictions on travel. These latter policies resulted in a significant 'flattening of the curve' that was evident by early April. This trend continued into early June, with daily cases declining to less than 10 new cases per day, compared to a high of 460 daily cases on 28 March. The states and territories thereafter eased internal restrictions, but several maintained their respective state border closures.

Australia's relative success in controlling the spread of the virus occurred despite notable administrative failures, including the disembarkation of some 2,700 passengers from the Ruby Princess cruise liner in Sydney on 19 March 2020 without undergoing quarantine (Walker 2020). From early June, a second wave of infections became apparent, peaking in late July and early August at a high of 721 cases on 30 July. The vast bulk of these new cases were concentrated in the city of Melbourne due to another policy failure, this time involving the use of poorly trained private security guards to monitor the state's hotel quarantine system.

The Victorian Government initially responded to the second wave through localised lockdowns focused on particular infection clusters in Melbourne and elsewhere, but these measures were not effective and in early August 2020 movement restrictions were implemented throughout the state, with even more severe restrictions imposed in Melbourne, including a controversial nightly curfew. These measures reduced the number of daily cases substantially, such that by mid-November no new cases had been reported for the previous 10 days (Department of Health and Human Services (Vic) 2020). During this period the Victorian Government had relaxed restrictions only very cautiously, giving rise to considerable controversy within the state as well as disagreements with both the Prime Minister and the Lord Mayor of the City of Melbourne.

The Australian Government initially framed its policy response around the goal of flattening the curve (Department of Health 2020b), based on models aimed at suppressing the virus in order to maintain health-care capacity (Moss et al. 2020). Some argued, however, that Australia should aim to eliminate the virus altogether, calling for an 8- to 12-week shutdown. Others responded that a sustained lockdown would have detrimental effects not only on the economy but on mental health as well as the diagnosis and treatment of other serious diseases, many of them more lethal than Covid-19. There was also debate about the effectiveness of particular measures, such as lockdowns, border closures and masking (Chaudhry et al. 2020; Hopman and Mehtar 2020), which gave rise to competing petitions by medical experts about what should be done.

Although the Australian response was relatively well coordinated between jurisdictions, differing assessments of the relative importance of these factors in the light of differing understandings of appropriate policy responses were at the heart of policy disagreements between the Commonwealth and the states and among the states themselves. The argument advanced by the Commonwealth's Deputy CMO that eradication was, in any case, an unrealistic goal (Coatsworth 2020) seemed to be vindicated as the second wave enveloped the State of Victoria through the winter months.

On 18 February 2020, the Commonwealth issued an emergency response plan for the Covid-19 pandemic, setting out a national approach designed to guide the Australian health sector's response to the pandemic (Department of Health 2020a). The plan, among other things, was meant to enable the state and Territory health systems to provide the highest quality medical care and to guide the efficient allocation and use of resources. Among its stated aims was to develop a whole-of-government framework at Commonwealth, state, territory, and local levels that protects Australia's social functioning and economy and minimises the outbreak's impact on the health of Australians. The plan was specific as to the particular responsibilities of the Commonwealth and the states and territories, and indicated several responsibilities to be undertaken jointly.

As noted, at a meeting of COAG on 13 March 2020, the Commonwealth, state, and territory governments agreed to establish a new National Cabinet, consisting of the Prime Minister, Premiers and Chief Ministers, which would meet at least weekly to coordinate the country's response to Covid-19. The Prime Minister sought to constitute the new body as a Cabinet Office Policy Committee operating in accordance with the conventions of the Commonwealth cabinet, among them the guiding principles of collective responsibility, solidarity, and confidentiality. The body is not a 'cabinet' in the ordinary sense of the word, however, because its members are not collectively responsible to the one parliament but individually responsible to their respective parliaments, and it is not clear how the usual conventions of cabinet responsibility, solidarity, and confidentiality could apply to it. Its success has depended on the commitment of the Prime Minister, Premiers, and Chief Ministers and their willingness to implement the National Cabinet's collective decisions within their respective jurisdictions. Despite its general effectiveness, considerable debate attended its unique and novel features and the likelihood of its continued operation once the crisis has passed (see Section 16.4.5).

16.4.2 Commonwealth action

The Commonwealth's actions fall into three categories: firstly, the leading role it took in coordinating government responses to the crisis; secondly, its primary fiscal role in implementing economic stimulus packages and providing additional funding to the states and territories to meet the needs of the emergency; and, thirdly, its attention to matters falling specifically within its responsibilities under the Constitution. As noted, although the powers available to the Commonwealth under the Biosecurity Act are vast, they were used only in relation to matters broadly of national interest or concern, including overseas travel, retail outlets at international airports, remote indigenous communities, cruise ships, the 'Covid Safe' app, and the distribution of 'essential goods' such as face masks and hand sanitiser. The Commonwealth parliament had a mostly passive role during the crisis. During a one-day sitting on 23 March 2020, however, it passed an Omnibus Bill approving, among other things, a stimulus package of AUD 66 billion and an amendment to the Biosecurity Act enabling biosecurity control orders to be issued by public service employees in the Health Department.

The Commonwealth's financial assistance measures included an additional fixed 'Coronavirus Supplement' payment added onto existing welfare scheme payments, more relaxed income and assets test standards for the existing JobSeeker scheme (welfare payments for unemployed job hunters), introduction of a new JobKeeper wage subsidy to keep at-risk employees from losing their jobs and a JobMaker Hiring Credit scheme to incentivise businesses in employing additional young employees, as well as certain measures aimed at preventing termination of commercial leases and relieving company directors from personal liability for insolvent trading by their companies.

Many of the deaths from Covid-19 in Australia were associated with aged-care facilities. Under the Constitution, responsibility for such matters ordinarily falls to the states and territories, but over time the Commonwealth has become increasingly responsible for their funding and regulation (Tracey and Briggs 2019: 42–46). The Commonwealth provided guidance and additional funding to aged-care facilities throughout the Covid-19 crisis (Pagone and Briggs 2020: 4–6). However, a recent Royal Commission report identified significant short-falls in the system, including conflicting advice provided by Commonwealth and NSW officials in relation to the movement into hospital of infected aged-care residents and failures to properly manage the outbreak of infections in Victorian aged-care facilities. The Royal Commission recommended the establishment of a national aged-care advisory body, promulgation of clear protocols regarding Commonwealth and state responsibilities, and appointment of trained infection-control officers in elderly care facilities (Pagone and Briggs 2020). These recommendations were accepted by the Commonwealth (Colbeck 2020).

The Commonwealth also provided support to the states and territories through the provision of large numbers of Australian Defence Force (ADF) personnel to help with quarantine compliance, contact tracing, border controls, and similar tasks. This became a point of political controversy following Victoria's bungling of its hotel quarantine program when it emerged that the Prime Minister's offers of ADF assistance had been ignored or refused by the Victorian Government. It was alleged that the poorly trained security guards employed to monitor hotel quarantine had engaged in sexual relations with persons under quarantine, contributing to the second wave of infections that required a second shutdown of the state. The scandal led to the resignation of the Minister for Health. The Victorian Government established a board of inquiry to investigate the actions of government agencies, hotel operators, and private contractors (Coate 2020).

16.4.3 State and territory action

The state and territory emergency management and public health laws allow declarations of emergency to be made and enable emergency powers to be exercised. These powers have been described as 'both extensive and highly elastic': they include the power to compel individuals in a broad range of ways and confer wide discretion on the relevant decision-maker (Carter 2020: 117, 127). In 2020, all jurisdictions except NSW declared a public health emergency, while Tasmania, Western Australia, South Australia, and Victoria also declared a state of emergency under their emergency management laws. In Victoria, a state of disaster declaration was not made until 2 August 2020, at which point it was deemed necessary as a response to a uniquely aggressive second wave of infections.

The particular measures taken by each state and territory were formulated within the National Cabinet framework. The latter enabled each jurisdiction to implement agreed policies in ways considered suitable to local conditions and to adopt specific measures to respond to particular challenges. These measures were ramped up when Covid-19 infections increased in March 2020, relaxed after they declined in April and May, ramped up again as infections increased, especially in Victoria, in July and August, and gradually relaxed in September and October. At the height of the second wave of infections, restrictions in Victoria were much more extensive than those in other states. By mid-November, in Queensland there were only relatively minor restrictions on gatherings, businesses and other activities and travel within the state, whereas in Victoria masks still had to be worn in public and gatherings in homes remained restricted (Victorian Government 2020).

All states except Victoria imposed strict border controls. The extent of these restrictions varied over time, ranging from 14-day quarantine requirements and targeted restrictions on travel by infected persons from particular hotspots to blanket bans with only minor exemptions. In response to prolonged border closures in states such as Western Australia, Commonwealth government ministers emphasised the importance of inter-state trade for the national economy, with the NSW Premier criticising the Queensland Government for imposing unrealistic conditions on the reopening of its borders. Apex business bodies criticised the 'patchwork of inconsistent state and territory-based rules that ignore the reality of the way small and large businesses operate across borders and Australians live their lives' (Ferguson et al. 2020). Similar tensions emerged about the maintenance of strict lockdown requirements in Victoria for indefinitely long periods without a sufficiently transparent set of criteria and timetable for their relaxation (Wells et al. 2020). In response to criticism by the Commonwealth Health Minister, the Victorian Premier argued that Victorian health officers and politicians have a better understanding of conditions within the state. However, similar complaints were made by local government leaders in regional Victoria, who expressed concerns about the state government's failure to understand or take into consideration conditions in regional areas.

The organisational structure of the state and territory health departments was also significant. In NSW, a decentralised system of local area health districts enabled the state to implement a relatively effective system of contact tracing from the outset, whereas in Victoria a highly centralised health department had to build contact-tracing capacity from a very limited local base, with much less success. The devolved public health units in NSW already had well-established links with local health providers and community leaders and were in a better position to understand the local social and cultural factors that determine the spread of the disease and the human response to government requirements (Bennett 2020).

The border restrictions gave rise to legal challenges on the basis that they contravene the constitutional requirement that inter-state 'trade, commerce and intercourse' must be 'absolutely free' (Constitution, section 92). This protection was seen by the framers of the Constitution as an essential element of the federal compact between the states (Aroney et al. 2015: 310–13). The expression of this protection in such sweeping and unqualified terms – 'absolutely free' – is extraordinary, especially given the otherwise precise and often technical language used in the Constitution. However, the High Court has found ways to restrict the apparently unlimited scope of section 92 (*Cole v. Whitfield* (1988) 165 CLR 360). The Court has accepted that laws can validly impose burdens on both trade and commerce and personal movement across state borders provided that such laws pursue a legitimate objective in a proportionate manner (*Cunliffe v. Commonwealth* (1994) 182 CLR 272).

The critical question is how to determine whether a law is proportionate, for such questions require the Court to weigh the competing public interests. Part of the reason why it has been difficult to predict the result of the constitutional challenges to the state border closures is that the exact test to be applied to determine their validity is not entirely settled. This uncertainty is then compounded by the complexity of the issues raised by government attempts to limit or prevent the spread of Covid-19 in the community.

The one sustained challenge to the border closures was brought by mining billionaire Clive Palmer against the border regime implemented by the State of Western Australia. Although Palmer wished to travel from Queensland to Western Australia to manage his Perth-based business, he did not classify as an exempt traveller under the Western Australia Directions and therefore was prohibited from entry into the state. His case depended on expert evidence concerning the reasonable need for and efficacy of the closure of the state border. On 25 August 2020, a Federal Court judge found that border controls are an accepted and effective component of the public health response to the control of infectious disease outbreaks. Notably, this finding was based on evidence provided by epidemiological and public health experts and did not take into consideration the economic, social, and individual impacts of the border closures, even though these factors could be relevant to a determination of whether the measures were reasonably proportionate.

However, on 6 November the High Court resolved the case on what may be called technical grounds (*Palmer & Anor v. The State of Western Australia & Anor* [2020] HCATrans 180). It determined that the relevant sections of the statute under which the Directions had been made complied with the requirements of section 92 of the Constitution and that the question of whether the Directions were validly authorised by those sections did not raise a constitutional question.

16.4.4 Local government action

As noted, local government is a creature of the states and its responsibilities are relatively limited. However, a role for local government was envisaged by the Commonwealth's emergency response plan (Department of Health 2020a: 2.4, 4.2.1). According to this plan, local government responsibilities are mostly supportive rather than regulative, although they do include representing the interests of local communities in broader planning processes and providing feedback on the effectiveness of government activities. Some local government researchers observed that these functions go beyond anything that local government has recently been expected to perform (Zierke 2020: 3). However, it can also be noted that several of them are already recognised functions of local government in the various state local government Acts.

The governments of Australia's three most populous states (NSW, Victoria, and Queensland) established dedicated websites with information and guidance for local governments. A survey of initiatives taken by the local councils of Australia's three most populous cities (Sydney, Melbourne, and Brisbane) located in these three states suggests they sought to communicate health-related information from their respective health departments; assist state authorities in contact tracing and encouraging testing and wearing of masks; implement measures to support businesses and facilitate economic recovery; and support physical and mental health and maintain community connection (City of Melbourne 2020; City of Sydney 2020; Queensland Government 2020).

However, this is to focus attention on the largest and most urbanised population centres in the three largest states. In the local government field, questions are being asked about whether government handling of the crisis illustrates problems associated with excessive centralisation of decision-making at state and federal levels vis-à-vis local government, especially in remote regions. A persistent criticism of state government lockdowns and border closures has been that they have tended to adopt state-wide policies focused on containment of the virus within large cities without sufficient adaptability or flexibility for regional and remote areas where the incidence of the virus is minimal or non-existent. This is partly a consequence of the perceived need for urgent and extreme action, but it is also an artefact of a centralised decision-making process driven by urban-based experts. It is an open question whether local governments in regional and remote areas would have made the same policy decisions for their particular communities based on the same information about the incidence, spread, and impact of the virus available to decision-makers at a state level.

Other issues that particularly affected local governments were pressures placed on local recreational areas and parks and local-government-managed caravan parks, which were under increased pressure during lockdowns and as a result of border closures (Zierke 2020: 8–11). In the October 2020 budget, the Commonwealth expanded the existing Local Roads and Community Infrastructure program with an additional AUD 1 billion for councils to immediately upgrade local roads, footpaths, and street lighting, complemented by the availability of an AUD 1.2 billion wage subsidy programme for trainees and apprentices and several other funding initiatives.

16.4.5 Intergovernmental relations

Most of Australia's responses to the Covid-19 crisis took place in the context of a coordinated all-of-government approach led by the Commonwealth but cooperatively agreed to by the states and territories within the newly developed National Cabinet process. While each jurisdiction exercised its constitutional powers independently and with important dimensions of diversity, this occurred within an agreed framework.

In making its risk assessments and policy decisions, the National Cabinet was informed primarily by an array of expert bodies that developed guidelines intended to provide nationally consistent advice to public health units concerning case management and contact tracing (Communicable Diseases Network Australia 2020). Other bodies were responsible for identifying issues to be addressed, assessing the resources and capabilities required to mitigate impacts, and coordinating activities with stakeholders in sectors such as education, public safety and policing, banking, transport, food, and agriculture in the development of public–private partnerships for anticipating and mitigating the social and economic effects of the pandemic (Department of Home Affairs (Cth) 2020).

On 29 May 2020, the National Cabinet took the further step of agreeing to the formation of the National Federation Reform Council (NFRC) and the cessation of COAG as the primary forum of intergovernmental relations (Department of the Prime Minister and Cabinet 2020). The Prime Minister claimed that the NFRC would change the way in which the Commonwealth, states, and territories address emergent issues requiring reform, with the intention that the new model would streamline processes and thus enable improved collaboration, communication, and effectiveness. A degree of continuity would be preserved, however, with particular COAG taskforces continuing to address their assigned matters.

By the end of 2020, the National Cabinet continued to function as the apex intergovernmental body coordinating the Commonwealth, state, and Territory responses to the crisis. The outcomes of its meeting of 23 October 2020 illustrate its capacity to facilitate cooperative federalism while also reflecting underlying tensions. On the one hand, the Commonwealth and seven of the states and territories agreed to a new framework for 'national reopening' (i.e., relaxation of restrictions), but with the notable disagreement of Western Australia, which was unwilling to 'cede control' over its border (McNeill 2020). On the other hand, all nine jurisdictions accepted the recommendations of a review of the old COAG councils and ministerial forums which was highly critical of inefficient and often ineffective, convoluted, and over-bureaucratised arrangements (Conran 2020: 2).

Noting the way in which the National Cabinet processes had enabled ministers and chief executive officers to cut through issues to agree on nationally coordinated responses, the report recommended disbanding numerous ministerial forums and rationalising others, greater ministerial control over agendas, and substantial reductions in administrative staffing (Conran 2020: 5–8). The implications of these and other changes may prove significant. To what extent do they signal a lasting change in Australian intergovernmental relations?

While described as a 'council', COAG was more in the nature of an occasional summit meeting of Australia's heads of government. It never 'existed' as a standing body established constitutionally or by legislation. Instead, it was an intermittent forum in which Australian political leaders met to discuss and adopt coordinated policies on issues of public importance. Its meetings were infrequent, fleeting, bureaucratised, and often politicised. In its early days, COAG was a collaborative body that achieved significant reforms, but its agenda and processes became increasingly dominated by the Commonwealth. At times it enabled significant intergovernmental cooperation, but it was also the site of acrimonious disagreement and contributed to 'executive federalism' in which democratic accountability and parliamentary responsibility are side-lined (Aroney 2017: 199).

Several structural features of the National Cabinet distinguish it from COAG. Firstly, while the National Cabinet plans to continue meeting monthly after Covid-19, COAG generally met only biannually. Secondly, the membership of COAG and the National Cabinet are not identical. While the National Cabinet is composed solely of the executive heads of each state, territory, and the Commonwealth, COAG's final membership also included representation of local government through the President of the Australian Local Government Association (ALGA). Under the new arrangements it appears the ALGA will be represented only at the annual meeting of the NFRC.

Thirdly, while COAG facilitated coordination of a wide range of matters, the old intergovernmental councils and ministerial forums will be drastically reduced under the National Cabinet scheme to several of the most important, such as education, energy, environment, health and infrastructure (Conran 2020: 5). Fourthly, whereas COAG processes were highly bureaucratised, it is intended that councils and ministerial meetings will be radically streamlined (Conran 2020: 7). Fifthly, in accordance with its establishment as a Cabinet Office Policy Committee, it is proposed that National Cabinet processes will be subject to cabinet secrecy and its decisions released only if the Prime Minister decides to do so. By contrast, COAG decisions were expected to be made public within the week of their being made.

The future of the National Cabinet is unknown and difficult to predict. The underlying political conditions for cabinet solidarity are not present because its members are drawn from and responsible to different parliaments and represent competing political party platforms and interests. The potential for division and disagreement was illustrated early on when, following the National Cabinet meeting of 22 March 2020, the NSW and Victorian Premiers and the Chief Minister of the Australian Capital Territory (ACT) appeared to break ranks by recommending that parents keep their school-aged children home from school, whereas the Federal Government maintained that schools should remain open.

This need not be seen as a weakness but rather a strength of the system, for the National Cabinet deliberately identified areas of coordinated action, leaving each jurisdiction free to make its own determinations about how best to implement those decisions and what other policies might be appropriate or necessary to meet the specific conditions and needs of each locality. As Cheryl Saunders (2020: 4) has observed, disagreements among the jurisdictions 'did not detract from the National Cabinet as an effective, genuinely intergovernmental process, responding to an urgent public need in ways the public could trust'.

Nonetheless, as Saunders also points out, a key ongoing question is whether the National Cabinet will continue to embody a form of executive federalism, or whether ways will be found to accommodate the important roles of the state and territory parliaments and cabinets in the system of intergovernmental relations in Australia (Saunders 2020: 4). Too many reform efforts in the past have served only to underscore the 'governmentality' of the Australian system, with changes that were supposed to improve accountability to the people resulting actually in increased accountability of the states and territories to Commonwealth bureaucrats (Aroney 2010: 75, 81).

16.4.6 Intergovernmental fiscal relations

The Commonwealth took a lead role in providing the very substantial funding required for emergency medical supplies and economic stimulus during the crisis. Early on, on 12 March 2020, it announced an AUD 17.6 billion stimulus package to protect jobs, which was soon followed on 22 March with a second stimulus package of AUD 66 billion. In addition, at the COAG meeting of 13 March 2020 a new 50–50 shared-funding deal between the Commonwealth, states, and territories was announced to support more effective assessment, diagnosis, and treatment of people with the coronavirus. By the time of the federal budget in early October 2020, the Commonwealth had spent or committed a total of AUD 198 billion to economic stimulus and health measures. These measures are significant because, while the states and territories own and run their own public hospital systems, they are dependent upon the Commonwealth for about 50 per cent of their funding.

Despite the radical nature of the reforms associated with the newly evolving National Cabinet system, it appears that the Council on Federal Financial Relations (CFFR), which consists of the treasurers of the Commonwealth, states, and territories, will continue to play a central role. This role includes reviewing all funding agreements between the Commonwealth and the states with a view to rationalising and consolidating them, as well as acting as the 'gatekeeper' for new agreements (Conran 2020: 18, 28). The long-term implications for federal-state financial relationship remain to be seen.

16.5 Findings and policy implications

Governmental responses to policy crises are shaped by institutional structures and decision-making processes. In unitary states, decision-making power is constitutionally concentrated in a single locus of governmental authority, whereas in federations it is constitutionally distributed. Federations thus enable democratically accountable governance to be conducted at the relatively smaller scale as well as on a whole-of-federation basis. This allows state governments to be more responsive to the needs and expectations of their respective populations. However, local governments in Australia are subordinate institutions: their powers and responsibilities are dependent and derivative; they lack constitutional self-determination and their jurisdiction is determined by state legislation.

A disease like Covid-19 does not respect national, state, or local boundaries. The spread of the disease in Australia has depended on patterns of human interaction, spreading most rapidly among mobile and concentrated populations in the major cities and large towns, while having less impact in regional centres and very little in rural areas. Governmental responses were obviously needed, but the pattern of the disease required different measures at national, state, and local levels. Very restrictive measures were instituted among concentrated populations, but the application of such measures in places where the impact of the disease was minimal or non-existent may have been excessively restrictive and could have resulted in an inefficient allocation of resources. Given the need for both general coordination and localised flexibility, how well has the particular federal configuration of governmental power in Australia facilitated a policy response that achieves both of these objectives?

Australia was relatively well prepared for the Covid-19 crisis. Legislation was in place at Commonwealth, state, and territory levels, and several policy documents detailed system-wide coordinated response plans for an array of emergency situations, including an influenza pandemic. While the powers available to the Commonwealth under the Biosecurity Act are extensive, they were used sparingly and only in relation to matters generally outside of the states' areas of primary responsibility. As might have been expected, the Commonwealth was the major financier of the coordinated response, whereas most of the regulatory measures were implemented by the states and territories pursuant to their respective laws, with important administrative and policy differences in each jurisdiction.

This did not mean that the jurisdictions acted independently. Rather, their actions were coordinated by the newly minted National Cabinet. This enabled a coordinated government response, based on shared expert advice, with each government implementing particularised policies within this framework based on the specific conditions and needs of its jurisdiction. Much of it was remarkably cooperative, but there were also political disagreements and disputes between the Commonwealth and the states and territories, as well as among the states themselves.

The relative success of the National Cabinet has depended on the political goodwill of the Prime Minister, Premiers, and Chief Ministers. However, considerable debate has attended its novel features and the likelihood of its continued effective operation once the crisis has passed. The jury is still out as to whether it will facilitate genuinely improved collaboration, effectiveness, and accountability in the long term. While substantial reforms have been implemented, there are also signs that cooperation is waning and 'politics-as-usual' may be returning.

Furthermore, while a whole-of-government approach was adopted, there are questions whether centralised decision-making at state level allowed sufficient adaptability or flexibility for regional and remote local government areas where the incidence of the virus was minimal or non-existent. Moreover, NSW's devolved public health system enabled it to implement a more effective contact-tracing regime than Victoria's more centralised system, and the exclusion of local government representation from the regular meetings of the National Cabinet was a point of contention. Nonetheless, in spite of occasional significant policy failures and administrative errors, the Australian response was remarkably effective in controlling the spread of the virus, suggesting the capacity of the Australian federal system to respond to a global crisis in a manner which is both centrally coordinated and regionally differentiated.

References

Aroney, Nicholas. 2010. 'Reinvigorating Australian Federalism', in Michael White and Aladin Rahemtula (eds), *Supreme Court History Program Yearbook 2009*, pp. 75–87. Brisbane: Supreme Court Library Queensland.

Aroney, Nicholas. 2017. 'Reforming Australian Federalism: The White Paper Process in Comparative Perspective', in Mark Bruerton et al. (eds), *A People's Federation*, ch. 12. Annandale: The Federation Press.

Aroney, Nicholas. 2020. 'What Remains of the Engineers Case? A Centenary Appraisal', *Australian Law Journal*, 94: 684–98.

Aroney, Nicholas, et al. 2015. *The Constitution of the Commonwealth of Australia: History, Principle and Interpretation.* Melbourne: Cambridge University Press.

Bennett, Catherine. 2020. 'Where Did Victoria Go So Wrong with Contact Tracing and Have They Fixed It?', *The Conversation*, 13 October, https://theconversation.com/where-did-victoria-go-so-wrong-with-contact-tracing-and-have-they-fixed-it-147993 (accessed on 23 November 2020).

Brenker, Stephanie. 2020. 'An Executive Grab for Power during COVID-19?', *Australian Public Law Online*, May 13, https://auspublaw.org/2020/05/an-executive-grab-for-power-during-covid-19/ (accessed on 15 August 2020).

Carter, David J. 2020. 'The Use of Coercive Public Health and Human Biosecurity Law in Australia: An Empirical Analysis', *University of New South Wales Law Journal*, 43(1): 117–54.

Chaudhry, Rabail et al. 2020. 'A Country Level Analysis Measuring the Impact of Government Actions, Country Preparedness and Socioeconomic Factors on COVID-19 Mortality and Related Health Outcomes', *EClinicalMedicine*, 25: 100464.

City of Melbourne. 2020. 'Coronavirus (COVID-19)', City of Melbourne, https://www.melbourne.vic.gov.au/community/health-support-services/health-services/Pages/novel-coronavirus.aspx (accessed on 7 November 2020).

City of Sydney. 2020. 'Covid-19 pandemic', City of Sydney, https://www.cityofsydney.nsw.gov.au/covid-19 (accessed on 7 November 2020).

Coate, Jennifer. 2020. 'COVID-19 Hotel Quarantine Inquiry: Interim Report and Recommendations', Victorian Government Printer, November 6.

Coatsworth, Nick. 2020. 'Deputy Chief Medical Officer's Press Conference about COVID-19 on 23 April 2020', Department of Health, April 23, https://www.health.gov.au/news/deputy-chief-medical-officers-press-conference-about-covid-19-on-23-april-2020 (accessed on 7 November 2020).

Colbeck, Richard. 2020. 'Government Welcomes Aged Care Royal Commission's COVID-19 Report Recommendations', Media Release, October 1, https://www.health.gov.au/ministers/senator-the-hon-richard-colbeck/media/government-welcomes-aged-care-royal-commissions-covid-19-report-recommendations (accessed on 7 November 2020).

Communicable Diseases Network Australia. 2020. 'Coronavirus Disease 2019 (COVID-19) CDNA National Guidelines for Public Health Units', Version 3.10, October 28.

Conran, Peter. 2020. 'Review of COAG Councils and Ministerial Forums – Report to National Cabinet', Australian Government – Department of Prime Minister and Cabinet.

Council of Australian Governments. 2011. 'National Health Reform Agreement', Council of Australian Governments, https://www.federalfinancialrelations.gov.au/content/npa/health/_archive/national-agreement.pdf (accessed on 7 November 2020).

Department of Health (Cth). 2019. 'Australian Health Management Plan for Pandemic Influenza (AHMPPI)', Australian Government – Department of Health, https://www1.health.gov.au/internet/main/publishing.nsf/Content/ohp-ahmppi.htm (accessed on 7 November 2020).

Department of Health (Cth). 2020a. 'Australian Health Sector Emergency Response Plan for Novel Coronavirus (COVID-19)', February 18.

Department of Health (Cth). 2020b. 'Impact of COVID-19: Theoretical Modelling of How the Health System can Respond', https://www.health.gov.au/sites/default/files/documents/2020/04/impact-of-covid-19-in-australia-ensuring-the-health-system-can-respond-presentation.pdf (accessed on 7 November 2020).

Department of Health (Cth). 2020c. 'Coronavirus (COVID-19) Current Situation and Case Numbers', https://www.health.gov.au/news/health-alerts/novel-coronavirus-2019-ncov-health-alert/coronavirus-covid-19-current-situation-and-case-numbers (accessed on 17 October 2020).

Department of Health and Human Services (Vic). 2020. 'Victorian Coronavirus (COVID-19) Data', Victorian Government – Department of Health and Human Services, https://www.dhhs.vic.gov.au/victorian-coronavirus-covid-19-data (accessed on 7 November 2020).

Department of Home Affairs (Cth). 2020. 'About Emergency Management: National Coordination Mechanism', Australian Government – Department of Home Affairs, https://www.homeaffairs.gov.au/about-us/our-portfolios/emergency-management/about-emergency-management/national-coordination-mechanism# (accessed on 7 November 2020).

Department of the Prime Minister and Cabinet. 2020. 'COAG becomes National Cabinet', Media Release, June 2, https://www.pmc.gov.au/news-centre/government/coag-becomes-national-cabinet (accessed on 4 August 2020).

Fenna, Alan. 2020. 'Coping with COVID: An Encomium to Australian Federalism', UACES Territorial Politics, June 12, https://uacesterrpol.wordpress.com/2020/06/12/coping-with-covid-19-an-encomium-to-australian-federalism/ (accessed on 7 November 2020).

Ferguson, Richard, Rebecca Urban and Adeshola Ore. 2020. 'Business Demands Action on Borders', *The Australian*, August 24, https://www.theaustralian.com.au/news/coronavirus-australia-live-news-australia-hk-embassy-bars-kiwi-spouse-from-queensland-return/news-story/4be362ea73f7197278c8f16666bbfdcf (accessed on 7 November 2020).

Hopman, Joost and Shaheen Mehtar. 2020. 'Country Level Analysis of COVID-19 Policies', *EClinicalMedicine* 25: 100500.

Lee, H. P., et al. 2018. *Emergency Powers in Australia*, 2nd ed. United Kingdom: Cambridge University Press.

McNeill, Heather. 2020. 'Other Interstate Border Policies are Working to Stop COVID-19, Despite WA Chief Health Officer's Advice', *WA Today*, October 26, https://www.watoday.com.au/national/western-australia/other-interstate-border-policies-are-working-to-stop-covid-19-despite-wa-chief-health-officer-s-advice-20201023-p5683y.html (accessed on 7 November 2020).

Moss, Robert, et al. 2020. 'Modelling the Impact of Covid-19 in Australia to Inform Transmission Reducing Measures and Health System Preparedness', https://www.medrxiv.org/content/10.1101/2020.04.07.20056184v1 (accessed on 05 March 2021).

Pagone, Tony and Lynelle Briggs. 2020. 'Aged Care and COVID-19: A Special Report', Royal Commission into Aged Care Quality and Safety, October 1.

Queensland Government. 2020. 'Border Restrictions', Queensland Government – Restrictions in Queensland, https://www.qld.gov.au/health/conditions/health-alerts/coronavirus-covid-19/current-status/public-health-directions/border-restrictions (accessed on 10 October 2020).

Saunders, Cheryl. 2020. 'A New Federalism? The Role and Future of the National Cabinet'. *Governing During Crises Policy Brief*, University of Melbourne.

Tracey, Richard and Lynelle Briggs. 2019. 'Interim Report: Neglect, Volume 1', Royal Commission into Aged Care Quality and Safety, October 31.

Victorian Government. 2020. 'Coronavirus (COVID-19) Reopening Roadmap: Third Step – Victoria', https://www.coronavirus.vic.gov.au/coronavirus-covid-19-reopening-roadmap-third-step-victoria (accessed on 10 November 2020).

Walker, Brett. 2020. 'Report of the Special Commission of Inquiry into the Ruby Princess', Special Commission of Inquiry into the Ruby Princess, August 14.

Wells, Geoffrey et al. 2020. 'Open Letter – Alternative Response to COVID-19 for Victoria', Australian Doctors Federation, August 31, https://ausdoctorsfederation.org.au/2020/09/03/open-letter-alternative-response-to-covid-19-for-victoria/ (accessed on 7 November 2020).

Zierke, Merle. 2020. 'Covid-19 and Local Government in Australia', Briefing for LGiU Australia, April 1.

PART V
Africa

17

CONTROLLING PUBLIC HEALTH EMERGENCIES IN FEDERAL SYSTEMS

The case of Ethiopia

Zemelak Ayitenew Ayele and Yonatan Tesfaye Fessha

17.1 Introduction

It was merely a day after the World Health Organization (WHO) declared the coronavirus disease (Covid-19) a global pandemic that Ethiopia recorded its first case of infection. On 12 March 2020, a week after entering the country from Burkina Faso, a 48-year-old Japanese national presented himself at a public health centre in the capital city, Addis Ababa, and was diagnosed as having Covid-19. The number of cases in Ethiopia's estimated population of 110 million climbed steadily in the following months, and by the end of October some 96,000 people were infected in what is one of the most populous countries in Africa.

According to official statistics, the infection rate reached its peak when 2,000 new cases were reported in August 2020, after which it began to decline. This was, however, not necessarily because the prevalence of Covid-19 decreased; it was because the government cut back on its daily testing for the disease. In August, it had been conducting more than 20,000 such tests a day; from the beginning of September, it reduced them by three-quarters to 5,000 (FDRE Ministry of Health 2020). It was little wonder that infection rates seemed to have dropped – here, as elsewhere in a country as vast and diverse as this, matters were not as straightforward as they appeared on the surface.

Located on the Horn of Africa, Ethiopia's territory of 1,104,300 km² is host, if not always home (increasingly a point of contention), to more than 80 ethnic groups, which gives the country a multifaceted character amply reflected in the complexity of its history. In the modern era, Ethiopia became a republic in 1974 when a popular revolt against the monarchy culminated in a coup that ousted Haile Selassie I and led to a period of military government and unitary state-hood. A 17-year-long civil war ensued, in which the ruling junta, the Derg, were defeated by the Ethiopian Peoples' Revolutionary Democratic Front (EPRDF),

DOI: 10.4324/9781003166771-23

a coalition of ethnic-based rebel groups. After this victory, Ethiopia became a federation in 1995 and would be ruled by the EPRDF for most of the next 30 years.

However, a three-year public protest that started in 2015 against what many described as the EPRDF's authoritarianism saw Dr Abiy Ahmed Ali emerge as Prime Minister in April 2018. He oversaw various reforms with the declared aim of transforming Ethiopia into a democratic state, among which was the amalgamation of the EPRDF coalition into a single party, the Ethiopian Prosperity Party (EPP). The sixth national elections, scheduled for August 2020, were meant to be a litmus test of whether the country was moving towards democratisation and a peaceful transition, but they were postponed due to the Covid-19 pandemic – events which, at the time of this writing, culminated in federal military intervention in one of the states.

Clearly, then, Covid-19's arrival in Ethiopia was especially inopportune, coming as it did when the country was at a political crossroads and the federation under heavy strain. This chapter argues that the 2020 pandemic further complicated the political entanglements that beset the federal system, in the process deepening the communal divisions that already threaten the country with disintegration.

17.2 The federal constitutional and legislative framework

17.2.1 Federal structure

The Federal Democratic Republic of Ethiopia is composed of a federal government and 10 states, demarcated along ethnic lines, and two self-governing cities, Dire Dawa and Addis Ababa; the tenth state, Sidama Regional State, was created in June 2020.[1] As Ethiopia has a parliamentary system of government, the executive is headed by a Prime Minister who governs the country together with the Council of Ministers. The federal parliament is a bicameral one in which only the lower house, the House of Peoples' Representatives (HPR), exercises legislative powers; the upper house, the House of Federation (HoF), exercises non-legislative functions that include resolving constitutional disputes.

At the state level, elected legislatures exercise powers over state matters. The highest executive authority in the state lies with the chief administrator (sometimes referred to as president), who presides over the state cabinet. In terms of the Constitution's dual court system, each state has a judiciary of its own to administer justice based on state law.

Local government is not explicitly recognised as an autonomous level of government; as such, its establishment is left within the exclusive competence of the state (Constitution, article 50(4)). In practice, states have formed ethnic local government (composed of special zones and special *woredas*) and regular local government (composed of *woredas* and city administrations) (Ayele and Fessha 2012). Dire Dawa and Addis Ababa, both of which are answerable directly to the federal government, are included in the category of local government (Ayele 2014).

17.2.2 Division of powers: Federal competences

Ethiopia has a dual federal system in which competences are divided between the federal and state governments. Local government is not part of the power division. Article 51 of the Constitution contains a list of 20 functional areas that usually fall under the exclusive competences of the federal government, including foreign affairs; defence; printing money; borrowing; immigration; and air, rail, waterway, and sea transport, as well as major roads linking two or more states. The powers of the federal government also extend to functional areas that are mentioned directly or indirectly in other parts of the Constitution (Fiseha 2007). The Constitution contains a short list of state competences (article 52(1)). Residual powers are left to state governments.

The federal government has broad powers in the area of public health. It has the power to 'establish and implement national standards and basic policy criteria for public health' (Constitution, article 51(3)). This implies that the federal government has the competence to develop policies and framework legislation for containing pandemics. However, a global pandemic like Covid-19 is not solely a public health issue, but also involves issues linked to, inter alia, the national economy, social services, international relations, and national security.

That makes the long list of powers of the federal government outlined in article 51 of the Constitution relevant, in one way or another, in the event of a global pandemic. For example, inasmuch as cooperation with other states is necessary to contain the spread of viruses, a pandemic has implications for foreign affairs. The immigration-related powers of the federal government are also implicated in that travel bans are a major way of containing pandemics. What is more, pandemics have economic repercussions which may require that the federal government use its power of regulating the national economy to minimise them.

The federal government's emergency powers are relevant too, since combating a pandemic may require restricting freedoms and liberties and then using coercive power to enforce these restrictions. Accordingly, Ethiopia's federal government not only has the power to declare a state of emergency but the competence to 'establish and administer national defence and public security forces as well as a federal police force' (Constitution, article 51(6)).

17.2.3 Division of powers: State competences

The Constitution does not expressly provide the states with competence in regard to public health. However, the federal government's power to 'establish and implement national standards and basic policy criteria' (Constitution, article 51(3)) in the area of public health implies that it is expected to restrict itself to setting the standards and defining the minimum requirements to which states have to adhere; this leaves room for states to come up with their own detailed policies based on the national standard (Fiseha and Ayele 2017). By implication, public health is a concurrent competence of the federal and state government in the mould of 'framework concurrency'.

Moreover, article 52(1)(2)(c) provides that the states can 'formulate and execute their own social and development policies, strategies and plans'. Arguably, public health is a social matter with respect to which the state could formulate its own policies. This, together with the reading above of article 51(3), would entail that states have competences in the area of containing the spread of a global pandemic such as Covid-19. The inference is bolstered by the fact that the Constitution expressly authorises the states to declare a 'state-wide state of emergency should a natural disaster or an epidemic occur' (article 93(1)(b)).

17.2.4 Local government competences

The role and power of local government in public health are not evident from the federal constitution, as it is silent on the functional competences of local government (article 50(4)). The state constitutions also tell us little about the role local government could play in public emergencies in general and the Covid-19 pandemic in particular. A brief survey of them finds that *woredas* and cities are authorised simply to implement their own plan on local social and economic matters; none of the state constitutions define the specific social and economic matters that are within the competences of local government (Ayele 2014).

In practice, local governments in Ethiopia play a robust role in matters of public health. They are responsible for providing basic utilities such as primary health care (by establishing health stations and clinics), drinking water, primary education, and security maintenance (ibid). The relevance of these competences, especially primary health care, in the fight against Covid-19 is self-evident.

17.3 Preparedness for a national disaster: The institutional framework

Long before Covid-19 emerged, various federal and state institutions were tasked to deal with emergencies, including public health emergencies. Among these institutions are the Federal Ministry of Health (MoH), the Ethiopian Public Health Institute (PHI), and the Ethiopian Food and Drug Control Authority (EFDCA).

The MoH has the primary duty of dealing with public health matters in general and public health emergencies in particular. Under article 27(6) of the Proclamation to provide for the definition of powers and duties of the executive organs of the Federal Democratic Republic of Ethiopia 1097 (2018), it has the duty to 'devise and follow up the implementation of strategies for the prevention of epidemic and communicable diseases'. Additionally, it has the mandate to 'take preventive measures against events that threaten the public health; in the events of an emergency situation coordinate measures of other stakeholders to expeditiously and effectively tackle the problem' (article 27(7)). As per Public Health Proclamation 200 (2000), the MoH also has the power

> to restrict movements to certain countries, or to the areas where there is epidemic, or to close schools or recreational areas, or to remove workers with communicable diseases from their working places, and to take other similar measures whenever an epidemic occurs.
>
> *(article 17(3))*

The main responsibility of the PHI is to undertake research to detect and prevent public health emergencies. It is expected to create early warning systems that enable other concerned organs, including the MoH, to take appropriate and timely measures. The EFDCA's main responsibility is to ensure that foods, medicines, and medical devices that are imported or produced in the country and distributed at national level are of appropriate quality and do not pose a risk to public health. The EFDCA had the additional authority of controlling ports of entry, enforcing laws and combating pandemics. This included quarantining or denying entry into the country to travellers suspected of being infected with communicable diseases. By way of Food, Medicine and Health Care Administration and Control Proclamation 661 (2009) and 1112 (2009), this power was transferred to the PHI in 2009.

Other federal agencies dealing with health emergencies are the Ethiopian Revenue and Custom Authority and the Ethiopian Civil Aviation Authorities, which are mandated to report, through their posts at ports of entries, individuals suspected of infection with a communicable disease to the relevant authorities so that the country's quarantine rules can be enforced (Council of Ministers Regulation 299 (2013), articles 45 and 46). Another federal institution with an important role in combating pandemics is the National Disaster and Risk Management Commission (NDRMC), which is charged with storing food and non-food items for use in cases of emergency.

States seem to organise their executive and administrative agencies in such a way that there is a counterpart to a federal agency at the state level, despite the absence of hard and fast rules requiring them to do so. Thus, as a counterpart to the MoH, there is a bureau of health at the state level and an office of health at the local level. State bureaus of health have the power to deal with public health emergencies. There are also state-level public health institutes and disaster and risk management commissions.

These state agencies work (or at least are expected to work) in coordination with their federal counterparts. In the absence of strong, formalised forums for intergovernmental relations (IGR), federal ministries or agencies interact on an ad hoc basis with their counterparts at state level. Thus, the MoH interacts with state bureaux of health, while the federal PHI interacts with state PHIs.

The blame for the ad hoc nature of these interactions can be laid at the door of the EPRDF, which controlled eight of the nine states and operated on the basis of democratic centralism: since IGR issues were addressed within the party structure, this practice stifled the emergence of formal IGR forums. When Covid-19 broke out, however, the EPRDF was no more and, in the absence of established IGR forums, the only mechanism for coordinating efforts to contain the pandemic was cooperative engagement among federal and regional sectoral offices with complementary mandates.

17.4 Rolling out measures to contain the pandemic

The response to Covid-19 was dominated by the federal government. The state governments took little or no initiative: with a few exceptions, outlined below, they were passive and merely followed federal instructions. This can be explained by the fact that the Ethiopian federation operates within a dominant-party state that reduced state governments to implementing agents of the federal government (Fessha 2019). At the same time, the effort to combat the pandemic took place in the context of major political developments that undermined the ability of the federal government to dictate to state governments, that prompted unusual defiance among state governments, and that saw the emergence of inter-communal conflicts across the country.

17.4.1 Taking the initiative

The spread of the coronavirus was initially slow, and almost all the confirmed cases were from Addis Ababa: from March to May 2020, the daily confirmed cases were less than 10. The virus nevertheless continued to spread throughout the country in subsequent months, even though Addis Ababa remained the epicentre and accounted for two-thirds of infections. By October 2020, there were close to 100,000 confirmed cases, and it was suspected, moreover, that the actual number of infected individuals was much higher than what was officially reported.

All eyes were on the federal government after the outbreak of the coronavirus in Wuhan, China, was reported in January 2020, even so before a global pandemic was declared. This was because only the federal government could have prevented its entry into Ethiopia, given that it is the level of government charged with controlling ports of entry into the country. There were public demands on mass and social media for the federal government to close borders and suspend flights, especially Ethiopian Airline's flight to and from China; concerns were heightened by the fact that Bole International Airport, located at the heart of Addis Ababa, is one of the largest and busiest airports in Africa as well as home to Ethiopian Airlines, the largest airline on the continent. The federal government initially rejected the demand for the suspension of flights and closure of the country's borders.

However, it did start taking precautionary measures even before the first case of Covid-19 was confirmed. On 27 January 2020, prior to the WHO's declaration of a global pandemic, the Council of Ministers 'activated' a National Public Health Emergency Preparedness Centre and began preparations to deal with a potential outbreak of Covid-19, with control mechanisms at ports of entry requiring anyone entering the country to undergo a temperature check. In the same period, the NDRMC established a National Coordination Centre (NECC) in which various sectoral agencies were represented (Public Health Emergency Operation Centre (PHEOC), Ethiopia: Weekly Bulletin 2020). The NECC was formed on the understanding that Covid-19 was not only an imminent health disaster but posed numerous risks, especially humanitarian ones that called for a multisectoral response. Accordingly, this body set up quarantine centres and food banks in various areas.

A few days after the first case of Covid-19 was confirmed, the Council of Ministers banned all public gatherings and sports events. It also ordered schools, including universities and colleges, to close and placed restrictions on religious gatherings. The decision was to be applicable at the national level. This was followed by a decision on 20 March 2020 requiring anyone entering the country to stay in quarantine for up to 14 days. One could be quarantined in designated hotels if one could cover the cost, or remain in other quarantine facilities at the expense of the government. The Council also ordered the closure of bars and clubs. Federal and state security organs were charged with enforcing these decisions.

Moreover, the Council of Ministers ordered that Ethiopian Airlines cease flights to 30 selected cities (surprisingly, cities in China were not on the list). On 24 March 2020, it decided that, from 25 March, all federal employees were to work from home, except those designated by each ministry and federal agency as essential workers. Likewise, the president of the Federal Supreme Court declared that federal courts would remain partially closed from 19 March to 2 April. The restrictions were imposed without a state of emergency having been declared.

The heavy hand of the federal government was evident in the early days of Covid-19. There was little initiative by the states to use their competences in the fight against the pandemic – their attitude seemed to be to wait and see what the federal government would do. However, some of them of their own accord took measures with the declared purpose of containing the pandemic, albeit that most of these measures were less than comprehensive. For instance, on 31 March 2020, the states of Oromia, Amhara, and the SNNP for two weeks banned public transport from entering or leaving them. The states took even more restrictive measures in some of the cities within their jurisdiction. For example, on 31 March, the Amhara state ordered a total lockdown and banned any movement of public transportation for two weeks in four cities, among them the state capital, Bahr Dar (Fana Broadcasting Corporation 2020). However, Addis Ababa, the country's capital, did not impose a complete lockdown despite its being the epicentre of Covid-19.

There was one major exception. Tigray National Regional State declared a state of emergency on 25 March 2020, long before similar action was taken by the federal government. As part of the emergency measure, the state government introduced several restrictions. It forbade any travel to and from rural areas within the state. It also required the closure of cafés, restaurants, bars, and clubs and banned all social activities including weddings. Anyone entering the state had to stay in quarantine for two weeks. It should be noted, though, that Tigray's declaration of a state of emergency was not simply an exercise of a constitutionally allocated power in the interests of the greater good. It is to be seen in the light of the prevailing political tension between the federal and state government (discussed in the next section).

17.4.2 Federal action

As the spread of the virus increased in terms both of numbers infected and area covered, the Council of Ministers resolved on 8 April 2020 to impose a state of emergency. As per article 93 of the Constitution, the proclamation by which it was declared was adopted by Parliament on 10 April.

The State of Emergency Proclamation (3/2020) was short and composed of a preamble and eight articles. The preamble explained that the state of emergency was necessary as Covid-19 had become a global pandemic that could not be controlled by regular methods of law enforcement. The adverse political, social, and economic impacts of the pandemic and the need to mitigate the ensuing humanitarian crises, said the preamble, warranted 'coordinated' decision-making and implementation, which in turn necessitated the state of emergency. The proclamation, which had nationwide application, superseded contrary federal and state laws. It also imposed a criminal penalty on those acting or failing to act in accordance with its provisions. The penalty was up to three years' imprisonment, or a fine of between ETB 1,000 and 200,000. The state of emergency remained in force for five months, starting on 8 April 2020.

On the basis of article 4 of the State of Emergency Proclamation, the Council of Ministers issued a regulation (Regulation 466 (2020)) detailing measures to contain the virus. The regulation banned some activities entirely and others partially. Among the activities that were banned entirely were gatherings of more than four people regardless of the purpose, shaking hands, teaching and learning in schools, and sports activities; clubs, bars, theatres, cinemas, and the like were ordered to close. Public transport, including buses and trains, was allowed to operate at half of its usual capacity. Cafeterias, restaurants, and hotels were required not to serve more than three people at a single table and to ensure sufficient space between tables. International borders were closed, although Ethiopian citizens were allowed to enter the country if and when the Council of Ministers permitted it.

Various rights and freedoms were thus restricted for the duration of the emergency. Freedom of expression was limited, as the regulation barred the media from reporting Covid-19 news in a way that could 'cause terror and undue distress among the public' (article 3(27)); in addition, factual information about

Covid-19 could be communicated only in a centralised manner (article 3(16)). Freedom of movement was restricted in that travellers from abroad had to be quarantined for 14 days. The regulation required everyone to wear masks in public.

Furthermore, the rights of property owners were restricted inasmuch as they could not evict tenants or increase rental fees. An owner of a vehicle, apartment, hotel, or other property could be required by the Ministerial Committee, established by the regulation, to submit his or her property to be used in the fight against the pandemic. Employers could not dismiss employees except in accordance with a protocol issued by the Ministry of Social Affairs. The regulation also placed obligations on certain service providers by requiring them not to discontinue their services during the state of emergency. This included electricity, water, and telecom service providers, along with, inter alia, banks, construction workers, and cleaners.

The pandemic created major economic challenges. Close to half a million jobs were lost due to Covid-19; many businesses closed down, while others suffered a significant loss of earnings as demand for goods and services plummeted. This resulted in a 4 per cent drop in growth in gross domestic product (GDP), dragging more than 2 million people under the national income poverty line. About half of urban and rural households experienced income loss (Dabalen and Paci 2020). In addition, the arrival of the virus during the rainy season led to poor agricultural productivity, as a result of which the country saw a 30 per cent rise in food inflation (World Food Programme 2020).

In response, the federal government sought to mitigate these impacts by, among other things, giving tax exemptions to affected companies and cancelling interest and penalties for unpaid taxes that had been due between 2015 and 2018. Moreover, it introduced price controls on basic commodities. The National Bank injected liquidity to the value of ETB 15 billion (USD 450 million) into private banks so that they could provide grace periods or 'debt relief and additional loans to their customers in need' (Samuel 2020). State and local governments also extended tax exemptions to small traders and businesses.

The federal government decided not to renew the state of emergency when it expired in September 2020; many of the restrictions were subsequently lifted. Although the rate of infection appeared to decrease from September and onwards, this was mainly because the MoH substantially reduced testing for the virus as it was running out of test kits.

17.4.3 State government action

After the federal government declared a state of emergency, the states adopted a more structured approach to Covid-19, given that the federal proclamation and its regulation, which had nationwide application, provided the necessary framework for state action. The states were responsible mainly for enforcing the state of emergency. They established quarantine centres and transported patients to and from these centres. They also mobilised health extension workers, who provided various services 'including immunization, at the community level and educated members of the communities on how to prevent the spread of the virus' (Getachew 2020).

As it was responsible for the area most heavily affected by Covid-19, the Addis Ababa city government took a number of measures to contain the pandemic. It established quarantine centres in various locations, including at the Millennium Hall, a venue usually used for music festivals. To curb the spread of the virus without hampering food supply to residents, the city government relocated Atkilt Tera, the largest fruit and vegetable market, to Jan Meda, an open space ordinarily used for sports and religious activities.

There was, however, one exception to the practice of state governments' limiting their role to enforcing the decisions of the federal government. The state of Tigray declared a state of emergency long before the federal government declared a nationwide state of emergency. Thereafter, in April 2020, Tigray undertook 'a state-wide door-to-door Covid-19 screening testing campaign' (Addis Fortune 2020). After the campaign, the state government eased the measures imposed by its state of emergency by lifting restrictions on public transport, cafés, restaurants, bars, and the like and allowing them to provide services subject to conditions. Tigray eased its restrictions two weeks after the federal government imposed its state of emergency – this did not necessarily violate the federal state of emergency since the remaining restrictions were as severe as those imposed by the federal government.

17.4.4 Local government action

Woredas and cities took measures to prevent the spread of the virus, albeit in an unstructured manner. As early as March 2020, some cities in Oromia imposed a partial lockdown, while those in the Amhara state, including the capital, imposed a complete lockdown (Fana Broadcasting Corporate 2020). Although this was done at the behest of the respective state governments, it was undertaken without a clear legal framework.

In April 2020, the Addis Ababa city government launched what it called 'door-to-door screening' in which more than a thousand health workers went from door to door to take temperature checks and isolate people showing the symptoms of Covid-19 (Ethiopian News Agency 2020). In the SNNP, some local government units attempted to impose restrictions to contain the spread of the virus. For instance, the Gurage zone government barred people from travelling to the zone for the Islamic holiday, Arafa, during which members of the Gurage community traditionally travel to the zone to celebrate the holiday and get married.

After the federal government declared a state of emergency, local governments were expected to play a key role in enforcing the emergency regulations, including the requirement that masks be worn in public spaces and that cinemas, bars, and so on be closed.

17.4.5 Intergovernmental relations

Although Ethiopia adopted a federal constitution in 1995, IGR has never had more than academic relevance in how its federal system operates (Fessha 2020). As an aspect of federalism, it was ignored in the past mainly because the EPRDF, which acted on the basis of 'democratic centralism' and controlled all levels of government, dealt with intergovernmental issues through party channels; federal agencies and their counterparts at state level interacted with each other, if at all, on an ad hoc basis (Fiseha 2009). As noted, the EPRDF has transformed itself into a new party, the EPP, which now controls nine of the country's 10 states. The EPP, unlike the EPRDF, is not a coalition of ethnic-based state parties but a single national party with state branches legally and politically accountable to the centre. Its party structure remains the most important mechanism for coordinating federal and state relations in Ethiopia – not much has changed in this respect.

There was, nonetheless, an attempt to formalise IGR, and to this effect a policy document on it was adopted in May 2018 by the HoF, the institution which is supposed to play a major role in facilitating federal-state relations, though it had not been implemented at the time of writing. A draft proclamation on IGR, prepared under the auspices of the HoF, was only recently endorsed by the HPR (Anberbir 2020). In the interim, the relevant federal and state agencies interacted with each other to coordinate their efforts in the fight against Covid-19. The MoH in particular was in regular contact with state bureaus of health, among other things making test kits available for them, receiving their reports, and consolidating these in nationwide test results that were published daily.

It might not be accurate to say nothing much has changed in federal-state relations: for the first time in three decades, a major intergovernmental dispute has arisen in Ethiopia. Although Covid-19 was not the main cause of the dispute between the federal government and the state government of Tigray, there is no doubt that it played a role in escalating the dispute.

The pandemic, as mentioned, broke out when the country was in political turmoil thanks to a split in the EPRDF, one precipitated by three years of countrywide protests against the party's authoritarianism and the country's ever-rising corruption. Abiy Ahmed, who assumed chairmanship of the EPRDF and premiership of the country after Haile Mariam Dessalgn resigned as Prime Minister, reconstituted the ethnic-based EPRDF into a single, formally non-ethnic party with a new name, EPP, and new ideology, that of '*medemer*', an Amharic word roughly translatable as 'convergence' (Ayele 2021). The Tigray People's Liberation Front (TPLF) – the founder, nucleus, and most influential member of the coalition – did not join the new party.

In April 2018 and thereafter, disgruntled members of the TPLF, including former ministers, Members of Parliament, and senior government officials in the federal government, left Addis Ababa and retreated to Mekelle, the capital of Tigray; the dispute between the Tigray state and the federal government soon began to unfold. The altercation worsened when it became clear that, due to Covid-19, the sixth general elections would not be held in August 2020 as per the schedule prepared by the National Electoral Board of Ethiopia (NEBE). The NEBE itself declared that it would not be able to administer free and fair elections in the context of Covid-19. At the same time, the term of the current Parliament was due to expire on 5 October 2020, so it was unclear how and by whom the country would be governed after the expiry and until elections could be held.

The government then sought the advice of the HoF, which, as noted, has the power to interpret the Constitution. The HoF, based on the recommendation of the Council of Constitutional Interpretation, the institution that assists it in discharging its mandate of constitutional interpretation, decided to extend the term of Parliament and all state councils until the next elections are held (FDRE Council of Constitutional Inquiry 2020; FDRE House of Federation 2020).

In response, the TPLF declared the HoF's decision unconstitutional. Furthermore, it decided to hold its own state elections by establishing its own electoral board and adopting its own electoral law (Addis Standard 2020a). This was constitutionally problematic since the power to administer any elections in the country exclusively belongs to the NEBE. Nevertheless, on 9 September 2020, the Tigray state went ahead with the elections, defying repeated warnings by the federal government against such actions.

Having conducted the elections and forming a new government, the Tigray state declared that, post-5 October 2020, when the terms of Parliament and the incumbent administration would have expired were it not for the term extension by the HoF, it would not recognise Abiy Ahmed's government as legitimate and have any relationship with it (Addis Standard 2020b). The federal government, for its part, declared the elections in Tigray null and void, refused to recognise the state government as legitimate, and said it would not have relations with it.

Intergovernmental tension was exacerbated when the HoF decided to suspend federal revenue transfers to the Tigray state government. Tigray reacted by making public its intention to withhold all federal taxes collected in the state. The federal government then declared its intention to bypass the state government of Tigray and interact directly with local authorities, including in the transfer of funds. Those were constitutionally suspect measures (Ayele 2020) and added a financial dimension to the already strained relations.

The actions and reactions of the two governments revealed the limits of the law's ability to dampen intergovernmental tensions. The state of Tigray labelled the federal government as illegitimate even though the bodies with the ultimate power to interpret the Constitution, the Council of Constitutional Interpretation and the HoF, allowed the federal government to stay in power until the next elections were held. Some aspects of that decision are arguably problematic (especially with regard to the extension of the terms of state governments). Nevertheless, those were the final words of the body given the power to interpret the Constitution and were expected to be respected as such. While a state government probably has the right to hold state and local elections, the Constitution envisages a single national body that administers elections.

Eventually, the federal government invoked its constitutional power of federal intervention and, at the beginning of November 2020, launched a military offensive against the government of the state of Tigray.[2] At the time of this writing, the federal military had removed the state government and the federal government had installed a transitional government in its place.

These disturbing developments highlight the absence of traditions and institutions of intergovernmental dialogue that allow for peaceful resolution of disputes. Indeed, what is striking, tragically so, is that there was not a single report of the federal government and government of Tigray having met behind closed doors to engage in intergovernmental dialogue. Instead, matters that should have been resolved by intergovernmental negotiation conducted away from the public arena were allowed to fester in a war of words. That is extremely concerning. The developments clearly indicate that Ethiopians are living in an era when they have to take the federal experiment seriously, a stance that should include an intent commitment to a culture of intergovernmental dialogue and negotiation.

17.4.6 Intergovernmental fiscal relations

The duality of the Ethiopian federal system is evident in the way that fiscal powers are divided between the federal and state government. The principle governing their fiscal relations is, as provided under article 94(1) of the Constitution, that 'federal government and the states respectively bear all financial expenditures necessary to carry out all responsibilities and functions assigned to them by law'; this also explains why 'the financial expenditures required for the carrying out of any delegated function by a state [are] borne [by the federal government]'. An exception to the principle is that the federal government could 'grant to states emergency, rehabilitation and development assistance and loans'. This suggests that, if it so wishes, the federal government can grant financial assistance to the states to deal with public health emergencies, including the Covid-19 pandemic.

In practice, the federal government makes two types of financial transfers to the states. The first, commonly known as block grants, are unconditional financial transfers. These comprise a little more than 36 per cent of the federal budget. The Constitution does not specifically mention this type of revenue transfers. The second type is specific-purpose grants (SPGs), which are conditional grants.

The outbreak of Covid-19 bore financial consequences both for the federal and the state governments. In particular, the federal government saw a massive drop in the revenue it usually collects. According to Ahmed Shide, the Minister of Finance, '[a] slowdown of economic activities and exports, because of COVID 19, affected the government's revenue ... [for] the budget year'

(Wondwosen 2020). He added that the collection of indirect taxes, including value-added tax (VAT) and excise taxes, decreased by close to 15 per cent in March 2020 compared to revenue collected in the same period in the previous year. Federal government estimates show that, between March and July, more than ETB 11 billion (USD 294 million) of revenue that could have been collected in the form of federal taxes had been lost.

On the expenditure side, the federal government incurred additional expenses of ETB 15 billion in buying personal protective equipment, medicines, and the like. Covid-19 also resulted in humanitarian challenges, including a growing need for emergency food assistance. This required the immediate purchase of more than 600,000 metric tons of wheat, costing billions of Ethiopian birr. The humanitarian situation was worsened by floods during the country's rainy season (June–September) and the invasion of much of north-eastern and south-eastern Ethiopia by desert locusts. These together put an estimated 15 million people or more in need of food assistance (Fikade 2020). To deal with the emergencies, the HPR in May 2020 adopted a supplementary budget of ETB 48.5 billion (USD 1.2 billion).

As for the states, even under normal circumstances they have never been financially self-sufficient and depend on federal transfers to cover in excess of 70 per cent of their annual budgets; as such, the transfers are used mainly to cover the current expenditure of the state and local governments. The pandemic aggravated the situation in two respects, however. In the first place, it led to a reduction in the revenue they could collect from taxes and service fees. Numerous businesses closed down due to Covid-19, while others requested tax relief from their respective state governments to avoid going bankrupt and keep paying salaries to employees. The states had no choice but to grant these requests.

Secondly, states' expenditure increased since they had to take a variety of measures to contain the virus, including opening and operating quarantine centres. In this regard, they received federal assistance both in cash and in kind. In the latter case, the federal government purchased and disbursed personal protective equipment and other medical equipment – for instance, it distributed more than 50 million masks to the states for subsequent distribution to returning students. It should be noted that most of the states ceased virtually all capital investments and used their full resources to deal with the economic and humanitarian consequences of the pandemic; this increased their dependence on federal government handouts in order to carry out their expenditure responsibilities.

17.5 Findings and policy implications

Although Ethiopia has a federal constitution, it functions largely as a centralised system. This meant it was taken for granted that efforts to manage the threat of Covid-19 would be driven by the centre. Conversely, state and local government were not expected to take separate initiatives to control the virus and manage its socio-economic impacts: as implementers of the decisions of the national government, they were required to follow directions given by the federal government. Indeed, this is exactly what happened.

The federal government dominated efforts to manage Covid-19, with state governments acting as implementers and local governments playing a peripheral role. There was no report of health ministers across the two levels of government engaging in dialogue to ensure coordination and protect citizens from the spread of Covid-19 across the country – even the breadth of the pandemic's impact did not prompt governments to engage in regular intergovernmental dialogue. This is no doubt linked to the fact that subnational governments acted as implementers of the federal government's decisions. They are, in other words, yet to be seen by the federal government as equal partners that need to be consulted through an intergovernmental mechanism.

There was one important exception, however. The state of Tigray took the initiative to declare a state of emergency within its territory, doing so long before the federal government declared a nationwide state of emergency. We cannot think of any other situation where a state in Ethiopia took a decision that departed from federal government action, let alone one that preceded it. Nevertheless, Tigray was acting within the limits of the Constitution.

Its decision to take actions independently of the federal government was an encouraging development as far as the federal experiment is concerned. Yet it was unavoidable to conclude that the action of the Tigray state was motivated largely by its desire to demonstrate its distinctiveness and autonomy from the federal government; put differently, it was hardly based on any specific assessment of Tigray's epidemiological status. The use of the pandemic to score political points against the federal government was clear. After all, this was the same state that, on the one hand, seemed to have taken Covid-19 with great seriousness, but, on the other, emerged as the fiercest opponent of the decision – made in response to Covid-19 – that allowed the federal government to postpone the national election.

From the foregoing, it is clear that the pandemic did not alter the way the federation operates; it did, however, serve as an opportunity to amplify the tensions that ensued after the election of Abiy Ahmed as Prime Minster and the reconfiguration of the ruling party that displaced the TPLF as the dominant member of the coalition. Indeed, the tensions that Covid-19 exacerbated can be read as harbingers of the intergovernmental disputes that are bound to emerge as the country transitions from a federation that operated under a dominant-party system. Developments during the Covid-19 pandemic exposed the absence of traditions and institutions of intergovernmental dialogue that allow for peaceful resolution of disputes within the federation. Ethiopians, it was clear, find themselves living in an era when they must take the federal experiment seriously and, in particular, make a commitment to entrenching a culture of intergovernmental dialogue and negotiation.

Notes

1 The original nine are Afar, Amhara, Benishanul-Gumuz, Gambella, Hareri, Oromia, Southern Nations, Nationalities and Peoples (SNNP), Somali, and Tigray. The new Sidama state seceded from the SNNP.

2 The offensive began on the night of 4 November 2020 when the Prime Minister, alleging that the TPLF had attacked military bases of the Northern Command of the Ethiopian National Defence Force, ordered armed intervention in the state. Many characterised the armed conflict between the two entities as a 'civil war'; for its part, the federal government described it as a surgical operation intended to enforce the rule of law in the Tigray state and conducted under the rules of federal intervention. The HoF ordered the Prime Minister to abolish the Tigray state government and appoint a transitional administrator once the federal government secured the TPLF's military defeat and gained full control of the state.

References

Addis Fortune. 2020. 'Tigray State to Start Door-to-Door Screening for COVID-19', 11 April, https://addisfortune.news/tigray-state-to-start-door-to-door-screening-for-covid-19/ (accessed on 20 January 2021).

Addis Standard. 2020a. 'Tigray State Council Approves Appointment of Regional Electoral Commission Officials', 16 July, https://addisstandard.com/news-tigray-state-council-approves-appointment-of-regional-electoral-commission-officials/ (accessed on 21 November 2020).

Addis Standard. 2020b. 'Tigray Region Says It Will Defy Federal Laws Enacted as of Oct. 05; EDP Calls for Transitional Gov't, Inclusive Dialogue & Reconciliation', 29 September, https://addisstandard.com/news-tigray-region-says-it-will-defy-federal-laws-enacted-as-of-oct-05-edp-calls-for-transitional-govt-inclusive-dialogue-reconciliation/ (accessed on 21 November 2020).

Anberbir, Yohannes. 2020. 'A Policy Framework Which Is Meant to Institutionalise IGR Has Been Sent to Parliament', *The Reporter*, 6 May, https://www.ethiopianreporter.com/article/10242 (accessed on 21 March 2020).

Ayele, Zemelak. 2014. *Local Government in Ethiopia: Advancing Development and Accommodating Ethnic Minorities*. Baden-Baden: Nomos Verlag.

Ayele, Zemelak. 2020. 'Far-sighted Federal Solidarity, Not Power Politics and Legalism, Is Needed to Solve Tigray Dispute', *Ethiopian Insight*, 9 October, https://www.ethiopia-insight.com/2020/10/09/far-sighted-federal-solidarity-not-power-politics-and-legalism-is-needed-to-solve-tigray-dispute/ (accessed on 20 January 2021).

Ayele, Zemelak. 2021. 'Constitutionalism and Electoral Authoritarianism in Ethiopia: From EPRDF to EPP', in Charles M. Fombad and Nico Steytler (eds), *Democracy, Elections, and Constitutionalism in Africa*, pp. 186–217. Oxford: Oxford University Press.

Ayele, Zemelak and Yonatan Fessha. 2012. 'The Place and Status of Local Government in Federal States: The Case of Ethiopia', *African Today*, 58(4): 89–109.

Dabalen, Andrew and Pierella Paci. 2020. 'How Severe Will the Poverty Impacts of Covid-19 Be in Africa?', *World Bank*, 5 August, https://blogs.worldbank.org/africacan/how-severe-will-poverty-impacts-covid-19-be-africa (accessed on 7 August 2020).

Ethiopian News Agency. (2020). 'Ethiopia Launches Door-to-Door COVID-19 Screening', 13 April, https://www.ena.et/en/?p=13832 (accessed on 19 February 2021).

Fana Broadcasting Corporate. 2020. 'It Has Been Decided That There Will Be a Complete Lock Down in Four Cities in the Amhara State, Including Bahr Dar' (translated),

31 March, https://twitter.com/addisstandard/status/1244992734911488001?lang=en (accessed on 14 December 2020).

FDRE Council of Constitutional Inquiry. 2020. Recommendations on Constitutional Issues that the House of Peoples Representatives Sent to the CCI in Relation to the Postponement of to the 6th General Elections due to COVID-19.

FDRE Ministry of Health. 2020. http://www.moh.gov.et/ (accessed on 19 February 2021).

FDRE House of Federation. 2020. The Permanent Committee for Constitutional Interpretation and Identity Affairs Draft Resolution on the Constitutional Interpretation by the Council of Constitutional Interpretation (CCI) on the Constitutional Issues Arising from the Postponement of the Sixth General Elections on Account of the Emergence of the COVID-19 Pandemic.

Fessha, Yonatan. 2019. 'A Federation without Federal Credentials: The Story of Federalism in a Dominant Party State', in Nico Steytler and Charles Fombad (eds), *Decentralization and Constitutionalism in Africa*, pp. 133–50. Oxford: Oxford University Press.

Fessha, Yonatan. 2020. 'The State of Ethiopian Federalism 2018–2019: Taking Intergovernmental Relations Seriously?' in Melaku G. Desta et al., *Ethiopia in the wake of political reforms*, pp. 403–21. Los Angeles: Tsehai Publishers.

Fikade, Birhanu. 2020. 'In May 2020, the HPR Adopted ETB 48.5 Billion ($1.2 Billion) Supplementary Budget in Order to Deal with the Financial Implications of Covid-19', *Ethiopian Reporter*, 23 May, https://www.thereporterethiopia.com/article/council-approves-second-supplementary-budget-four-months (accessed on 27 October 2020).

Fiseha, Assefa. 2007. *Federalism and the Accommodation of Diversity in Ethiopia: A Comparative Study*. Nijmegen: Wolf Legal Publishers.

Fiseha, Assefa. 2009. 'The System of Intergovernmental Relations (IGR) in Ethiopia: In Search of Institutions and Guidelines', *Journal of Ethiopian Law*, 23: 96–113.

Fiseha, Assefa and Zemelak Ayele. 2017. 'Concurrent Powers in the Ethiopian Federal System', in Nico Steytler (ed.), *Concurrent Powers in Federal Systems: Meaning, Making and Managing*, pp. 214–60. Leiden: Brill Nijhoff.

Getachew, Feven. 2020. 'Health Extension Workers Mobilized to Fight COVID-19 in Ethiopia', *UNICEF*, 29 June, https://www.unicef.org/ethiopia/stories/health-extension-workers-mobilized-fight-covid-19-ethiopia/ (accessed on 20 January 2020).

Public Health Emergency Operation Centre (PHEOC), Ethiopia: Weekly Bulletin. 2020. 'COVID-19 Pandemic Preparedness and Response in Ethiopia', 03 May, https://www.ephi.gov.et/images/novel_coronavirus/EPHI_-PHEOC_COVID-19_Weekly-bulletin_1_English_05042020.pdf (accessed on 20 January 2020).

Samuel, Gelila. 2020. 'State Avails Stimulus Package to Rescue Banking Industry', *Addis Fortune*, 28 March, https://addisfortune.news/state-avails-stimulus-package-to-rescue-banking-industry/ (accessed on 7 September 2020).

Wondwosen, Muluken. 2020. 'Parliament Approves Additional Budget to Fight Covid-19', *Capital Ethiopia*, https://www.capitalethiopia.com/featured/parliament-approves-additional-budget-to-fight-covid-19/ (accessed on 21 November 2020).

World Food Programme. 2020. 'Ethiopia WFP: Ethiopia Market Watch – May 2020', https://reliefweb.int/sites/reliefweb.int/files/resources/WFP%20Ethiopia%20Market%20Watch%20-%20May%202020.pdf (accessed on 8 September 2020).

18

SOUTH AFRICA

Surfing towards centralisation on the Covid-19 wave

Nico Steytler, Jaap de Visser and Tinashe Chigwata

18.1 Introduction

When the Covid-19 pandemic reached its shores between February and March 2020, South Africa was already in a vulnerable situation – socially, economically, and politically. Although the country's population, estimated at 59.6 million in 2020, is two-thirds urban, thus facilitating the spread of the virus, its age cohorts mitigated against Covid-19's devastating impact – 28.6 per cent of the population is below 15 years old, and only 9.1 per cent is 60 years and older. Nevertheless, other factors placed the country at heightened risk.

More than half of the population is poor, and the unemployment rate stands at 42 per cent (Statistics South Africa 2020); in South Africa, one of the most unequal countries in the world, the poor and unemployed are predominantly black. In 2018, social grants were, after salaries, the second main source of income for 45.2 per cent of households, with about 13.1 per cent of households living in informal dwellings. Most households with no or limited access to basic services, such as water, are found in townships, informal settlements, and rural areas – places which are inhabited mainly by black South Africans and where poverty tends to be extreme. In 2019, the public health system, which has been neglected for years, served more than 71 per cent of households, while only 16.4 per cent of the population had medical insurance cover for private health care (Statistics South Africa 2019). Moving out of these severe socio-economic conditions has been difficult, given that the South African economy had been in a downward spiral and was in a technical recession in March 2020.

Facing the tidal wave rolling in from abroad was a multilevel system of government comprising a national government, nine provinces and 257 local governments, the latter two characterised by great diversity in territorial size, population, and, eventually, infection rates. The two provinces with the highest

DOI: 10.4324/9781003166771-24

level of urbanisation – Gauteng and the Western Cape – became infection hot-spots, although two more rural provinces – KwaZulu-Natal and the Eastern Cape – followed close on their heels. The Northern Cape, the province with the largest territory and lowest population, sported the lowest infection rate. As for South Africa's municipalities, these range from large urban conglomerates – such as Johannesburg Metropolitan Municipality (population 5.7 million) in Gauteng and the City of Cape Town (3.4 million) in the Western Cape – to sparsely populated rural local municipalities.

These state institutions were governed largely by the African National Congress (ANC), which experienced deep in-fighting between the country's president, Cyril Ramaphosa, and a faction supportive of former president Jacob Zuma. In the 2016 local government elections, the party lost its majority in key metropolitan municipalities such as Johannesburg, Tshwane, and Nelson Mandela Bay and shed some electoral support to opposition political parties, namely, the official opposition, the Democratic Alliance (DA), representing mainly white and coloured voters, and the Economic Freedom Fighters (EFF), a split-off from the ANC with a radical Africanist and economic agenda. However, after the 2019 national and provincial elections, the ANC was firmly back in the saddle, remaining in control of both houses of Parliament, eight of the nine provinces and most of the 257 municipalities (including seven of the eight metropolitan councils). At the start of 2020, the ANC was therefore still the country's main political actor and facilitated coordination efforts when the pandemic broke out domestically.

South Africa recorded its first confirmed case of Covid-19 on 5 March 2020 and first Covid-19-related death on 27 March. By the end of May, it was in the top five in the world in terms of confirmed infections, with a total of 493,183, but in terms of Covid-19-related fatalities, the number was significantly low, at 8,005 (Department of Health 2020). After reaching a peak during June and July, case numbers dropped substantially, only to rise again in October when a second wave of infection gained momentum. By 31 October 2020, 725,452 infections had been recorded and 19,276 deaths (John Hopkins University 2020). These were much underreported figures: the number of natural deaths between 5 May and 10 November 2020 in excess of the anticipated number (so-called excess deaths) was 51,473, and in all probability linked to Covid-19 (Bradsaw et al. 2020).

The response to Covid-19 by South Africa's system of multilevel government entailed a centralisation of power that made the subnational governments' implementers rather than partners within the constitutional framework of cooperative government. The majority of provinces and municipalities were ill suited to manage the pandemic adequately due to incapacity, incompetence, and corruption. The possible benefits of a differentiated approach to decentralisation, in terms of which the well-functioning provinces and municipalities could have shown more initiative, were provided for but never explored. Unity, and not diversity, was the key word.

18.2 The federal constitutional and legislative framework

South Africa's Constitution of 1996 establishes a multilevel system of governance that may be described as a hybrid federal system (Steytler 2013). The provinces have exclusive powers over a short list of peripheral responsibilities (including ambulance services) but concurrent powers over a long list of significant ones, among them disaster management, education excluding tertiary education, health services, trade, and welfare services (Constitution, schedules 4 and 5). As both the national parliament and provincial legislatures have complete legislative powers over the concurrent responsibilities, conflicts are readily resolved in favour of national legislation on the basis of a qualified override clause. Local government's constitutionally protected set of responsibilities includes municipal health services, trading regulations, water and sanitation services, cemeteries, public places, refuse removal, and solid waste disposal (Constitution, schedules 4B and 5B). These functions may be regulated, however, by both the national and provincial governments. Any functional area not listed – such as international travel, policing, and the judiciary – falls under the residual powers of the national government.

An emergency such as the Covid-19 pandemic cuts across the listed responsibilities and involves all three levels of government, necessitating coordination and cooperation. The Constitution indeed instructs all three levels of government to adhere to the principles of intergovernmental relations and strive towards cooperative governance (sections 40 and 41). A formal and rule-bound system of intergovernmental relations (IGR) has been developed to support this. The Intergovernmental Relations Framework Act 13 of 2005 establishes the President's Coordinating Council (PCC), a forum for matters of national interest that comprises the President, deputy president, four national ministers, the premiers of the nine provinces, and a representative of organised local government (South African Local Government Association (Salga)). A national minister of a line department with a mandate falling within the list of concurrent functional areas may establish an IGR forum comprising the minister (Min) and members of the provincial executive council (MEC) responsible for that functional area – hence the forum's name of MinMEC. A representative of Salga must also be included if a matter affects local government.

The law also provides for two statutory MinMECs that are pivotal in the management of pandemics. The first is the Intergovernmental Committee on Disaster Management (discussed below). The second, comprising the national minister and the MECs for education, is the Council of Education Ministers, which is mandated to 'co-ordinate action on matters of mutual interest to the national and provincial governments' (National Education Policy Act 27 of 1996, section 9).

Given that states of emergency were used for political repression in the apartheid past, restrictions on such declarations were imposed by the 1996 Constitution. It provides that '[a] state of emergency may be declared only in terms of an Act of Parliament and only when … the life of the nation is threatened by war, invasion, general insurrection, disorder, natural disaster or other public emergency'; furthermore, the declaration has to be 'necessary to restore peace and order' (section 37(1)). It is subject to strict constitutional guarantees and is valid only for 21 days, unless the National Assembly approves its extension by a majority and then for not more than three months at a time.

The national executive decided not to use its emergency powers under the Constitution to manage the Covid-19 pandemic. Instead, it opted for using the framework of the Disaster Management Act 57 of 2002, which obviates the need for parliamentary approval.

18.3 Preparedness for a national disaster: The institutional framework

When measured in terms of the availability of law, policy, and plans, South Africa ought to have been well-prepared for Covid-19. The Disaster Management Act contains an impressive framework of national, provincial, and local institutions and mechanisms to manage disasters. Key features are a designated national minister, a National Disaster Management Centre, nine provincial disaster management centres, and 52 municipal disaster management centres (one for each district and metropolitan municipality), a dedicated intergovernmental committee, and an array of advisory forums, plans, and frameworks. The Act contains rules for the declaration of local, provincial, and/or national disasters.

The designated national minister is the Minister of Cooperative Governance and Traditional Affairs, the very same minister who oversees the functioning of the IGR system. Nationally, the Minister may declare a disaster if existing legislation and contingencies do not adequately equip the national government to deal with the disaster or other special circumstances warrant it. This then empowers the Minister to issue regulations on a vast array of matters. The overall purpose of the regulations must be to assist and protect the republic, provide relief, protect property, combat corruption, or deal with the destructive and other effects of the disaster.

The Act also provides for an Intergovernmental Committee on Disaster Management (mentioned above), which is the primary intergovernmental structure to oversee disaster management. When it was eventually established in 2016, it was a top-heavy forum comprising 20 national ministers, nine MECs and two Salga representatives (Presidency 2016).

18.4 Rolling out measures to contain the pandemic

When President Ramaphosa announced South Africa's lockdown regulations in March 2020, political parties across the board showed their solidarity with his strong stance, a sentiment shared by the broad public and various civil society formations. Nevertheless, as the first three weeks of lockdown turned into five weeks and another month of lockdown was announced until the end of May, and the impact of the regulations began hitting home in a dramatic rise in unemployment and poverty, the public's mood rose against the lockdown. The official opposition party, the Democratic Alliance (DA), also changed position, challenging the constitutionality of the Disaster Management Act and the regulations made thereunder; however, its approach to the Constitutional Court for direct access to that Court was denied (Mailovich 2020).

The crisis painfully revealed the deep schisms that run through South African society. In what is one of the most unequal countries in the world, the poor (largely synonymous with the black majority) felt the effects of the pandemic in two vital areas: access to health services and increased unemployment and poverty. Moreover, compliance with severe lockdown regulations highlighted the two different worlds in South Africa. Orders to observe social distancing and stay at home could be complied with (and was readily done so) in suburbia, but it was far less possible to heed them in the cramped living conditions in townships and informal settlements.

18.4.1 Taking the initiative

The first and main response to the coronavirus came from the national government when it declared a national state of disaster on 15 March 2020. The initial measures, promulgated on 18 March, included a travel ban on foreign nationals from high-risk countries, the prohibition of non-essential travel by government officials outside the country, the closure of all borders, and the screening of travellers. On 23 March, the President announced further, more drastic, measures centred on a national lockdown, which became effective on 27 March. In support of the national measures, particularly the call for social distancing, the City of Cape Town took the initiative to close its beaches from 24 March, three days before the lockdown came into effect. South Africa's lockdown was seen as one of the harshest in the world which included a ban on the sale of tobacco and alcohol, and the security forces enforced its regulations in a heavy-handed fashion.

From the outset, the national government adopted a centralised approach despite the fact that provinces have a concurrent responsibility for disaster management. The usual IGR structures were sidelined, in one fell swoop, by the announcement of a specialised disaster management structure at national level – the National Coronavirus Command Council (NCCC), an informal council established by the President and comprising, at first, a select number of cabinet ministers and, later, the entire cabinet. The NCCC's functioning was shrouded in secrecy.

18.4.2 National government action

The national government managed the pandemic chiefly by issuing regulations and directions under the Disaster Management Act after approval by the NCCC.

The first set of regulations, those of 18 March 2020, sought to (1) isolate South Africa from contagion by closing its international borders, (2) prevent the spread of the virus internally, and (3) manage the infected. Measures included the identification of places of quarantine and isolation by all three spheres of government, restriction of gatherings, closure of schools, restrictions on the sale and movement of alcohol and tobacco, and emergency procurement.

The second set of regulations, issued on 23 March 2020, ordered a 21-day national lockdown, effective from 27 March, that entailed severe prohibitions on freedom of movement and assembly. The regulations corralled, top-down, all subnational government structures into becoming facilitators and implementers of the national effort:

> For the duration of the state of disaster for Covid-19, all Premiers, Members of Executive Councils responsible for local government in the provinces, the President of the South African Local Government Association, all Executive Mayors/Mayors and institutions of Traditional Leadership shall take all reasonable measures to facilitate and implement the measures [against Covid-19].
>
> *(Direction 6(1) Disaster Management Act, 25 March 2020)*

In addition, all spheres of government and their agencies were directed to implement precautionary measures to mitigate employee health and safety risks. There were also directions aimed specifically at provincial and local governments. For instance, provinces were directed to work with municipalities in identifying quarantine and isolation facilities, to avail resources to disaster coordinative or management structures at the local level, to establish a special disaster management structure, to adopt Covid-19 response plans, to monitor the impact of the national government's Covid-19 interventions, and to report regularly to the national government.

The economic bite of the lockdown was felt immediately, and so a third set of measures focused on ameliorating the lockdown's economic and social impact (National Treasury 2020). On 21 April 2020, President Ramaphosa announced a ZAR 500 billion economic package providing for, among other things, the extension of lines of credit to small businesses. Food relief programmes, grants for the unemployed, funds for the health sector, and financial support for municipalities were also announced.

Shortly afterwards, on 23 April, came the exit plan from the lockdown – a 'risk-adjusted strategy' for managing the pandemic by means of five levels of lockdown, with alert level 5 the most stringent (imposing 'hard lockdown') and 1 the most relaxed. The country moved to alert level 4 on 1 May with a slight relaxation of the restrictions on movement. The strategy made provision for the possible imposition of different alert levels for different provinces and municipalities depending on infection rates. However, this differentiated approach was never adopted during the period under review.

After South Africa's infection numbers peaked in June and July 2020, the government moved to alert level 2 from 18 August to 30 September, a change that saw, inter alia, the lifting of restrictions on interprovincial travel and tourism-related activities. On 1 October, the country was on alert level 1, with the economy having been reopened fully and nearly all restrictions lifted, barring those on gatherings, sports events, and international travel, among other things.

Given the immediacy of the threat the pandemic posed, there was a strong shift to executive rule during the initial stages of the lockdown. Decisions taken by the NCCC and ratified by the cabinet were implemented without oversight from the legislature. Indeed, parliamentary proceedings were temporarily suspended, in line with lockdown regulations that prohibited in person sessions, but returned partially in May (Waterhouse 2020).

In the absence of a robust parliament holding the executive to account, civil society and political parties turned, as they had done before, to the courts to vindicate their rights and demands for good governance. The courts were, on the whole, not inclined to upset the apple-cart by invalidating regulations. As noted, the Constitutional Court gave the DA the cold shoulder when it contested the constitutionality of the Disaster Management Act itself. An attack on the legality of the regulations because of the 'unconstitutional' role of the NCCC was also rejected (*Esau and Others v. Minister of Co-operative Governance and Traditional Affairs and Others* [2020] ZAWCHC 56 (26 June 2020)). More successful was a civil society attack on the constitutionality of the declaration of a National State of Disaster and regulations made under it; a High Court found that while the declaration was constitutional, a number of regulations (the ban not allowing people to visit those dying of Covid-19, the ban on the operation of fisheries, hairdressers etc., and the restricted hours in which people could exercise) were irrational and thus invalid (*De Beer and Others v. Minister of Cooperative Governance and Traditional Affairs* [2020] ZAGPPHC 184 (2 June 2020)), a decision that became moot when these regulations fell away. The attack on the ban on the sale of tobacco also floundered as the High Court found that this regulation was rational as there was a link between the measure (tobacco ban) and its purpose (saving lives) (*Fair-Trade Independent Tobacco Association v. President of the Republic of South Africa and Another* [2020] ZAGPPHC 246 (26 June 2020)).

Unlike the European Union, the Africa Union (AU) in practice has a limited legal impact on South Africa in general and on combating Covid-19 in particular. However, South Africa played a part in formulating a comprehensive continent-wide strategy against the pandemic. Soon after the World Health Organization (WHO) declared Covid-19 a pandemic, the AU adopted its Africa Joint Continental Strategy for Covid-19 Outbreak which provided for the coordination of anti-Covid-19 efforts on the continent by AU member states, AU agencies, the WHO and other international agencies (AU and Africa CDC 2020).

As a member of the AU, South Africa was expected to implement the strategy and other measures of the AU, all the more so since President Ramaphosa, the incumbent chairperson of the AU, was leading the coordination of the continent-wide response to Covid-19, including the establishment of supply chains for shared resources, such as personal protective equipment (PPE).

18.4.3 Provincial action

With the response to Covid-19 being driven by the national government, provinces acted as supporting and implementing structures. To begin with, prior to the pandemic, no province had adopted provincial legislation on disaster management, despite it being a concurrent competency. Furthermore, during the pandemic, they did not take any legislative measures, with their policies and actions falling largely within the broader national Covid-19 strategy.

Within the scope of that strategy, provinces played an important role in three concurrent areas – health, education, and social welfare. First, provinces are responsible for both primary and secondary health care (i.e. for all hospitals and clinics). From the start, given that the objective of the lockdown was to flatten the curve of infections, provinces had to upgrade their health systems in preparation for the surge. This involved equipping existing hospitals and constructing field hospitals. They also conducted testing and contact tracing, monitored infection rates, and ran campaigns raising awareness about Covid-19.

Secondly, provinces implemented the national strategy with respect to the closure and opening of schools. For instance, when the national government announced the decision to reopen schools under level 3 (from 8 June 2020), provinces had to ensure that the schools were Covid-safe and educators and learners had the necessary PPE. Thirdly, within the broader strategy of minimising the harsh impact of the pandemic and the lockdown on livelihoods, provincial governments had to administer food relief programmes.

The provincial response to Covid-19, as prescribed by the national government, had to be uniform, but the actual performance was highly uneven. The Eastern Cape is the extreme example, but not the only case of incompetence mixed with corruption. Even several weeks into the lockdown, the provincial administration, in particular its health department, had not put adequate measures in place to respond to the pandemic. As a result, it failed to treat Covid-19 patients effectively or undertake testing and contact tracing, a situation that contributed to a high rate of viral transmission for a rural province. The national government was forced to provide support and oversight of the province in a manner that resembled a national-level intervention in a province, with the national Minister of Health bringing in a team of managers to assist the province in revamping its health system; medical personnel from the defence force were also deployed to augment the provincial health personnel. Less prominent but equally poor were health services in Mpumalanga and Limpopo.

Another common problem was poor recording of cases and deaths by provincial authorities. For example, for a period of 19 days an Eastern Cape health district that coincides with the Nelson Mandela Bay Metropolitan Municipality

(Port Elizabeth) reported no mortalities – notwithstanding that the metro managed 76 Covid-related burials in the same period (*Legal Brief* 2020a).

By contrast, the provincial governments of Gauteng and the Western Cape fared well in addressing the country's two main zones of infection. The Western Cape adopted innovative health measures. It put together a team of experts who produced large datasets to inform the province's response to Covid-19 in matters such as testing in hotspots and contact tracing. The Western Cape also established the country's first set of field hospitals for treating Covid-19 patients, for which it received accolades from the national Minister of Health.

Doing something contrary to national policy met with national disapproval. KwaZulu-Natal's attempt to impose a stricter lockdown regime by making quarantining in state institutions compulsory did not get far (*Legal Brief* 2020a). Being less restrictive than the national government was also frowned upon, but the Western Cape's MEC for education persisted in not toeing the line. In the initial lockdown, all government schools were closed, as were their school nutrition schemes. The Western Cape, however, continued to operate the scheme, though without meeting much central opposition.

The second skirmish evoked more reaction. The national Minister of Education gave a directive that schools should open on 1 June for Grade 7 and 12 learners, based on the condition that the schools would be Covid-safe. After petitions by most of the provincial departments of education for a delay because their schools were not yet ready, the Minister informally announced the postponement of the opening date by a week. The Western Cape MEC for education refused to comply, arguing that there was no need for the delay as 98 per cent of the schools in her province were Covid-safe; she instructed that schools reopen as originally scheduled by the Minister.

Condemnation came from several quarters. The Gauteng MEC for education, instead of supporting a provincial colleague, lashed out:

> The *misbehaviour* and the attitude of the Western Cape Government to think that they're a federal state or they're a government on their own and they can defy national government and open schools when we are told not to open schools must be rejected.
>
> *(Nicolson 2020, emphasis added)*

The MEC berated the Western Cape government further by saying '[they] don't support the need to ensure that all children are treated equally', and claiming the action would benefit the rich and prejudice the poor (Nicolson 2020). The same sentiment was shared by the South African Human Rights Commission and teachers' unions, who said that 'the Western Cape going alone undermined the unitary nature of our education system' (Nicolson 2020).

There was thus no space for a better-performing province to advance education: the overriding notion was that of solidarity where the pace is set by the slowest provinces. However, this reaction may only be partially concerned with federal politics; underlying it is antagonism towards the DA and the history of racial inequality in education. Representing mainly minority groups and, after the 2019 national and provincial elections, alienating and shedding most of its African leadership, the DA is perceived as promoting largely white interests.

Provinces cooperated in a number of areas, such as the management of inter-provincial traffic, movement of people between provinces, and the transportation of deceased persons across provincial boundaries. For instance, the Western Cape and Eastern Cape, which share a provincial boundary, entered into cooperative agreements to manage the movement of seasonal farm workers and deceased persons between the two provinces during the lockdown period.

Like the national parliament, provincial legislatures were not active in the early stages of the lockdown, seeing as their proceedings were temporarily suspended in line with national regulations prohibiting in-person sessions. The provincial response to Covid-19 was thus led and driven during this period by provincial executives operating without oversight by legislatures.

Overall, given their limited constitutional space, provinces in general did not push the boundaries of their autonomy but willingly accepted their role as implementers acting under national direction. They became in effect administrative agents of the national government, which funded their response to the pandemic. Few of them, however, excelled in their administrative role.

18.4.4 Local government action

The role played by local government was principally reactive. Municipalities generally positioned themselves as loyal partners in the national government's response; although they were closely monitored by provincial governments, they were ultimately left to their own devices to absorb the cost of the crisis.

The declaration of a national disaster was followed immediately by a range of detailed directions for local government. Among other things, municipalities were instructed to ban all public meetings, close public amenities and markets, sanitise public places, raise awareness, and increase water delivery to informal settlements. They were instructed as well to develop response plans, report regularly to their provincial governments, and set up and participate in the new district 'command councils' tasked to coordinate the government's response. The national government also ordered municipalities to ban all council and committee meetings, an instruction later amended to a blanket command to meet virtually. Municipalities were directed, furthermore, to abandon their internal delegations and allow the mayor, in consultation with the municipal manager and chief financial officer, to conduct emergency procurement to respond to the crisis (De Visser and Chigwata 2020a).

The impact of pandemic response on municipalities was threefold. First, a range of existing local government responsibilities was suddenly intensified and redirected. Municipal police and law enforcement were tasked with helping the South African Police Service and the army to enforce the lockdown (Beukes

2020). Water tanks needed to be delivered to settlements without access to water; street traders had to be furnished with special permits, public transport facilities, sanitised, and the like. Municipalities were also tasked with identifying infection hotspots and assisting in the identification of quarantine sites.

Secondly, a number of new responsibilities emerged, the most controversial one being the delivery of food parcels. Food assistance falls within the remit of the national and provincial departments of social development and education, which manage these two concurrent functions. However, in the chaos of the government's initial response to the hardship of the lockdown, municipalities became involved in the identification of recipients and even the funding of food parcels. This led to reports of councillors abusing the intervention for political ends and municipalities incurring unauthorised expenditure (Payne 2020a).

Thirdly, the lockdown had an immediate and devastating impact on municipal revenue, with collection of property rates dropping almost instantly. They were facing the prospect of fewer paying utility users and a reduction in intergovernmental funding (Davis 2020). For instance, although the national government promised them assistance to the value of ZAR 20 billion (National Treasury 2020: 7), this was woefully inadequate.

The fact that municipalities adopt their own budgets enabled them to pass adjustment budgets and redirect funds. Similarly, because they have considerable policy discretion to determine, and collect taxes and service fees, some were able to ameliorate the impact of the lockdown. For example, Stellenbosch Local Municipality introduced relief from property rates for individuals and companies that suffered losses as a result of the lockdown (Stellenbosch Local Municipality 2020). This was not a widespread practice, as most municipalities were too cash-strapped to follow suit. Other municipalities at least eased off on their debt collection and reconnected households whose services had been discontinued. There was innovation, too. Municipalities were thrust into a practice of holding online council meetings and experimenting in forms of public engagement that avoided the somewhat tired town-hall approach (De Visser and Chigwata 2020b).

Although the regulations provided for differentiated responses to the pandemic, local deviation from the national norms was not tolerated. The request of Ethekwini Metropolitan council to remain at level 5 when the rest of the country moved to level 4 found no national support (OFM 2020). By all accounts, the national government, unwavering in its initial response to the pandemic, centralised power in respect of local government and in the process also meddled in the provinces' oversight role.

First, it conscripted local government through measures that upended the constitutional status of local government. The initial blanket prohibition of all municipal council meetings was almost certainly unconstitutional; as for the subsequent instruction to all of them to meet virtually, this may have been overbroad, ignoring differences in size and ability to have responsible physical, or hybrid, meetings. The instruction to abolish internal checks and balances and centralise procurement in the mayor's office may not only have been constitutionally impermissible but also may have contributed to the corruption in PPE contracts that later engulfed the country.

Secondly, further centralised planning emerged through the 'command councils' that were set up to coordinate at each district and metropolitan level. These coincided with the roll-out of a new national government programme to improve intergovernmental alignment, the so-called District Development Model (DDM). The DDM is predicated on positioning the eight metropolitan municipalities and 44 district municipalities as the pivots for all intergovernmental planning (Department of Cooperative Governance and Traditional Affairs 2019). The DDM provides nothing that has not been tried before. However, bolstered by the momentum of district-led coordination of the Covid-19 response, it may end speculation about abolishing the much-maligned district municipality, the 'upper tier' of local government.

Thirdly, a similar trend emerged when national politicians assumed the role of mentoring local government. The President initiated an informal scheme of deploying senior ministers and their deputy ministers (also elected politicians) as 'mentors' to metros and key district municipalities. For example, the Minister of Trade and Industry, Pravin Gordhan, was sent to Tshwane Metropolitan Municipality (Pretoria) to assist a highly unstable council (Pijoos 2020). The significance of this initiative is that a national minister leapfrogged over the province that bears the primary responsibility of monitoring and support.

18.4.5 Intergovernmental relations

Throughout the pandemic, a strong centralised system and ethos prevailed, coming to the fore as well in the sidelining of pre-existing IGR forums and processes. The President's Coordinating Council (PCC) could have played a pivotal role in coordinating a whole-of-government approach. Instead, the PCC was pushed to the margins, with dictates coming mainly from the informal NCCC, on which there was no provincial and local representation.

There was some consultation with the provinces, however. When President Ramaphosa announced the first lockdown, he noted, after referring to the decision of the NCCC to that effect, that the decision was made after consulting the provincial premiers. Although the NCCC was the driving force in the country's pandemic response, in the initial phase of the lockdown the PCC did meet weekly, in contrast to its previous twice-yearly get-togethers. Anecdotal evidence suggests, though, that these meetings were a conduit for information and instructions rather than a platform for negotiation. Before the move to level 3 on 1 June 2020, it was reported that the President had a virtual meeting with the premiers and mayors *following* his announcement of the easing of restrictions (*Daily Maverick* 20 May 2020), which suggested that no *prior* consultation had taken place.

Although a top-heavy Intergovernmental Committee on Disaster Management had been established in 2016, it faded into obscurity and did not re-emerge during the lockdown. This by-passing of the Committee is in a sense a transgression of the spirit, if not the letter, of the Disaster Management Act: a dedicated, intergovernmental structure bringing together all three spheres of government to advise the cabinet, was replaced by an ad hoc structure consisting exclusively of national government ministers.

The Council of Education Ministers (CEM) fared better, emerging as a cooperative institution making joint decisions on key issues on schooling during the lockdown. In March 2020, prior to the lockdown, it reached agreements on matters such as the timetable for final-year examinations and the school calendar for 2021 (Motshekga 2020a). After the lockdown and closure of schools, the CEM held frequent meetings in an effort to save the school year. The national Minister, Angie Motshekga, also couched major decisions as those of the CEM (see Motshekga 2020c). However, such decisions were funnelled to the NCCC, which then affirmed even the school opening calendar (Motshekga 2020b).

The role of formal IGR forums also receded, with IGR consultations becoming more informal and direct. Ahead of a move to a level 4 lockdown, the Minister of Cooperative Government asked for input from the provinces (Meyer 2020), yet without using the Intergovernmental Committee on Disaster Management for that purpose. As the decision-making process at the national level was murky, it is not clear whether such inputs had any impact and whether the regulations were ever the product of agreements. Also, it would appear that provinces (and municipalities) preferred to direct specific requests directly to the President rather than work through IGR forums which did not allow space for individual provinces.

For example, after restrictions on liquor sales were eased for the first time in three months, the Eastern Cape premier asked for the reinstatement of the ban because of an increase in violence-related casualties at hospitals (Dayimani 2020). With the support of the Minister of Police, the President sprung a surprise on the country by re-imposing the liquor ban after a mere three weeks. By contrast, few of the requests from the Western Cape and the City of Cape Town seemed to find a receptive ear.

18.4.6 Intergovernmental fiscal relations

At the beginning of 2020, the South African economy was already in a technical recession. Moody's, the last of the rating agencies to do so, downgraded South Africa in March 2020 to junk status, making borrowing costlier. This was bad news, as the February 2020 national budget deficit as a percentage of gross domestic product (GDP) was 8.1. The biggest contributors to the problem were the major state-owned enterprises, which, thanks to years of maladministration and corruption, were deeply mired in debt. Moreover, due to past maladministration of the country's tax authority the revenue collection forecast for the 2020–2021 financial year fell substantially short of target. Consequently, the

Division of Revenue Bill of February 2020 contained cuts in the transfers to both the provinces and municipalities.

The lockdown, having closed most economic activities in the second quarter of 2020, brought further destruction to this ailing economy, which contracted in that period by 51 per cent; the official prediction for the year as a whole was that it would contract by 8.1 per cent. By the time the national Special Adjustments Budget was tabled at the end of June 2020, the budget deficit had nearly doubled to 15 per cent of GDP. Thus, while the economy was delivering less taxes, demands on government services and support escalated dramatically.

The provinces' increased responsibilities were not covered by transfers determined in February 2020 — transfers upon which provinces are almost totally dependent, given that only 3 per cent of their revenue is own revenue. Municipalities' own revenue fell by 60 per cent on average, and in the case of metros, by 30 per cent. The poor performance prompted Moody's to push two metros deeper into junk status in September 2020. By the end of June, more than half of the municipalities owed more to creditors than they had cash in the bank.

The National Treasury responded with a number of measures that provinces and local government had to adopt. First, provinces had to reprioritise their expenditure to meet pandemic-related needs. In the main, the reprioritised funds came from infrastructure spend on public works, roads, and transport. Secondly, spending cuts were sought, including breaching a three-year wage agreement that in 2020 would have given above-inflation wage increases to the civil service (including provincial officials) — a move vehemently opposed by labour unions.

Thirdly, equalisation transfers (i.e. each province and municipality's equitable share of the revenue raised nationally) were slightly reduced for provinces, but slightly increased for local government. Conditional grants for infrastructure development were suspended or reprioritised for Covid-19 spending.

Fourth, the shortfall in revenue drove the national government to take the politically contested step of borrowing money from the International Monetary Fund (IMF); the ANC's alliance partners — the trade union COSATU and the South African Communist Party — saw the spectre of losing national sovereignty to IMF structural adjustment programmes.

Despite these measures to save money, the national government did not hesitate to shoot itself in the foot by banning the sale of tobacco, thereby forsaking billions of rands in excise duties in exchange for a possibly marginal reduction in the pressure on hospitals. The ban on alcohol sales also contributed generously to the loss of 'sin taxes'.

The patrimonial state is firmly embedded in the fabric of the ANC and the governments they control, notwithstanding Ramaphosa's ascendency as president of the ANC and the country on an anti-corruption ticket and his subsequent actions in this regard. Financial accountability to Parliament, provincial legislatures and municipal councils is weak overall, a state of affairs not helped by the clampdown on oversight by provincial legislatures and municipal councils.

Indeed, the pandemic merely provided new feeding opportunities for the patrimonial state.

The saddest evidence was the looting by officials, politicians and their cronies of funds earmarked for Covid-19 relief, including for buying PPE using procurement procedures that had been relaxed given the urgency of the situation. In the Eastern Cape, for example, the number of provincial employees doing business with the provincial government jumped from 29 prior to the lockdown to 565 during it (*Legal Brief* 2020b). The shamelessness of the feeding frenzy was heightened by the fact that the Zondo Commission into State Capture was holding hearings at the same time on the financial depravity that characterised the Zuma presidency; moreover, in November 2020 the Secretary-General of the ANC was arrested on corruption and racketeering charges stemming from the Zuma years.

As far as national oversight of local finances was concerned, the Budget Forum, an IGR forum comprising the Minister of Finance and the nine MECs for finance, resolved that the National Treasury would take the lead in municipal financial matters while the Department of Cooperative Governance would keep an eye on governance and service delivery (Mkentane 2020). This clarification of roles in an area notorious for messy oversight overlaps may be one of the few financial positives to have come out of the lockdown.

18.5 Findings and policy implications

The Covid-19 pandemic and response to it touched the constitutional core of the multilevel government system – namely, the concurrent functions of disaster management, health services, social welfare and education – and thereby also brought the need for cooperative government to the fore. The national government, leading the charge against the pandemic, could have declared a state of emergency, but chose the unencumbered powers that the Disaster Management Act provides. Despite the existence of a system of cooperative government erected by the Constitution and legislation, powers were sucked up not only to the centre but also within the national government, in the form of the NCCC. Even where IGR forums worked cooperatively, such as with the CEM, their decisions had to be sanctioned by the NCCC. The end result was that the measures taken to combat the Covid-19 pandemic emphasised and enhanced the centralised nature of the South African system of multilevel government.

Provinces and municipalities were in effect corralled into being implementers of nationally determined measures. They did so willingly, but often not competently. The majority were mired in maladministration and corruption, although some provinces, notably Gauteng and the Western Cape, which contended with the two largest hotspots of infections, were capable of being efficient and even of developing innovative measures. Generally, the inhabitants of the Eastern Cape, for instance, fared poorly under their provincial government.

In the face of this unevenness, the question of whether subnational governments helped or hindered pandemic management cannot be answered with an unequivocal yes or no. To add to this equivocation, it is hard to speculate if the national government might have done better in their stead, since it is scarcely a paragon of good governance either.

Both provinces and local government lost some of their autonomy during the lockdown. Will this surge in centralisation have long-term implications for the current system of multilevel government? The great tidal wave of the Covid-19 pandemic, it is argued, may well send a state already tottering atop an upheaval of problems seemingly beyond its capacity to quell, towards centralisation.

First, one of the perennial reasons for centralisation is the poor performance of the majority of provinces and municipalities. The poor performance of most of the provinces during the pandemic deepened the pre-pandemic trend of incapacity, maladministration, and corruption. Although capacity is not in abundance in the national government, popular faith still rests at that level. The good performance of Gauteng and the Western Cape in dealing effectively with the highest rates of Covid-19 infections in the country is not likely to steer the national ship towards differentiated decentralisation. The same applies to municipalities: a steady decline in their performance prior to the pandemic was exacerbated by the lockdown.

The second reason for the further drift towards centralisation is the absence of a 'federal spirit' in the body politic. The federal spirit espoused by Michael Burgess (2012) refers both to tolerance of diversity among constituent units as well as to the celebration of innovative measures for better governance. The absence of this spirit within the ruling party and sections within society became glaringly conspicuous in the *contretemps* over a trifling practical but policy-laden decision by the Western Cape government to start schooling a week before the rest of the country. Doing something different from the rest of the provinces was attacked by the other well-performing province, Gauteng, as 'misbehaviour', on the ground that all provinces had to obey the national direction even though it was not couched in binding law.

The third reason for the continuing drift towards centralisation relates to the country's dire financial situation, acutely felt by subnational governments. In a context in which there is less public money, where provinces perform poorly and municipalities go bankrupt, expenditure controls will intensify in order to ensure better use of dwindling resources. Unlike the 2008 financial crisis – which did not much affect multilevel government in South Africa, a country that at the time had enjoyed a period of economic growth (Steytler and Powell 2010) – the Covid-19 crisis was far more severe in impact and afflicted an already-ailing economy. The national purse strings are thus likely to reign in autonomy.

Is it all bad news for decentralisation? Perhaps not. As the economic crisis, deepened by the lockdown, came to dwarf the fading Covid-19 health challenge, the national government's focus shifted to stimulating economic growth through infrastructure spending. Differentiated decentralisation, so argued the Gauteng and Western Cape governments, could be a further measure towards enhancing economic growth (Payne 2020b). Gauteng, the economic and financial hub of the country, argued that it should be allowed to raise its own revenue and to attract investments, while the Western Cape sought a much broader empowerment deal to provide a better governance infrastructure necessary for economic growth, including powers over policing, rail, and energy supply. The same arguments could be made by the main metropolitan governments.

Out of sheer desperation, the national government may well consider empowering the two provinces and the key metros to facilitate economic growth. A careful step in this direction was taken in 2020 when electricity laws were amended to enable municipalities to develop their own power generation projects, thus reducing their dependence on Eskom, the troubled national electricity utility. While anti-federal mindsets and political complexities tell against it, the prospect of differentiated decentralisation, though slight, is not remote.

References

African Union (AU) and the Africa Centres for Disease Control and Prevention (Africa CDC). 2020. *Joint Continental Strategy for Covid-19 Outbreak*.

Beukes, Jennica. 2020. 'Khosa v. Minister of Defense: Municipalities Warned on Enforcing the Lockdown', *Local Government Bulletin*, 15(2), https://dullahomarinstitute.org.za/multilevel-govt/local-government-bulletin/vol-15-issue-2-june-2020/khosa-v-minister-of-defense-municipalities-warned-on-enforcing-the-lockdown (accessed on 16 November 2020).

Bradsaw, Debbie, et al. 2020. 'Report on Weekly Deaths in South Africa 1 January–17 November 2020 (Week 46)', SA Medical Research Council, https://www.samrc.ac.za/sites/default/files/files/2020-11-25/weekly17November2020.pdf (accessed on 29 November 2020).

Burgess, Michael. 2012. *In Search of the Federal Spirit: New Theoretical and Empirical Perspectives in Comparative Federalism*. Oxford: Oxford University Press.

Davis, Gay. 2020. 'Extended Lockdown Could See Municipalities Lose R14bn in Revenue, Warns SALGA', *Eye Witness News*, https://ewn.co.za/2020/05/13/extended-lockdown-could-see-municipalities-lose-r14bn-in-revenue-salga (accessed 16 November 2020).

Dayimani, Malibongwe. 2020. 'Mabuyane Wants Alcohol Ban until Level 1 in Eastern Cape, Hits back at "Irresponsible" Critics"', *Media24*, 10 June, https://www.news24.com/news24/southafrica/news/mabuyane-wants-alcohol-ban-until-level-1-in-eastern-cape-hits-back-at-irresponsible-critics-20200610 (accessed on 28 November 2020).

De Visser, Jaap and Tinashe Chigwata. 2020a. 'Municipalities and COVID-19: A Summary and Perspective on the National Disaster Management Directions', *Local Government Bulletin*, 15(1), https://dullahomarinstitute.org.za/multilevel-govt/local-government-bulletin/volume-15-issue-1-march-2020/municipalities-and-covid-19-what-the-national-disaster-management-directions-mean-for-municipal-governance (accessed on 16 November 2020).

De Visser, Jaap and Tinashe Chigwata. 2020b. 'Municipalities and COVID-19: What the National Disaster Management Directions Mean for Municipal Governance',

Local Government Bulletin, 15(1), https://dullahomarinstitute.org.za/multilevel-govt/local-government-bulletin/volume-15-issue-1-march-2020/municipalities-and-covid-19-what-the-national-disaster-management-directions-mean-for-municipal-governance (accessed on 16 November 2020).

Department of Cooperative Governance and Traditional Affairs. 2019. *Towards a District Coordinated Development Model*.

Department of Health. 'Update on Covid-19 (31st July 2020)', https://sacoronavirus.co.za/2020/07/31/update-on-Covid-19-31st-july-2020/ (accessed on 2 October 2020).

John Hopkins University. 2020. 'South Africa', https://coronavirus.jhu.edu/region/south-africa (accessed on 30 October 2020).

Legal Brief. 2020a. 'Covid-19 Crisis: Municipalities Want Funding for Services, Too', *Legal Brief*, 28 April.

Legal Brief. 2020b. 'AG Reveals Scale of Procurement Corruption', Legal Brief Covid-19, 2 September.

Mailovich, Claudi. 2020. 'Constitutional Court Denies DA's Bid to Challenge Disaster Management Act', *Business Live*, 1 July, https://www.businesslive.co.za/bd/national/2020-07-01-constitutional-court-denies-das-bid-to-challenge-disaster-management-act/ (accessed on 5 October 2020).

Meyer, Warda. 2020. 'Só Sal Meer Kan Werk met Vlak 4', *Die Burger*, 29 April, p. 6.

Mkentane, Luyolo. 2020. 'Treasury to Keep Closer Eye on Municipal Finances', *Business Day*, 25 August, p. 2.

Motshekga, Angie. 2020a. 'Statement Delivered by the Minister of Basic Education, Mrs Angie Motshekga at a Media Briefing Following the Meeting of the Council of Education Ministers Held in Pretoria', 9 March, https://www.gov.za/speeches/meeting-council-education-ministers-9-mar-2020-0000 (accessed on 5 October 2020).

Motshekga, Angie. 2020b. 'Basic Education Sector Recovery Plans for the Reopening of Schools, Following the Coronavirus Covid-19 Lockdown Adjustment of Regulations', 20 April, https://www.gov.za/speeches/minister-angie-motshekga-basic-education-sector-recovery-plans-reopening-schools-following (accessed on 5 October 2020).

Motshekga, Angie. 2020c. 'State of Readiness for the Opening of Schools', 7 June, https://www.gov.za/speeches/minister-angie-motshekga-state-readiness-reopening-schools-7-jun-2020-0000 (accessed on 5 October 2020).

National Treasury. 2020. *Economic Measures for COVID-19*, http://www.treasury.gov.za/comm_media/press/2020/20200428_COVID_Economic_Response_final.pdf (accessed on 16 November 2020).

Nicolson, Greg. 2020. 'Panyaza Lesufi: Western Cape Is Undermining the Poor by Opening Schools', *Daily Maverick*, 2 June, https://www.dailymaverick.co.za/article/2020-06-02-panyaza-lesufi-western-cape-is-undermining-the-poor-by-opening-schools/ (accessed on 5 October 2020).

OFM. 2020. 'Parts of KZN May Remain on Level 5 Lockdown', OFM, 27 April, https://www.ofm.co.za/article/sa/287655/parts-of-kzn-may-remain-on-level-5-lockdown (accessed on 16 November 2020).

Payne, Suné. 2020a. 'Western Cape Councillors Barred from Food Distribution', *Daily Maverick*, 14 May, https://www.dailymaverick.co.za/article/2020-05-14-western-cape-councillors-barred-from-food-distribution/ (accessed on 16 November 2020).

Payne, Suné. 2020b. 'Give Us More Power to Boost Economic Recovery, Say Gauteng and Western Cape', *Daily Maverick*, 2 October, https://www.dailymaverick.co.za/article/2020-10-02-give-us-more-power-to-boost-economic-recovery-say-gauteng-and-western-cape/ (accessed on 16 November 2020).

Pijoos, Iavan. 2020. 'Pravin Gordhan Deployed to Lead Tshwane's Fight against Covid-19', *Timeslive*, 20 July, https://www.timeslive.co.za/politics/2020-07-20-pravin-gordhan-deployed-to-lead-tshwanes-fight-against-covid-19 (accessed on 16 November 2020).

Presidency. 2016. 'President Zuma Appoints Intergovernmental Committee on Disaster Management', 24 August, http://www.thepresidency.gov.za/content/president-zuma-appoints-intergovernmental-committee-disaster-management (accessed on 6 October 2020).

Statistics South Africa. 2019. 'Statistical Release P0318: General Household Survey 2018'.

Statistics South Africa. 2020. 'Quarterly Labour Force Survey, Quarter 2: 2020', http://www.statssa.gov.za/?p=13652&gclid=Cj0KCQiAh4j-BRCsARIsAGeV12DSlNx0tXjcgCAHyyUcbmcxb4eERyd67BgbsOBA0UhOmuU6yDK0dNEaApnNEALw_wcB (accessed 28 November 2020).

Stellenbosch Local Municipality. 2020. 'COVID-19 Relief Measures for Residents: Stellenbosch Tackles Challenges Head-On', 26 March, https://stellenbosch.gov.za/2020/03/26/corona-virus-update/ (accessed on 16 November 2020).

Steytler, Nico. 2013. 'South Africa: The Reluctant Hybrid Federal State', in John Loughlin, Wilfried Swenden and John Kincaid (eds), *The Routledge Handbook of Regionalism and Federalism*, pp. 442–54. London and New York: Routledge.

Steytler, Nico and Derek Powell. 2010. 'The impact of the global financial crisis on decentralised government in South Africa', *L'Europe en Formation*, 358: 149–72.

Waterhouse, Samantha. 2020. 'Now is Not the Time to Suspend Parliamentary Oversight', *Daily Maverick*, 7 April, https://www.dailymaverick.co.za/article/2020-04-07-now-is-not-the-time-to-suspend-parliamentary-oversight/ (accessed on 16 November 2020).

19
MANAGING COVID-19 IN A 'FAÇADE FEDERALISM'
The case of Nigeria

Lukman Abdulrauf

19.1 Introduction

On 27 February 2020, Nigeria, one of Africa's major federations, recorded its first case of Covid-19. The pandemic struck at the peak of its political, economic, and social challenges. The country had just emerged from a bitter election further polarising it along ethno-religious lines; economically, it was battered by a sharp fall in oil prices, a huge infrastructural deficit, and corruption. Indeed, at the turn of 2020, it was in its second recession in four years, with unemployment and soaring poverty rates a cause for grave concern.

Nigeria's population is estimated at 208 million, making it the largest country in Africa and seventh largest in the world (WPR 2020). Most of its people are concentrated in a few cities, with Kano in the lead with about 14 million, followed by Lagos with 13 million (NBS 2018). The population is not only large but diverse. More than 500 ethnic groups are spread across different regions that together span an area of 923,768 km^2, a fact pointing to the reasons that the country adopted federalism.

Politics in Nigeria – a country divided into a Federal Capital Territory (FCT) and 36 states that comprise 774 local governments – is heavily influenced by ethnicity and religion. Of its two main parties, the People's Democratic Party (PDP) was the dominant party until its defeat in the 2015 elections by the All Progressives Congress (APC), which is currently the ruling party at federal level, albeit not without serious opposition from the PDP. Much of the North and South-West are controlled by the APC; the PDP controls the East and South-South.

Health care has long been a campaign priority for political parties, yet there is little to show for it. Nigeria's average life expectancy of 54.5 years is one of the lowest in West Africa, while rates of HIV-AIDS, poliovirus, and child and

DOI: 10.4324/9781003166771-25

maternal mortality remain high, with one out of every five children dying before the age of 5 (WPR 2020). The weaknesses this indicates in the public health system were further exposed by the Covid-19 pandemic. After the country's first case was recorded, the federal government re-assessed the system and admitted that until then it had never realised the extent to which health care in Nigeria is in decay.

The rate at which the coronavirus began to spread in Lagos and FCT was alarming. The first 30 days after the first confirmed case showed an elitist disease distribution in that most of the infected persons were returnees from abroad (NCDC 2020a). When it became obvious that community transmission had started, it was the Lagos state government that took the first concrete step of imposing a lockdown in the state.

By August 2020, Nigeria reached the peak of its infections and, with cases declining, the government began a phased reopening of the country and a roll-out of economic recovery measures. By the beginning of October, however, a second wave of infection and lockdown was anticipated, particularly in the light of country-wide protests against police brutality, but this did not come to pass, as the total number of confirmed cases by the end of the month remained low at 62,853, with 1,144 fatalities (NCDC 2020a).

For a country with an ailing health-care system, these statistics may look impressive. Yet while some have commended the country's response, others argue that the figures do not bespeak success for reasons such as inadequate reporting and low rates of testing. There is hence no clear picture yet of the state of the pandemic in Nigeria or how effectively it was addressed.

This chapter contributes to an evolving understanding of the situation by examining the multilevel government response to Covid-19 in Nigeria until the end of October 2020. Its key findings are that federalism in Nigeria is dysfunctional, that this had an impact on a coordinated response to the pandemic, and that states and local government are consigned a diminishing role while otherwise having to keep up the pretence of 'façade federalism'.

19.2 The federal constitutional and legislative framework

The Constitution of 1999 delineates the role of each of Nigeria's three tiers of government. The federal government has exclusive powers over issues in the Exclusive Legislative List, while matters in the Concurrent List are shared between it and state government (sections 4(2), (4), (7)); states have exclusive powers over matters in the 'residual list'. Local government authorities (LGAs), or councils, also have powers set out in the Constitution.

While each tier is expected to function independently based on its legislative competence, the federal government's powers have preponderance over the others. For instance, in terms of section 4(5), federal legislation overrides state legislation where there is potential conflict between them. The disequilibrium between state governments and LGAs is more pronounced in that the latter depend on the former for their existence and structure (section 7).

As health care is not in the exclusive or concurrent lists, logically it is a residual matter within the competence of state government (Nwabueze 2014: 380). This inference is fortified by the fact that the Constitution stipulates that the 'provision and maintenance of health services' is one of the functions in which LGAs participate in state governance (Fourth Schedule, section 2(c)). Other health-related LGA services include sanitation and refuse disposal. In the case of health care, then, it is the responsibility of the state government, which is supported in this regard by LGAs.

In the case of disaster management, however, the position is not as straightforward. While the Constitution vests the power to declare a state of emergency in the event of disasters solely in the federal government, the National Emergency Management Agency Act 50 of 1999 (NEMA Act) seems to establish a joint regime comprising both the federal government and states. It is thus arguable that disaster management, unlike health care, is supposed to be their shared responsibility, with the federal government playing the leading role.

Moreover, in the event of a pandemic that can be considered a natural disaster, the federal government can declare a state of emergency 'in the federation or any part thereof' (Constitution, section 305). This is an exclusive power of the President; the governor of a state can only 'request' that the President declare a state of emergency in a state (section 305(4)). The President, though, has overriding powers 'if a State fails within a reasonable time to make a request' (section 305(5)).

Importantly, Nigeria's Constitution, unlike that of many other countries, does not distinguish between a state of national disaster and a state of emergency. In Nigeria, states of emergency have been declared in states several times, for instance in response to terrorism by Boko Haram. States of emergency have not been declared before for health emergencies, however, despite calls for this during the Ebola crisis. As with Covid-19, the government did not consider Ebola a sufficiently 'imminent danger' to warrant such a declaration (Abdulrauf 2020a).

Generally, state governments have powers to 'make laws for the peace, order, and good government of the State' (Constitution, section 4(7)). This means they can make emergency laws as well, so long as it is for the peace, order, and good government of the state and it is within their legislative competence. In case of public health emergencies, state governments can make regulations in the course of exercising emergency powers based on their public health laws. Such emergency regulations may also be justified by federal legislation, in this case by the Quarantine Act of 1926. Although quarantine is a matter within the federal Exclusive Legislative List, the Quarantine Act vests state governors with the powers to make emergency regulations if the federal government fails to do so (Quarantine Act, section 8).

It is on the basis of this legal framework that the Lagos state government issued the Infectious Disease (Emergency Prevention) Regulation 2020 which gave the governor powers, inter alia, to restrict movement and close internal borders. LGAs do not have any equivalent powers.

19.3 Preparedness for a national disaster: The institutional framework

The nature of the disaster determines the appropriate institution to respond to it. Generally, the National Emergency Management Agency (NEMA) is the primary agency responsible for disaster management. Established by the NEMA Act, its responsibilities are, among other things, to formulate policies on disaster management and coordinate the relevant plans and programmes. NEMA is an agency under the Federal Ministry of Humanitarian Affairs, Disaster Management and Social Development.

NEMA does not appear to be an intergovernmental body because other tiers of government are not represented in its membership. Moreover, phrasing in the Act suggests its distinctness from equivalent institutions at state level. The Act mandates states to establish a State Emergency Management Committee/Agency (SEMC/A) to 'respond to any disaster within the state' (NEMA Act, section 9(b)), albeit that, to date, only 25 states have SEMAs (Mashi et al. 2019: 8); at the national level, NEMA is only to 'liaise' with the state committees 'to assess and monitor' the distribution of relief material (NEMA Act, section 6).

On this basis, NEMA is, arguably, not established as an intergovernmental body, which means in turn that the federal government is solely responsible for disaster management at federal, or nation-wide, level.

Since Covid-19 is classifiable as a natural disaster, the role of one other agency is noteworthy: the Nigeria Centre for Disease Control (NCDC). It has the responsibility of coordinating the scientific response to epidemics and pandemics, with its main function being 'to lead the preparedness, detection, and response to infectious disease outbreaks and public emergencies' (NCDC 2020b). Formed in 2011, the NCDC first came to prominence during the West African Ebola virus epidemic of 2013–2016.

19.4 Rolling out measures to contain the pandemic

As countries worldwide began taking action to curb the pandemic, Nigeria followed suit with similar measures, chiefly the closure of international borders, restriction of movement, and development of relief interventions. At the federal level, the President introduced them formally in a national address on 30 March 2020. The ruling APC was in full support of the measures, while the PDP took a critical stance, castigating President Buhari's administration for having allowed the virus to get into the country in the first place and blaming this lapse on its 'negligence and laidback attitude to the governance and welfare of Nigerians' (Premium Times 2020). However, what drew the most heated criticism, particularly from opposition parties, was the unilateral way the central government imposed the lockdown on the federated states.

More widely, the diverse character of Nigerian society had an impact on the response to Covid-19. The degree of seriousness with which different regions took the pandemic varied and largely reflected the North-South divide. In most parts of the North, even the political class treated it with some levity. This was apparent in the initial response in such states as Kano, as well as among the population at large, where levity sometimes turned into violent resistance against the lockdown and social distancing orders. For example, youths in Katsina state (in North-Western Nigeria) set a police station ablaze because its officers, in enforcing these orders, prevented them from attending their mosque.

Similarly, the sense of marginalisation commonly felt by people in poor rural communities was deepened by the government's response measures. Many of them thought the pandemic was a hoax or a trick the government had pulled off to exploit them; others yet believed the pandemic affects only the rich and powerful, given the number of high-profile individuals who contracted the virus or went on to die of it (Ihonvbere 2020).

19.4.1 Taking the initiative

Initially, there was uncertainty about who should take the lead in responding to the pandemic. A first possible reason for this is that governments at all levels appear to have underestimated its potential harmfulness, so it took some time before they appreciated the magnitude of what was at stake and gave full focus to questions of who should respond and in what way. A second reason related to the conflict of legal frameworks regarding the pandemic. If Covid-19 were considered a natural disaster, it would fall under the NEMA Act and the response be driven by the federal government; however, if it were considered a health matter, it would be within the constitutional competence of state governments, with the support of LGAs.

After Nigeria reported its first confirmed case in February 2020, the federal government constituted the Presidential Task Force on Covid-19 (PTF) only on 9 March, two days before the World Health Organization (WHO) declared Covid-19 a pandemic. The PTF did not take any concrete steps immediately on being established. Since most cases then were imported, the federal government closed all air and land borders on 18 March. Thereafter, cases started to increase exponentially and it became clear that community transmission had set in.

Lagos State, initially the epicentre, witnessed the highest daily increase – unsurprisingly so, given that it is the country's commercial hub and has one of the busiest international airports in Africa. On 23 March, it also saw Nigeria's first coronavirus-associated fatality.

Thus, it was that on the following day, 24 March, the government of Lagos State took the first decisive steps in Nigeria towards domestic containment by imposing restrictions on social gatherings and certain businesses with effect from 26 March. The restrictions were formalised on 27 March in the Lagos State Infectious Diseases (Emergency Prevention) Regulation 2020, the essence of which is that it gives the state governor reactive emergency powers to curtail the spread of the virus. The Ekiti state government made a similar regulation.

With these states having got the ball rolling, the federal government awoke from its slumber and began taking charge. In a televised address on 29 March, President Buhari ordered a two-week lockdown of the FCT and the two states with the highest case numbers, responses that were formalised in a regulation of 30 March (Covid-19 Regulation No. 1); the latter was subsequently extended on April 14 (Covid-19 Regulation No. 2). After this intervention by the federal government, all the other states, excepting Kogi and Cross River, imposed restrictions of one form or another between March and May.

In a further address on 27 April 2020, the President announced that from 2 May there would be a 'phased and gradual' easing of lockdown measures in the states with federally decreed lockdowns in place. The other states with state-imposed restrictions followed suit and started to ease their lockdown measures.

19.4.2 Federal government action

As mentioned, the federal government's first formal step was to issue Covid-19 regulations pursuant to the powers of the President under the Quarantine Act of 1926 (sections 2–4). The first regulation, which was for an initial 14-day period, declared Covid-19 'a dangerous infectious disease' and outlined measures for curtailing the effects of the coronavirus. They included the suspension of air travel and restriction of movement in Lagos, Ogun, and the FCT. At the expiration of the term of the regulation, another regulation was made for a 14-day extension (Covid-19 Regulation No. 2 of 2020).

In the course of making these regulations, the President was criticised for intruding in state government with the unilateral declaration of lockdowns in Lagos and Ogun, and, later, Kano. This was said to be unlawful since no state of emergency was in place in terms of the Constitution and the President never provided any clear legal justification when the order was made in his national address – it was only on the day thereafter that the Quarantine Act was invoked to justify his actions. This issue thus touches on the larger conflict between the Quarantine Act, which is still an effective law, and the Constitution.

The army was deployed to provide support in enforcing lockdown orders, especially at the country's borders, but it played a broader role than this. According to an army memo, the army was to forcibly transfer the sick to hospitals and enforce lockdown orders by the President and state governors (TRT World 2020). It also leased equipment to the government for possible mass burials and deployed medical personnel (Punch Healthwise 2020a).

Socio-economic measures were adopted too, especially for the most vulnerable in society. The Ministry for Humanitarian Affairs, Disaster Management, and Social Development pledged to distribute food to vulnerable households. Furthermore, in terms of a conditional cash payments initiative launched in April 2020, NGN 20,000 would be paid to families in the National Social Register of Poor and Vulnerable Households, established in 2016 to combat extreme poverty. As of October, the Social Register contained 4.6 million poor and vulnerable households – arguably insignificant in a country where an estimated 83 million people, or 40 per cent of the population, live below the poverty line (NBS 2018). With regard to micro, small, and medium enterprises, the Central Bank of Nigeria announced that NGN 50 billion in credit facilities was being made available to support them (CBN 2020).

What is striking about these socio-economic measures is that they were all managed by the federal government and its agencies and that none were sufficient for meeting the needs of Nigeria's teeming population.

Towards the end of April, the pandemic seemed under control and the federal government began a phased reopening of the country under the direction of the PTF and NCDC. Curfews were relaxed and centres of worship reopened, albeit that the latter were still subject to hygiene and social distancing protocols. Airspace was opened to domestic travel on 5 July and international travel on 5 September, with international travellers having to use only two of Nigeria's international airports (Lagos and Abuja). Students in exit classes resumed school on 17 August, while those in other levels were to resume in October.

Since the exigencies of the pandemic called for swift action, executive rule held sway. The President took unilateral decisions without recourse to the legislature, as emergency powers under the Quarantine Act enable him to make regulations and orders without legislative intervention. The National Assembly played only three notable roles during this time. First, it 'advised' the federal government to urgently set aside a special intervention fund to curtail the spread of Covid-19. Secondly, the Senate Committee on Health and Private Healthcare and Communicable Diseases was to continue to engage with the Federal Ministry of Health and the PTF while the legislature was in recess due to the pandemic (Nwachukwu 2020). Thirdly, the House of Representatives (the lower legislative house) passed the Emergency Economic Stimulus Bill 2020 to provide economic relief to businesses and individuals (BKLC 2020).

Neither the legislature nor the judiciary served any substantial accountability function during this period. There were no cases before the courts on constitutional challenges relating to the federal system; as for the legislature, paradoxically, it sought to give the executive greater powers. It wished, in particular, to hurry into law the Infectious Diseases Bill of 2020, which gives the President, Minister of Health and Director-General of the NCDC extensive powers in managing infectious diseases (Abdulrauf 2020a). Controversy around the bill led to a court action – *Sen. Dino Melaye v. The Clerk of the National Assembly of the Federal Republic of Nigeria and 4 Others* – seeking its provisions declared authoritarian, undemocratic, and unconstitutional. In view of an outcry against the bill from state governments, civil society, and others, it was provisionally withdrawn.

The federal government's pandemic response was informed by the decisions and guidance of international organisations. First, it was guided by the Africa Joint Continental Strategy for Covid-19 Outbreak, which was jointly established by the African Union and Africa Centres for Disease Control and Prevention (African Union and Africa CDC 2020). The Director-General of the NCDC was co-chair of one of the working groups of the Africa Task Force for Coronavirus (AFTCOR), which is the coordinating body of the strategy. Secondly, Nigeria adhered to WHO guidelines on Covid-19. The WHO country representative in Nigeria was an active member of the PTF, which, as mentioned, is the coordinating structure in place for the management of Covid-19 in Nigeria. For its part, the Economic Community of West African States (ECOWAS) merely issued statements and provided updates with which the Nigerian response was already in alignment.

19.4.3 State government action

Given that the federal government monopolised the pandemic response, states had to align themselves with its strategy and directives. This was illustrated by its National Covid-19 Pandemic Multi-Sectoral Response Plan, in terms of which federal agencies were dominant and state agencies assigned only a subsidiary role. The Response Plan 'directed' states to establish a Covid-19 Taskforce to be chaired by their governors or the latter's designates and to establish a State Emergency Operation Centre (EOC) along the same lines as the federal NCDC's EOC (FG 2020: 20 and 21).

In view of their constitutional competence in health, state governments, with varying degrees of effort, upgraded their health-care facilities and set up isolation centres. With the support of the NCDC, state governments established greater numbers of molecular laboratories in order to scale up virus testing. Lagos State, the epicentre of the pandemic, erected the largest number of isolation centres in the country, an effort that included converting the state sports stadium into an isolation centre.

Within their constitutional spaces, state governors, as chief security officers, put in place and enforced lockdown orders. The latter was tricky in that the only police force is the federal police (Okeke 2020: 5) and, as such, state executives do not have direct control of the police without recourse to the federal government (Elaigwu 2005). Nevertheless, they found the means to work around this constitutional complexity. In the case of states controlled by the ruling party, they tried to ensure a harmonious working relationship with the police; as for states controlled by opposition parties, some established special taskforces to monitor their borders and thereby avoid alleged 'sabotage' by the federal police.

Despite the dominance of the federal government, various state governments still found the space in which to assert their autonomy. For example, when the federal government imposed a lockdown in the FCT and states of Lagos and Ogun commencing on 30 March 2020, the governor of Ogun postponed the start of the lockdown by five days to allow residents time to stock up on food and other necessities (Onwubiko 2020). Similarly, the Kano state government eased the centrally imposed lockdown even before its expiration date 'to enable people to move out and make some purchases' in preparation for the Muslim Ramadan fast (Mbah 2020).

Generally, however, states willingly complied with the federal government, especially those controlled by the ruling party. Their pandemic responses were, accordingly, crafted along the lines of the federal government's Covid-19 regulations of March and April 2020 and in adherence to the PTF. In expressing support for the federal government's supremacy, the governor of Lagos State mentioned on two occasions that, in regard to the curfew, only the President who declared the curfew can decide on it otherwise. Similarly, when the federal government relaxed restrictions on inter-state travel, the governor of Cross River State said the state had surrendered its sovereignty and duly opened its boundaries as per the federal order (Punch Healthwise 2020b).

Since the states generally aligned their responses with the federal government, few of them felt compelled to devise innovative means to deal with the virus within their constitutionally permitted spaces (Okeke 2020: 6). However, the Lagos state government was creative in regard to contact tracing and adopted a relatively effective house-to-house testing initiative; it also set up testing centres in all LGAs and supported this initiative with an intensive publicity campaign (Ihonvbere 2020). Similarly, the Lagos state legislature went above and beyond other state legislatures by enacting, on 26 March 2020, the Emergency Coronavirus Pandemic Law of 2020, which recommended penalties for defaulters of lockdown regulations and empowered the governor to declare an emergency for up to three months; the governor was also required to consult the legislature before issuing any regulations.

State governments undertook numerous initiatives to ameliorate the social and economic effects of pandemic control. For example, they gradually reversed lockdowns imposed by either themselves or the federal government. Because states had differing ideas about easing, there was no unified approach, albeit that they generally toed the federal line. Some were consequently quick to ease lockdowns, others, slower. The Oyo state government (controlled by the opposition PDP) began easing its lockdown in April even when infections were on the increase – the governor argued that 'the economic health of the state is more important than public health' and that this was in residents' best interests (Feyisipo 2020). Lagos State also began to ease lockdown regulations so as to mitigate economic hardships.

Another common initiative was to provide material relief to vulnerable groups. Lagos State, at the start of the lockdown, announced several poverty-alleviation packages (Shaban 2020). In one of these, it budgeted for 200,000 households – amounting to 1.2 million residents – to receive food rations. In another, it provided unconditional cash transfers to about 250,000 economically challenged persons listed with the Lagos State Residents Registration Agency (LASRRA); further initiatives included a school-feeding programme aimed at feeding more than 37,000 households in which school pupils were living. Other states, such as Kano, had similar initiatives in place (Murtala 2020).

Such efforts were supported by private donations to state governments and by the Coalition against Covid-19 (CACOVID), a private sector partnership with the federal government. Yet as laudable as they were, it was – to echo similar remarks in the discussion above of federal government action – scarcely conceivable that they could make any significant impact given the size of state populations. There were claims, too, that poverty-alleviation measures were deployed for political and/or corrupt purposes. For instance, in protests in April 2020 in Lagos and the FCT, the contention was that politicians were corruptly diverting relief-measure resources to their party loyalists or into their own pockets (Okon 2020).

There were indeed instances too where states obstructed the implementation of necessary preventative measures. A notorious example is provided by the Kogi state government, which denied the existence of Covid-19 when its governor declared that '[n]inety percent of the noise about Covid-19 is for political, economic, financial [or] material gain. The other 10% [is about] ordinary flu, like the common colds Nigerians generally suffer' (Offiong 2020). The governor went on to refuse to allow testing in the state, threatening to quarantine the PTF delegation sent to Kogi to provide technical support. When two cases were reported, he dismissed them as 'false allocations', all the while rejecting federal intervention; finally, when he had to put in place a state Covid-19 taskforce, he refused to fund it.

Kogi's case was all the more controversial because the state is located in the North-Central region and sits between states with a high number of infections. In a similar episode of state-level obstructionism, the Cross River state governor questioned the need for social distancing and cast doubt on scientific evidence regarding the coronavirus (Offiong 2020).

As at the federal level, the exigencies of the pandemic and need for speed meant that state-level accountability structures were relegated to the sidelines. State executives, like their federal counterpart, unilaterally took decisions where circumstances required. Although state legislative houses were closed in the early stages of the lockdown, they all reopened during its easing. Even so, they mostly played an insignificant role and rubber-stamped the actions of governors. Only in Lagos State was the legislature proactive in monitoring executive action.

It is worth noting, though, that even before the pandemic, state legislatures had long been under the thumb of too-powerful governors. Nor were the courts particularly useful either as accountability mechanisms: there were no cases challenging state government actions. While all state courts were closed for two weeks from 24 March 2020 – and thereafter indefinitely by the Chief Justice of the Federation, raising another concern for Nigeria's federalism – they were subsequently reopened.

The overall response among states was mixed. While most of them willingly followed the federal government, a few attempted to assert their autonomy – some for no good cause. State responses were also indirectly influenced by party-political dynamics, but, all in all, it was the federal government that called the tune and directed state responses.

19.4.4 Local government action

Local governments were not left out in the fight against Covid-19. In terms of the Constitution, LGAs are expected to participate in state matters concerning health services. However, they were not properly harnessed for this purpose, partly because LGA-maintained health care and basic education facilities are the worst in the country and notoriously corrupt (see Isa 2016).

Only in two areas were LGAs commonly used. First, they assisted states in the distribution of material support (mostly food packages), though not without criticism – Ihonvbere (2020) maintains that '[LGA] chairmen ... politicized the distribution by only favouring their political party members'. Secondly, LGAs were deployed to support state governments in conducting public education and awareness-raising campaigns in rural areas.

In Lagos State, LGAs participated more actively and widely in the state government response. They formed part of the state Covid-19 taskforce and were involved in sample-collection surveillance at grass-roots level, but even in this case, it is apparent that their role was merely a supporting one. The fact that 18 LGAs (out of 774) accounted for more than 60 per cent of confirmed cases in Nigeria at the time of this writing indicates that LGAs needed to be engaged substantively in the management of the pandemic.

As matters stood, they were generally underutilised by federal and state government alike. This led to occasions in which the federal government gave policy directions to LGAs directly – for example, the PTF threatened to impose a total lockdown on LGAs with high increases in confirmed cases. The implication is that the federal government was willing to bypass state governments, which are the entities constitutionally mandated to play a supervisory role over LGAs (Constitution, section 7(1)).

State governments generally have not allowed LGAs to flourish, a tendency motivated by the desire to reduce the costs associated with running LGAs. It is thus surprising that whereas the organised voice of this sector – the Association of Local Government of Nigeria (ALGON) – usually fights for the autonomy of LGAs, it was conspicuously silent when it came to Covid-19. Its Delta State branch appeared to be the only one seeking to ensure that the state's LGA chairpersons were united in enforcing social distancing in public schools (Igbekoyi 2020).

19.4.5 Intergovernmental relations

A distinctive feature of federalism in Nigeria is that there is no active structure for intergovernmental relations (IGR) on high-level policy matters (Osaghae 2015). The two constitutionally created IGR forums – the Council of State and the National Economic Council (NEC) – perform only advisory functions. The Council of State mainly advises the President on issues such as appointments and the prerogative of mercy, while the NEC, as its name indicates, advises on economic matters (Constitution, Third Schedule, Part I).

In terms of their composition, the NEC comprises the Vice President (VP), governors of all the states, and the governor of the Central Bank of Nigeria; the Council of State has a broader membership, including the President, all former presidents, and all governors. Neither forum has representation from LGAs (Ikeanyibe et al. 2019: 1044). The NEC meets monthly to review the nation's economic planning efforts; however, it was only in its meeting in May 2020 that Covid-19 was at the top of the agenda. On that occasion, the NEC set up a committee to advise on the reopening of the Nigerian economy, with its members consisting of a selection of governors and federal ministers. Its advisory role aside, the NEC has had to defer to the PTF when it comes to issues relating to linkages between Covid-19 and economic planning – a consideration that has not made it particularly useful as an IGR platform.

The implication of the foregoing is that the most authoritative body engaged in coordinating multilevel government response to the pandemic is the PTF. The PTF drew its membership from several ministries and parastatals. One of its key objectives is to '[p]rovide a coordinated and effective national and sub-national response to the COVID-19 pandemic', thereby fostering relations between the various levels of government (FG 2020: 6). Apart from its coordinating function, the PTF was also to report directly to the President and give a daily press briefing to members of the public. As crucial as the task of the PTF appears, the extent to which it was able to achieve effective IGR remains questionable for two reasons: state governments (or their taskforces) were not represented on it, and state governments were used only as implementers of federal policies.

The relationship between federal and state government in pandemic management was, overall, a lopsided one. Since the federal government, with the support of the Quarantine Act and Disaster Management Act, exercised overwhelming powers over states, most of them had no option but to quietly fall in line; the powers the federal government wields over public finance are a further instrument for subjugating state governments. So, while it is difficult to assess the relationship between the levels governments, it is probably safe to say that what existed before the pandemic was not improved by it and may well have deteriorated.

The coldness of this relationship is worse where the units of government belong to different political parties – in such case, conflicts abound. Two examples suffice. The first is the case of the governor of Oyo State, an opposition-held state, who, contrary to the PTF's stipulations and the advice of the medical community, organised a political rally on 19 March to spite the federal government and the ruling party (Babatunde 2020).

The second is the conflict between the federal government and the Rivers state government. The latter had imposed a state-wide curfew to curb the spread of the virus; meanwhile, the Federal Minister of Aviation authorised some helicopters to operate in the state, helicopters which violated the curfew.

The government of Rivers State, an opposition-held state, instructed the police to arrest the passengers and crew for violating the state-imposed curfew. In response, the head of the federal police force removed the state's commissioner of police for enforcing a state law (by arresting crew and passengers) against federal orders (Chukwu 2020).

States also cooperated with each other to carry out joint efforts, especially in matters such as border control. For example, in a statement after its monthly meeting of April 2020, the Nigeria Governors' Forum (NGF), an association of all 36 state governors, said, 'Governors unanimously agreed to the implementation of [a two-week] interstate lockdown ... to mitigate the spread of the virus from state to state' (Reuters 2020). They also agreed to set up Covid-19 regional committees comprising state commissioners of health and aimed at fostering a coordinated pandemic response. Significantly, the governors called for the 'decentralization of the Covid-19 response as the best chance of nipping the spread of the virus' (Olaniyi 2020).

What is also notable, though, is that various of the NGF's decisions appear so closely aligned with the imperatives of the federal government and PTF that they verge on the redundant and seem like mere affirmations purporting to suggest the NGF thought of them first. Still, some state governors jointly rejected certain federal measures. For example, the Northern States Governors' Forum came together to reject federal lockdown measures due to their economic impact, holding that each state should adopt an approach suitable to its setting (Abraham 2020).

Initially, the NGF was united as an IGR platform. State governors were unified in interacting with the federal government and among themselves, thereby fostering vertical and horizontal cooperation, respectively. However, once the federal government started allocating funds through its special intervention regime to support states' responses, there seems have been a rift. This was due to the perception that some states, notably Lagos, were treated more favourably than others in being awarded a larger share of funding; the federal government argued that Lagos had invested heavily in pandemic response and warranted it (see below).

19.4.6 Intergovernmental fiscal relations

Managing Covid-19 was an overwhelming fiscal venture in a country where the pandemic's impacts on the economy and public finances placed severe strain both on the federal government and on an already complicated fiscal framework.

Public finance is governed by the Constitution, which stipulates that all revenue raised by the nation is held in a federation account and shared via a formula approved by the National Assembly (Constitution, section 162). In 2020, the sharing formula was (in percentages) 53:27:20 for the federal government, state governments, and LGAs, respectively. However, the pandemic intensified interstate competition for the federation's overstretched resources.

As a result of Nigeria's heavy reliance on oil revenue and the absence of fiscal autonomy for the regions, state governments generally rely solely on their allocation of 27 per cent – only Lagos, Rivers, and Akwa Ibom states can sustain themselves without federal transfers. In view of the huge infrastructural deficit in their health and related sectors, states had to increase spending in order to cope with Covid-19 – at the same time at which the pandemic's impact on the economy led to a significant downturn in federal transfers. The result is that most states were sliding into bankruptcy, with a collective debt of more than USD 23.6 billion (DMO 2020).

The further result is that, in terms of Nigeria's fiscal federalism, the federal government had to attempt to bail out states. States turned to the federal government, which itself had to resort to taking out further loans to meet the demand – among other things, it sought, and on 28 April 2020 obtained, approval of an emergency International Monetary Fund (IMF) loan of USD 3.4 billion to provide support for states (Transparency International 2020).

The federal government augmented states' financial allocation by way of a Stabilisation Fund of USD 150 million and granted a moratorium on states' debts. Other major support was in the form of a Covid-19 Intervention Fund based on an amendment of the 2020 budget to include a fiscal stimulus of NGN 500 billion (USD 3 billion) (Ejiogu et al. 2020). Funds were allocated to states based on the extent to which they were affected by the pandemic and the amount they had spent on critical infrastructure. By and large, it appeared that there was no specific formula for disbursement, but it was the case that Lagos State, the hardest hit, received the lion's share.

As mentioned, this complicated IGR between federal and state governments, particularly given that the federal government denied Kano State's request for NGN 15 billion, saying it 'needs to be convinced by what it sees on the ground in the state to know how and what to support' (Bello 2020). Conversely, it said it had allocated NGN 10 billion to Lagos State 'only because it was satisfied that the government of Lagos started on the right footing, rolling out proper plans and mobilizing its fund to fight the pandemic' (ibid).

Apart from special intervention funds, the most notable source of finance for the various levels of government was CACOVID. This, as also previously noted, is a private-sector taskforce that partnered with the federal government, NCDC, and WHO to mobilise resources across industries and avail funding as well as technical and operational support – among other things, CACOVID provided medical facilities that included testing, isolation and treatment centres, intensive care units, and molecular testing laboratories. By the end of May 2020, it had raised more than NGN 28 billion of a target of NGN 120 billion. Under this initiative, the federal government was responsible for the distribution of monies to state governments – indeed, the partnership was led by the governor of the Central Bank of Nigeria and the funds were placed in a special account with the same bank.

Managing such large amounts of money will always arouse suspicion, especially in a country with pervasive corruption (Abdulrauf 2020b: 215). Consequently, two significant efforts were made to guarantee accountability in regard to the sums raised by CACOVID and other federal government interventions. First, the Finance Minister stated that to enhance transparency, the donations would be spent only after appropriation through a supplementary budget of the National Assembly (Moshood 2020). Secondly, the Independent Corrupt Practices and Other Related Offences Commission (ICPC) – one of Nigeria's anti-corruption agencies – noted that it was monitoring the management of these funds and had commenced auditing the state governments, agencies, and personnel that spent the funds (Moshood 2020).

Nevertheless, various state governments still made strong allegations of federal government's corruption and discrimination (in favour of the North) in the distribution of these funds.

19.5 Findings and policy implications

The Covid-19 pandemic has presented an opportunity for a holistic assessment of Nigeria's federal governance system, and in this regard arrived with perverse good timing at the height of clamour in the country for restructuring and questing after true federalism. Originally, federalism in Nigeria served the useful purpose of holding together diverse regions and ethnic groups, but recent events show that there are deeper issues which federalism should address yet which still hang in the balance. Indeed, the nature, structure, and design of Nigeria's federalism itself is a cause for concern. As Babalola (2019: 157) aptly remarks, 'the political framework established to "cure" the country's ills have become part of the illness'.

The handling of the pandemic has exposed the fault lines of Nigeria's federalism. It has shown that true federalism in Nigeria exists only in theory and that it is consequently not off the mark to refer to the current arrangement as 'façade federalism'. This term has been used by Wright (1982) to suggest the diminishing status and role of state and local government in a federal system. The more specific findings of the present study are enumerated below.

First, the federal government usurped state governments' health-care powers and exercised overwhelming control in the management of the pandemic. It used several policies and fiscal strategies to further denude state governments of autonomy.

Secondly, in most cases, state governments did not oppose this and rarely made creative use of their constitutional space: they were comfortable with the master-servant relationship. Those few states that tried to differ from the federal government did not do so to assert their autonomy in the best interests of combating the pandemic but rather for other reasons such as party-political affiliation.

Thirdly, within the narrow sphere of their operations, state governments further subjugated LGAs even though the Constitution grants the latter a supporting role in health matters. LGAs therefore played an insignificant role in responding to the pandemic.

Fourthly, the current fiscal framework in which state governments are heavily dependent on federal allocations has been further cause for states to maintain an inferior position in the federal arrangement.

Fifthly, in the absence of any formal IGR structure, no new IGR structure or practice emerged to help effectively coordinate the multilevel government responses. The Council of State and NEC did not have the formal constitutional powers to take on this role but existed merely as advisory bodies. The PTF that was established to coordinate multilevel responses did not function effectively as an IGR platform – it simply issued policy directions, indirectly through the President and directly to states without engaging with state governments.

Lastly, there was no federal spirit even in the National Assembly, where legislators sought to ensure continued centralisation of powers with the attempted enactment of the Infectious Diseases Act of 2020, which grants the federal executive overwhelming powers over states.

These findings have long-term implications for Nigeria's federalism. Two closing observations may be made in this respect. First, there were no strong voices or movements for greater autonomy and independence between the levels of government. All the previous calls for reforming the federal system fell still in this period, with few stakeholders recognising the potential long-term impact of highly centralised pandemic governance on Nigerian federalism at large. Secondly, and consequently, Nigeria moved ever-faster towards ever-greater centralisation, with the spirit of federalism all the while rapidly declining.

References

Abdulrauf, Lukman. 2020a. 'Nigeria's Emergency (Legal) Response to COVID-19: A Worthy Sacrifice for Public Health?', *Verfassungblog: On Matters Constitutional*, 18 May, https://verfassungsblog.de/nigerias-emergency-legal-response-to-covid-19-a-worthy-sacrifice-for-public-health/ (accessed on 30 November 2020).

Abdulrauf, Lukman. 2020b. 'Using Specialised Anti-Corruption Agencies to Combat Pervasive Corruption in Nigeria: A Critical Review of the ICPC and EFCC', *African Journal of Legal Studies*, 13(3–4): 215–41.

Abraham, James. 2020. 'We Can't Lockdown North – Northern Governor', Punch, 14 April.

African Union and Africa CDC. 2020. *Africa Joint Continental Strategy for COVID-19 Outbreak*, https://www.tralac.org/documents/resources/covid-19/regional/3219-africa-joint-continental-strategy-for-covid-19-outbreak-africa-cdc-march-2020/file.html (accessed on 30 November 2020).

Babalola, D. 2019. *The Political Economy of Federalism in Nigeria*. London: Palgrave Macmillan.

Babatunde, A. 2020. 'Gov. Makinde apologises for holding PDP rally amid coronavirus outbreak', Premium Times, 20 March.

Bello, Bashir. 2020. 'COVID-19: Why FG Ignored Ganduje's N15b Intervention Request', Vanguard, 7 May.

Brooks & Knights Legal Consultants (BKLC). 2020. 'Nigerian Emergency Economic Stimulus Bill: All You Need to Know', https://iclg.com/briefing/11493-nigerian-emergency-economic-stimulus-bill-all-you-need-to-know (accessed on 30 November 2020).

Central Bank of Nigeria (CBN). 2020. *Guidelines for the Implementation of ₦50 Billion Targeted Credit Facility*, https://www.cbn.gov.ng/Out/2020/FPRD/N50%20Billion%20 Combined.pdf (accessed 30 November 2020).

Chukwu, I. 2020. 'IGP Intervenes in Rivers' COVID-19 Wars, Orders Free Passage of Essential Workers, Foods', Business Day, 17 May.

Debt Management Office (DMO). 2020. *Sub-National Debts*, https://www.dmo.gov.ng/ debt-profile/sub-national-debts (accessed 30 November 2020).

Ejiogu, Amanze, O. Okechukwu and C. Ejiogu. 2020. 'Nigerian Budgetary Response to the COVID-19 Pandemic and Its Shrinking Fiscal Space: Financial Sustainability, Employment, Social Inequality and Business Implications', *Journal of Public Budgeting, Accounting & Financial Management*, 32(5): 919–28.

Elaigwu, Isawa J. 2005. 'The Federal Republic of Nigeria' Forum of Federations, http:// www.forumfed.org/libdocs/Global_Dialogue/Book_2/BK2-C08-ng-Elaigwu-en.htm (accessed on 30 November 2020).

Federal Government (FG). 2020. 'National COVID-19 Pandemic Multi-Sectoral Response Plan', https://statehouse.gov.ng/covid19/wp-content/uploads/2020/06/National-COVID-19-Multi-Sectoral-Pandemic-Response-Plan_May-19-2020_2.pdf (accessed on 30 November 2020).

Feyisipo, Remi. 2020. 'Coronavirus: There Will Be No Lockdown in Oyo, Says Gov. Makinde', *Business Day*, 27 April.

Igbekoyi, Felix. 2020. 'Covid-19: Delta ALGON in Trouble Over Double Standard', Independent, 23 March.

Ihonvbere, Julius. 2020. *Federalism and the COVID-19 crisis: Nigerian Federalism*, Forum of Federations, http://www.forumfed.org/wp-content/uploads/2020/04/NigeriaCOVID. pdf (accessed on 30 November 2020).

Ikeanyibe, Okechukwu Marcellus, Patrick Chiemeka Chukwu and Jide Ibietan. 2019. 'Model and Determinants of State-Local Governments' Relations in Nigeria', *Journal of Public Administration*, 53(6): 1040–66.

Isa, Muhammad Kabir. 2016. 'Nigerian Local Government System and Governance: Lessons, Prospects and Challenges for Post-2015 Development Goals', in Eris D. Schoburg, John Martin and Sonia Gatchair (eds), *Developmental Local Governance: A Critical Discourse in 'Alternative Development'*, pp. 107–26. London: Palgrave.

Mashi, Sani Abubakar et al. 2019. 'Disaster Risks and Management Policies and Practices in Nigeria: A Critical Appraisal of the National Emergency Management Agency Act', *International Journal of Disaster Risk Reduction*, 33: 253–65.

Mbah, Fidelis. 2020. '"Lockdown Made Everything Gloomy": Ramadan in Nigeria's Kano', Aljazeera, 13 May, https://www.aljazeera.com/news/2020/5/13/lockdown-made-everything-gloomy-ramadan-in-nigerias-kano (accessed on 30 November 2020).

Moshood, Yusuff. 2020, 'Despite over N25bn Donations for COVID-19, Isolation Centres Run Low on Bed Spaces', *Punch Healthwise*, https://healthwise.punchng.com/despite-over-n25bn-donations-for-covid-19-isolation-centres-run-low-on-bed-spaces/ (accessed on 30 November 2020).

Murtala, Abdulmumin. 2020. 'Nigeria: COVID-19 – 50,000 Poor Households Get Palliative in Kano', Vanguard, 23 April.

National Bureau of Statistics (NBS). 2018. *Demographic Statistics Bulletin – 2017*, https:// nigerianstat.gov.ng/download/775 (accessed on 30 November 2020).

Nigeria Centre for Disease Control (NCDC). 2020a. *An Update of COVID-19 Outbreak in Nigeria*, https://ncdc.gov.ng/diseases/sitreps/?cat=14&name=An%20update%20of%20 COVID-19%20outbreak%20in%20Nigeria (accessed on 30 November 2020).

Nigeria Centre for Disease Control (NCDC). 2020b. *About NCDC*, https://ncdc.gov.ng/ncdc (accessed on 30 November 2020).

Nwabueze, Remigius. 2014. 'The Legal Protection and Enforcement of Health Rights in Nigeria', in C. M. Flood and A. Gross (eds), *The Right to Health at the Public/Private Divide: A Global Comparative Study*. Cambridge: Cambridge University Press.

Nwachukwu, Onyinye. 2020. 'National Assembly Adjourns for Two Weeks as Coronavirus Fears Heighten across Nigeria', Business Day, 24 March.

Offiong, Adie. 2020. 'COVID-19: When a Governor Believes It's a Hoax and Ordinary Flu', *Good Governance Africa*, https://gga.org/covid-19-when-a-governor-believes-its-a-hoax-and-ordinary-flu/ (accessed on 30 November 2020).

Okeke, Remi Chukwudi. 2020. *Covid-19 Pandemic, Federalism and Nigeria's Leadership Challenges*, https://advance.sagepub.com/articles/preprint/COVID-19_PANDEMIC_FEDERALISM_AND_NIGERIA_S_LEADERSHIP_CHALLENGES/12127038 (accessed on 30 November 2020).

Okon, Desmond. 2020. 'Lamentation Still Trails Lagos, FG's Palliative Package as Middlemen Hijack Programme', *Business Day*, 19 April.

Olaniyi, Muideen. 2020. 'Nigeria: Governors Agree on 14 Days National COVID-19 Lockdown' *Daily Trust*, 22 April.

Onwubiko, Emmanuel. 2020. 'COVID-19 and Issues around Federalism', *The Nigerian Voice*, 21 April.

Osaghae, Eghosa. 2015. 'Nigeria: Struggling to Formalize and Decentralize Intergovernmental Relations', in Johanne Poirier, Cheryl Saunders and John Kincaid (eds), *Intergovernmental Relations in Federal Systems*, pp. 272–304. Oxford: Oxford University Press.

Premium Times. 2020. 'PDP Blames Buhari for Coronavirus in Nigeria', *Premium Times*, 28 February.

Punch Healthwise. 2020a. 'Military Supports COVID-19 Fight with Extra 220 Medical Personnel', *Punch Healthwise*, https://healthwise.punchng.com/military-supports-covid-19-fight-with-additional-220-medical-personnel/ (accessed on 30 November 2020).

Punch Healthwise. 2020b. 'Cross River Insists on Zero COVID-19 Infection', *Punch Healthwise*, https://healthwise.punchng.com/cross-river-insists-on-zero-covid-19-infection/ (accessed on 30 November 2020).

Reuters. 2020. 'Nigerian Governors to Ban Interstate Movement to Contain Coronavirus', *VOANews*, 23 April, https://www.voanews.com/africa/nigerian-governors-ban-interstate-movement-contain-coronavirus (accessed on 30 November 2020).

Shaban, Abdur Rahman. 2020. '"Close up" Social Distancing as Lagos Distributes Coronavirus Food Aid', *Africanews*, 3 April.

Transparency International. 2020. 'Nigeria, IMF and COVID-19' https://www.transparency.org/en/blog/nigeria-imf-covid-19# (accessed 30 November 2020).

TRT World. 2020. 'Nigerian Army Prepares for Coronavirus Lockdown', *TRT World*, https://www.trtworld.com/africa/nigerian-army-prepares-for-coronavirus-lockdown-34871 (accessed on 30 November 2020).

World Population Review (WPR). 2020. *Nigeria Population 2020 (Live)*, https://worldpopulationreview.com/countries/nigeria-population (accessed on 30 November 2020).

Wright, Deil. 1982. *Understanding Intergovernmental Relations*, 2nd ed. Wisconsin: Cole Publishing.

PART VI
Conclusion

20

GRAPPLING WITH THE PANDEMIC

Rich insights into intergovernmental relations

Cheryl Saunders

20.1 Introduction

The purpose of this chapter is to examine the theory and practice of intergovernmental relations in the light of the experiences of federations in dealing with Covid-19. To this end, this chapter draws on the information provided by 18 country case studies in this book, together with a study of the European Union. All cases have federal or quasi-federal systems of government. Otherwise, however, they are diverse in a wide variety of ways that include geographic and population size and configuration, economic development, political system, and the framework for federalism itself. Factors of these kinds influenced the ways in which each of these federations has responded to the pandemic, including, relevantly for this chapter, the role of intergovernmental relations.

All the case studies were finalised towards the end of 2020, with the result that neither they nor this chapter take account of subsequent developments in intergovernmental relations as the pandemic continued to play out. As they stand, the cases are a rich resource yielding new knowledge and understanding of intergovernmental relations in federal systems in a context in which governmental systems have been placed under extreme and unusual stress. The time limitation is relevant, nevertheless. As these chapters show, intergovernmental relations changed within federations in the course of 2020 in tandem with successive 'waves' of the pandemic and policy responses to it. That evolution can be expected to have continued into 2021, when governments were still struggling to manage the pandemic and vaccines began to be rolled out.

The challenges presented by the spread of the Covid-19 across the world were a test of federal systems generally and intergovernmental relations in particular. The pandemic created two types of crises, one with serious implications for

DOI: 10.4324/9781003166771-27

public health and the other affecting national and subnational economies. These two sets of issues were typically seen as in competition with each other, albeit on the understanding that if the health crisis were managed quickly and effectively, they could be reconciled. How the tension between the two played out in any federation depended on a mixture of ideological preferences, the federal division of powers, and the realities on the ground. In every case, however, these complex, interlinked crises, affecting the lives of communities in so many respects, required an exercise of authority by all levels of government. Each level of government had a role of some kind to play, even where formal emergency powers were invoked. Failure was all too obvious, placing a premium on capability and performance. More often than not, an effective response required coordination across jurisdictional lines, both horizontal and vertical, in ways that also preserved the potential for localised divergence.

In the analysis that follows, intergovernmental relations are understood broadly as covering all instances in which governments in a federal systems work together across jurisdictional boundaries in the common interest. The term thus refers to activity that, strictly speaking, might be described as intragovernmental inasmuch as an institution of one level of government is constituted to incorporate representatives of another: the German *Bundesrat*, comprising representatives of *Land* governments, is an example. The term also includes relations between governments that, from the standpoint of the formal constitutional scheme, are constitutionally or legally mandated, as well as those in which joint action is voluntary. In addition, it includes situations in which joint action is top-down and in effect coercive rather than 'cooperative', to invoke another term often used in this context.

A broad and inclusive understanding of the subject is necessitated by the variety of approaches to intergovernmental relations in this range of federal-type systems, approaches which are manifested not only in the practices that are adopted but in the ways in which intergovernmental relations are conceived and described. A narrower approach would risk a partial understanding of how governments interacted with each other in responding to Covid-19. Conversely, it may be, as I will argue, that analysis of the range of responses to Covid-19 enables a more nuanced, critical appraisal of intergovernmental relations which identifies practices that are more productive than others without necessarily excluding any from the field.

The rest of this chapter proceeds as follows. To aid comparison, the next section identifies and explains aspects of each federal-type system that have a bearing on intergovernmental relations. section 3 considers the purposes for which intergovernmental relations were used by different federal-type systems in responding to the pandemic, while section 4 examines the modalities through which intergovernmental relations took place. The final section highlights the most significant insights gleaned from the experience of Covid-19 and serves to inform future research in the field.

20.2 Contexts

The contexts in which federal-type systems operate differ in many ways that are relevant to an assessment of intergovernmental relations in response to Covid-19. This section draws attention to four of the most significant forms of differentiation: geophysical characteristics, economic development, the form and operation of government, and the multifaceted framework for federalism itself. Each of these aspects of context is significant in its own right; they also combine in different ways in different federations to create distinctive settings that need to be understood before general conclusions are drawn.

For present purposes, geophysical characteristics include the geographical size of a country, its distribution into federated units, patterns of population settlement, particularly around internal borders, and global location. The range can be grasped by comparing, for example, Switzerland and Austria with Canada and Australia. The former both have a relatively small land mass, divided into 26 cantons (Switzerland) and nine *Länder* (Austria). They have a population density of 219 and 109 persons per kilometre, respectively, and external land borders shared with other densely populated countries on all sides. Both Canada and Australia, by contrast, have a large land mass divided into 13 provinces and territories (Canada) and eight states and territories (Australia) and a population density of 4 and 3 persons per km^2, respectively. They are located far from the huge, interconnected Eurasian continent.

In geographically smaller federations like these, conditions relevant to managing the pandemic are less likely to vary significantly between units, while internal borders are likely to be porous, strengthening the case for harmonisation of policy settings and for cross-border cooperation. In geographically larger federations, however, the rate of infection and other conditions pertinent to the pandemic are more likely to vary between units, suggesting that intergovernmental arrangements should leave greater room for policy divergence around the country and increasing the importance of gathering information from localised sources. It may also be noted in passing that a larger number of units creates a different dynamic for multilateral intergovernmental relations than a smaller one, and may also have a bearing on the size and capabilities of individual units.

A second aspect of context is economic development. Less affluent countries have fewer options at their disposal to respond to the pandemic. Health systems are likely to be weaker and more readily overrun; resources are less likely to be available to support the isolation of those exposed to infection; supplies, including vaccines, may be hard and slow to obtain. These realities channel the policy choices available to governments individually or collectively. It may also be that, in circumstances of slow or recent economic development, all levels of government but, in particular, subnational levels, lack the capacity, in the sense of capability, to respond to the challenges of Covid-19 effectively. South Africa is a case in point, where the authors identify 'incapacity, incompetence and corruption' on the part of provinces and municipalities; problems that certainly also are experienced in federations elsewhere. The likelihood that the centre will dominate the Covid-19 response may be heightened in such cases by the federation's design, which typically concentrates power at the centre and provides authority for central intervention in unit affairs when major problems arise.

Thirdly, the form of government influences intergovernmental relations in ways that were relevant to responses to the pandemic. Most obviously, the distinction between parliamentary and presidential systems affected some modalities of intergovernmental relations in relation to Covid-19. Governments in parliamentary systems are more likely than those in presidential systems to use formal meetings of heads of government for the purposes of vertical coordination, if only because agreement between governments can lead easily enough to legislative action. Most of the parliamentary federations covered by the case studies used meetings of some kind between heads of government of the federation and federated units to coordinate aspects of their responses to the pandemic, although the frequency and significance of these meetings varied. By contrast, none of the six presidential systems (Mexico, Brazil, Argentina, Nigeria, Russia, United States (US)) recorded systematic vertical meetings between heads of government, although horizontal meetings between the governments of some or all units were common and informal, often bilateral, contacts between the president and governors sometimes took place.

More authoritarian styles of government also affected intergovernmental relations during the pandemic, doing so in the adoption of approaches that were top-down, less likely to be consultative, and more likely to mandate action of specified kinds by the federated units. Russia is an example where, nevertheless, the sheer size of the country ultimately required some local diversity as it responded to the pandemic. A tendency towards top-down central action also was present in other federations in which a single party is dominant across all levels of government. The syndrome is evident across both presidential and parliamentary systems, as the examples of Argentina, Mexico, Ethiopia, Nigeria, and South Africa show, although it manifests somewhat differently in each case.

The cases show that the distribution and strength of party-political allegiances affected the intergovernmental response to the pandemic in other ways as well. Generally speaking, parties broadly on the right were inclined to prioritise the economy and eschew restrictions on individual movement for infection control, while those broadly on the left were more likely to prioritise public health. The mix of parties in office in the various jurisdictions, combined with the distribution of federal powers and responsibilities, thus helped to shape the outcomes of intergovernmental negotiations.

For example, in Australia, operating through a newly established 'National Cabinet', the particular admixture of interests and power had the effect of softening extreme positions, leading to intergovernmental US, deep compromises that proved effective in minimising transmission. By contrast, in the ideological differences, both horizontal and vertical, served to deter effective intergovernmental arrangements altogether. Predictably, too, across a range of federations party allegiances variously resulted in favouritism towards particular units, notwithstanding formal intergovernmental arrangements; encouraged alliances between some units to the exclusion of others; and offered an alternative avenue to intergovernmental relations. Equally, however, the significance of party affiliation should not be overstated. The exigencies of responding to the pandemic were experienced by all jurisdictions in all federations and were capable of creating common cause across party lines, at least until the worst of the crisis had passed.

The federal distribution of powers or competences is another contextual factor that affected the form and operation of intergovernmental relations. It has at least three dimensions that are relevant for present purposes: the contrast between dual and integrated federations, the categorisation of legislative powers, and the distribution of the powers and competences on which responses to the pandemic drew.

The categories of dual and integrated federations refer, respectively, to federations in which each jurisdiction administers its own legislation and those in which subnational governments can, or must, implement some central legislation. During the pandemic, intergovernmental relations in federations with features of integration often took the form of policy-making through central legislation that was implemented by other levels of government – an option which typically is not available to federations with a dualist design. The US is an example of a country in which integration is precluded, or at least restricted by a decision of the Supreme Court invalidating the 'commandeering' of State officials by federal law (*Printz v. United States* (1997) 521 US 898 (1997)). Australia may be another.

However, there also are variations within each of these two models that affected intergovernmental relations. Some integrated federations, including Germany, have formal procedures for consultation with federated units about the laws they are to implement. Others, of which Germany also is an example, allow substantial discretionary scope to federated units in the course of implementation. Some dualist federations, of which Canada is an example, do not constitutionally preclude implementation of central law by the federated units, or vice versa, if agreed between jurisdictions, although the device was not used in responding to the pandemic.

A second dimension of the federal division of powers that contributes to contextual differences that could affect intergovernmental relations is the categorisation of allocated powers. One familiar point of distinction lies between concurrent and exclusive powers; less familiar are differences in the understanding of concurrency in different systems, differences that can also come into play in intergovernmental relations (Saunders and Dziedzic 2017). As a generalisation, there is a dividing line between federations in which concurrency is understood as involving joint action of some kind and those in which it merely involves identifying legislative powers which are potentially available for exercise by either level of government, subject to a rule about which law prevails if both seek to exercise the power. This difference in understanding may be attributable in part to the role played by concurrent power in the overall allocation of power. In some federations, of which Australia is an example, concurrency is used to categorise in a single list most of the powers available to the central legislature, without there necessarily being any implication of joint action. In other federations, including, for example, India and South Africa, concurrent power complements two other lists of exclusive powers by identifying powers that are shared.

Whatever the explanation, different understandings of concurrency emerge from comparative analysis of intergovernmental relations in federations during the pandemic. In some cases, of which Mexico, South Africa, and Italy are examples, concurrent power enabled the centre to provide a legal framework, of varying degrees of detail, within which federated units supplemented and administered the central legislation. In other cases, of which Australia is an example, both levels of government enacted and administered their own legislation by relying on aspects of the same concurrent power and taking legislative precautions against invalidation for unintended inconsistency.[1]

In many cases, this familiar format for the structure of the federal division of power was modified or embellished, sometimes in distinctive ways. So, for example, Mexico distinguishes 'coordination' from concurrency;[2] Argentina distinguishes 'shared' from concurrent power, describing the former as requiring 'joint decisions'; Brazil provides separately for 'concurrent' legislative powers and administrative powers that are held 'in common' (Brazil, Constitution, articles 23 and 24); Italy subjects 'shared' powers to principles prescribed in national legislation; and Austria specifically provides for the enactment of 'framework' legislation by the *Bund,* leaving 'more detailed implementation' to *Land* legislation (Austria, Constitution, article 15(6)). Some federations, including Belgium, rely entirely on exclusive powers and do not use concurrency at all. Notably, however, in Canada, where most powers also are characterised as exclusive some, of which public health is an example, have in practice become concurrent, in the sense of being shared.[3] These and other similar features of the framework for the federal distribution of powers inevitably shaped the specific form that intergovernmental relations took in the various federations.

The particular distribution of powers also mattered, inevitably. In most federations, the wide range of powers relevant to responding to the pandemic were distributed between two or, in some cases, three levels of government, providing the stimulus for intergovernmental relations with which this chapter deals. The precise formulation and mix of powers affected the dynamics, however. Federations in which significant relevant powers were vested in the federated units, such as Canada, operated differently to those in which a preponderance of power was exercisable by the centre, *de jure,* as in Austria, or de facto, as in Nigeria. In the context of the pandemic, moreover, the distribution of power to deal with emergencies was an additional consideration. In some federations, power to declare and respond to an emergency is conferred on the centre, directly or indirectly, expanding central power vis-à-vis the federated units, as occurred in Spain and Switzerland. In other federations, including Canada and the US, emergency power is distributed between the levels of government, requiring intergovernmental relations of some kind if coordinating action is required.

A final set of contextual factors involves federal culture rather than the technical requirements of the federal division of powers. Considerations of this kind are more abstract, but no less relevant to intergovernmental relations. Some have a foothold in the relevant constitution, where they may play a reflexive role in shaping culture (Frankenberg 2006). Certain federations, including Belgium, Italy, and Switzerland, expressly or implicitly prescribe a principle of loyalty or good faith which, in the context of the pandemic, had implications for cooperation and consultation, even if these played out in different ways. The European Union expressly acknowledges a principle of subsidiarity, which can affect the design of intergovernmental arrangements, generally and in application to the pandemic. The Constitution of South Africa prescribes principles for 'cooperative government', now given legislative shape in the Intergovernmental Relations Framework Act of 2005, which require, for example, coordination, consultation, mutual support, and good faith, all of which are relevant to the conduct of intergovernmental relations. The goals of intergovernmental relations are likely also to be affected by expectations in some federations about the equivalence of social conditions, expectations which have no counterpart in others. In Germany, for example, these have a foundation in article 72 of the Basic Law.

20.3 Purposes

In many, perhaps most, federations, the initial governmental response to Covid-19 came from individual constituent units, or even local authorities, when the virus began to pose a threat. Typically, the core public health and police powers necessary to combat the virus were located in any event at the subnational level. Some of these early, localised actions were well targeted and effective, anticipating strategies that ultimately would be adopted elsewhere. Early steps taken by the Indian states, with Kerala the standout example, involved a range of measures to prevent and track spread of the virus and illustrate the point.

As the virus spread, and the scale of the crisis became apparent, central governments intervened. In some cases, of which India again is an example, the intervention was comprehensive and top-down, severely restricting local discretion; in at least one other, the US, central involvement was limited and spasmodic to the extent that it existed at all. Most federations operated on a spectrum between these two extremes, varying their approach over the course of the year in the light of experience. Whatever approach was adopted, however, at whatever point in time, intergovernmental relations played a role of some kind once both levels of government were engaged.

The value of intergovernmental relations is often assumed, without there being a critical examination of the contribution it makes to multilevel government. Reliance on intergovernmental relations in federations across the world to deal with the complex challenges presented by Covid-19 offers a rare opportunity for such an examination in a practical context. This section considers the purposes for which intergovernmental relations were used during this period, as a means of better understanding their potential and their limits.

A familiar purpose of intergovernmental relations, also on display in the context of Covid-19, is 'coordination'. Coordination is too general a term for present purposes, however. It can be focused by asking what was coordinated, between whom and to what degree. In the collective experience of these federations, the subject matter of coordination ranged from the overall strategy for managing the pandemic, as it stood at one point in time to another, to particular aspects of it. The former typically encompassed where and how the balance was to be struck between limiting transmission and preserving the economy – an example might be the length and extent of a particular lockdown. In either case, the function of coordination sometimes was to harmonise different powers and capacities, whether legislative or administrative, across the levels of government, so as to secure an adequately holistic response. Alternatively, coordination served to harmonise the exercise of the same powers by the constituent units in the interests of meeting expected standards of equivalence or, sometimes, to enhance the simplicity of messaging. It follows that coordination was sometimes vertical, involving all levels of government, and sometimes horizontal, involving all or some of the constituent units. Even where a working relationship between the centre and the constituent units was undeveloped or ineffective, as in the US or Brazil, coordination between units in the same region or sharing a similar ideology was a common feature of intergovernmental relations in responding to the pandemic.

The extent or degree of coordination sought varied significantly between federations, ranging from uniformity at one extreme, through various forms of harmonisation, to what in Canada was described as a 'guidance framework', on the other. These choices were driven partly by the opportunities that were presented by the scope of the authority of the respective levels of government, de jure or de facto. In addition, however, they were driven by considerations of what was necessary for an effective response to the pandemic, an assessment that sometimes changed over the course of the year in the light of experience. Spain offers an instructive example for this purpose, although it was not the only one. The constitutional 'state of alarm' triggered by the Spanish government early in the year centralised power and resulted in a top-down approach to management of the pandemic during the first wave of infections, which exposed the limitations of what the centre could do effectively. When the second wave emerged later in the year, a state of alarm was again declared, but this time with the support of the autonomous communities and in a fashion that married coordination with significant decentralisation.

This example makes a broader point. Whatever degree of coordination was sought in response to the pandemic, in most federations some scope was left or taken for a level of local management in a form that assumed local diversity. Where this occurred, its potential advantages were to enable constituent units to respond to local conditions, to experiment with new approaches to a novel problem, and to strengthen accountability to local communities. This potential was not realised where local capability was weak, as in South Africa. In some federations, including Ethiopia and Nigeria, limited opportunity combined with low capability also resulted in considerable asymmetry in the extent of local initiative that was taken. Otherwise, however, while the scope for more localised diversity as an element of coordination varied significantly across federations, it was sufficiently prevalent to challenge the automatic equation of coordination with uniformity, at least in tackling problems of this kind.

A second, related purpose of intergovernmental relations during the pandemic was to provide a framework within which consultation might take place between jurisdictions and across levels of government. Notoriously, consultation can take different forms, which in the current context might range from some opportunity for feedback on a predetermined course of action to active engagement enabling perspectives to be shared as a basis for deciding on the action to be taken. The flow of information between jurisdictions in the course of the pandemic was patchy between federations. Even top-down communication was poor in some cases, causing unnecessary confusion: the failure of the government of India to communicate with the states before imposing the nationwide lockdown in March 2020 was an example. In other cases, too, consultation was perfunctory, to the extent that it existed at all. Criticism along these lines was made in regard to South Africa, Mexico, and Argentina, for example.

Nevertheless, there was sufficient use of active, multilateral communication to demonstrate its usefulness for responding to the pandemic and to suggest that it constitutes a significant purpose for intergovernmental relations, hard though it sometimes may be to achieve. At its best, in the course of the pandemic it enabled knowledge about local conditions to be fed into a federation-wide planning process; contributed to the dissemination of innovative ideas and good practice; and underpinned local ownership of intergovernmental solutions. Australia, Switzerland, and Spain provide examples. In some federations, consultation of this kind may be considered to be mandated by requirements of interjurisdictional loyalty. Equally significantly, however, in the context of the pandemic it was driven by the need to maximise the effectiveness of the governmental response.

Other purposes of intergovernmental relations that were revealed by responses to the pandemic can be dealt with more briefly but are equally significant. In some cases, intergovernmental relations were used to solve a shared problem. The arrangements between neighbouring states in Australia to create a 'bubble' to protect border communities from differential lockdowns and border closures are an example; the 'Atlantic bubble' in Canada is another. In other cases, intergovernmental arrangements involved the sharing of resources. The use of defence force personnel to monitor aspects of pandemic control in Canada is an example; the movement of scarce health equipment between states in the US, as needs rose and fell, is another. Another familiar purpose of intergovernmental relations during the pandemic was to achieve economies of scale or other economic benefits that flow from joint, usually central, action. Thus in many federations, response to the pandemic involved central procurement of, for example, personal protective equipment, intensive-care beds and vaccine supplies for distribution to the constituent units. Insofar as these supplies were sourced internationally, procurement by the centre was indicated as well.

It is sometimes suggested that a purpose of intergovernmental relations in federations is to manage disputes, particularly in the form of legal action between jurisdictions (South Africa, Constitution, section 41(1)(h)(vi)). Intergovernmental relations can be assumed to have played some role in this regard during the pandemic by providing a framework for joint action to deal with a shared problem, albeit that the speed with which the various crises developed may have inhibited interjurisdictional litigation as well. Disputes resulting in litigation nevertheless occurred, and might have been averted by more effective intergovernmental relations, even though many were instigated by private parties in federations where such procedures are available (Aroney and Kincaid 2017). This chapter on Argentina gives several examples of litigation over competition between provinces in the purchase of respirators and over the movement of medical personnel working in one province but living in another. In other federations, there were legal disputes over constitutional powers and responsibilities. Examples include India and Spain, where questions about the federal division of power were resolved by courts in favour of the centre and Brazil, where challenges to federal action were resolved in favour of the states. Judicial decisions of these kinds affected the dynamic of intergovernmental relations and, indirectly, altered the response to the pandemic.

Finally, intergovernmental relations were used in most federations to alleviate the financial pressures on governments created by the pandemic due to the collapse of economic activity and tax bases and the heightening of expenditure demands. While these effects were felt at all levels of government, the generally superior financial position of the centre typically meant that subnational governments were more exposed. The full magnitude of the economic consequences of the pandemic are yet to be realised, and may call ultimately for a more radical adjustment of existing federal fiscal arrangements. The point made here, however, is that extreme fiscal pressures in some federations, of which Brazil, Nigeria, and the United Kingdom (UK) are only some examples, were mitigated in the short-term in the course of the pandemic by forms of intergovernmental relations.

20.4 Modalities

Comparative studies of intergovernmental relations in federal-type systems across the world show that, at a level of generality, broadly similar types of arrangements, or modalities, are used (Poirier et al. 2015). They include legislative schemes of various kinds designed to achieve a desired level of coordination; meetings of political and other representatives of participating jurisdictions; agreements between jurisdictions, as a framework for future action; joint or shared institutions; and fiscal transfers (Poirier and Saunders 2015).

The actual design of institutions within each of these categories varies between federations, often significantly, depending on context. So does their scope. In federal experience, for example, intergovernmental arrangements may operate horizontally, vertically, or both; may involve bilateral or multilateral relations; and may include any two or more levels of government. Practice also varies in terms of the legal authority for intergovernmental arrangements. Some arrangements have a framework in the constitution or legislation, or both. South Africa offers a still relatively rare example of constitutional provision for intergovernmental relations that purport to be comprehensive (South Africa, Constitution, Chapter 3), but many constitutions make provision for particular intergovernmental institutions or practices. The Inter-State Council in India (India, Constitution, article 263), the procedure for intergovernmental agreements in Austria (Austria, Constitution, article 15(a)), and the requirement for loyal cooperation in Italy (Italy, Constitution, article 120) are examples. The jury is still out on whether the formalisation of intergovernmental relations enhances their effectiveness, although in principle it has advantages for transparency. Whether a legal framework exists or not, less formalised interaction between jurisdictions is a feature of almost all federations and is critical to understanding their operation in practice.

This section examines the modalities of intergovernmental relations used in the country case studies in dealing with the pandemic. It adopts the same broad categorisation of intergovernmental arrangements used in earlier studies, noting, however, that some intergovernmental practices during the pandemic also departed from previous experience in ways that may have legacies for the future. Where this occurred, it seems to be due to the nature of the challenges presented by the pandemic itself: a fast-moving, inadequately understood, dire threat to the lives and well-being of entire populations, demanding speedy and effective responses from governments. Whether this diagnosis is correct or not, the account that follows shows that some apparently established intergovernmental institutions were bypassed or modified and that some replaced altogether. It also sheds light on practices that worked or not and that offer indication of directions for future change.

Legislative schemes of various kinds typically frame and support intergovernmental action when an enforceable, normative base is required (Poirier and Saunders 2015: 455–57). Legislation also played a role in intergovernmental responses to Covid-19. In emergency conditions in which legislatures often were bypassed, however, many rules were laid down in subordinate rather than primary legislation or, sometimes, executive decrees, to the extent that constitutional systems allowed. Resort to 'guidance' rather than law was another, marked phenomenon in the response of many governments to Covid-19, one which also surfaced occasionally in intergovernmental arrangements. Thus in Canada, for example, 'guidance frameworks' were issued by the federal government, sometimes covering issues such as schools that are within provincial jurisdiction, but without the binding quality that would attract constitutional limitations.

One common use of legislation to coordinate the actions of jurisdictions during Covid-19 involved the enactment of primary legislation by the federal legislature as an umbrella for action by the constituent units and, sometimes, local government. In some cases, of which Austria and Mexico are examples, the ordinary competences of the federal legislature were sufficient to support this action; in others, including Spain, Switzerland, and Italy, federal competences were expanded by the emergency conditions. In some federations, some or all the constituent units supported federal leadership, actively or passively, even when the limits of federal competence were doubtful; others were critical of overcentralisation. In a distinctive example of support for central legislative action, the devolved legislatures of the UK gave consent to the enactment of the Coronavirus Act of 2020 by the Westminster Parliament in the form required by the 'Sewel' Convention (Institute for Government 2020).

The bases on which central legislation engaged the constituent units varied. In some cases, as in Germany, Switzerland, or South Africa, the constituent units were engaged through the usual process of implementing federal legislation. In others, including Mexico, Brazil, and Ethiopia, the constitutional scheme permitted the federal legislature to enact what in essence was framework legislation, within which constituent units could, or had to, act. In others, again, of which Russia and India were examples, the federal legislation was prescriptive, providing rules with which constituent units had to comply or mandating the action they were to take.

Whatever the legal basis for this form of joint action, key points of difference between federations in practice concerned the extent to which constituent units had discretion in applying and supplementing the federal law in local conditions; the extent to which units were consulted in relation to the form of the federal law and the action permitted or required to be taken under it; and whether units were accountable for their actions to their own communities or to the federal government. The spectrum ranged from Germany, where the *Länder* implemented federal legislation in their own right under article 83 of the Basic Law, had considerable discretion in doing so, and were consulted through the institution of the *Bundesrat* in addition to other means, to India, where the states acted within the boundaries of unilateral Union legislation on which they were not consulted at all. In the case of some federations, the scope of authority exercisable by constituent units expanded in the course of the year, as experience suggested that there was likely to be benefit in relying on rules and processes of administration that were locally informed and could be adapted to local conditions. Spain was a notable case in point, moving from centralised control under the first state of alarm to a form of 'co-governance' during the second.

More dualist federations typically do not involve the constituent units in the implementation of regular federal legislation. Where legislation is used for intergovernmental arrangements, the goal instead is to ensure that the legislation for which each jurisdiction is responsible is harmonised appropriately with that of all the others. Time did not permit the negotiation and implementation of elaborate legislative schemes of this kind during the pandemic. The technique was used nevertheless in several ways in Australia and, to a lesser extent, in Canada and the US.

Any agreement on coordination, whether vertical or horizontal, relied on voluntary compliance by the parties, through legislation, including delegated legislation, where necessary. Decisions of the 'National Cabinet' in Australia, for example, were given effect in that way, as was coordinated action between neighbouring constituent units in Canada and the US. Furthermore, in some cases, of which Australia again is an example, strategies or 'plans' for identifying the roles of the different levels of government in dealing with disasters generally and pandemics in particular had been developed in earlier years and had prompted implementing legislation that was coordinated to this extent. The use of plans is considered further below in the context of intergovernmental agreements. They could not have been expected to anticipate all the exigencies presented by the realities of the pandemic, but they offered at least a starting point.

Some of the practical difficulties of coordinating government action under the legislation of different jurisdictions are illustrated by an Australian controversy early in the pandemic. The critical issue was uncertainty about whether officers of the federal government or of New South Wales had been responsible for allowing infected passengers returning from an international cruise to enter New South Wales and travel to other parts of Australia. An official inquiry concluded that the responsibility lay with New South Wales, but neither level of government emerged from the Inquiry unscathed. The Commissioner recommended that both bureaucracies develop 'better levels of awareness of their own and each other's roles and responsibilities … and more formal protocols for … interaction and communication' (Special Commission of Inquiry 2020: 2.20).

A second core institution of relations between government comprises *interjurisdictional forums* of various kinds that involve two or more participating jurisdictions, whether operating vertically or horizontally (Poirier and Saunders 2015: 458–63). The most high-profile of such forums involve heads of government or line ministers, but many others involve bureaucrats at different levels or officeholders of various kinds across participating jurisdictions. This section focuses on intergovernmental forums involving political actors, while also noting the practical contribution of others in responding to the pandemic, some of which, including, for example, the Pan-Canadian Public Health Network, are identified in the case study chapters.

In some federations, a forum for political collaboration between jurisdictions is built into the central law-making process. The German *Bundesrat* is a prime example, but second chambers in other jurisdictions, including South Africa, are constituted so as to represent the constituent units and have some, if varying, potential to act in this way. Whether or not a federation has a second legislative chamber or equivalent that can contribute to effective coordination, other forums also may be used for the purpose that are more self-evidently intergovernmental in design. When the pandemic broke out, some federations had well-established intergovernmental forums through which political leaders could meet should they choose to do so. Examples include Australia, where a complex network of ministerial councils, with the Council of Australian Governments (COAG) at the apex, had existed since 1992; South Africa, where a President's Co-ordinating Council (PCC) and supporting councils of line ministers were established by legislation in 2005, implementing Chapter 3 of the Constitution; India, where an Inter-State Council (ISC) was established in 1990 by presidential order under article 263 of the Constitution; Switzerland, where a system of largely horizontal inter-cantonal conferences was complemented from 1993 by a Conference of Cantonal Governments (Schnabel and Mueller 2017); and Spain, where a Premiers' Conference was established by the central government in 2004.

One of the more interesting observations from the collective experience of federations during the pandemic was how much of the intergovernmental status quo was found wanting in the face of this sudden and novel threat. This was not the case everywhere. In Germany, for example, less formal meetings between the Chancellor and the first ministers supplemented the limitations of the *Bundesrat* to coordinate the actions of governments in an area where so much authority lay with the *Länder* and seem to have been adequate to the purpose. In other federations, existing arrangements proved less satisfactory in a variety of distinct ways.

Federations where intergovernmental forums were already weak or non-existent, as in Mexico, had no obvious vehicle to bring heads of government together, prompting calls for better intergovernmental architecture in the future. In Mexico, ad hoc arrangements were made for a meeting, but not until August, when the pandemic was well advanced. In Ethiopia, where such forums also were lacking, coordination took place through party connections, to the extent that it took place at all. In others, including the US, Brazil and Nigeria, horizontal meetings achieved some coordination to fill the gap partly, but typically these were not fully inclusive, bringing together governors connected by region or, sometimes, party affiliation.

More surprisingly perhaps, many federations in which intergovernmental forums were available altered them or did not use them at all. In some cases, they were bypassed in favour of bodies designed to coordinate action at the centre, initially with no constituent unit representation at all. Argentina, Italy, and Nigeria are examples. Relevantly for present purposes, however, in at least some cases, including Italy, intergovernmental forums were activated or reactivated in the course of the year in the light of experience with the pandemic. In a similar vein, in some cases, of which the UK and Belgium are examples, central coordinating bodies were supplemented, permanently or on an occasional basis, by representatives of the constituent units. Along the same lines again but in an example of a different kind, in India, while the formal intergovernmental forum, the Inter-State Council, did not meet, eight less formal online meetings are reported to have occurred between the Prime Minister and the state premiers in the period covered by this chapter in this study.

In some federations, experience with the pandemic proved a catalyst for change to intergovernmental forums. One phenomenon reported across several federations is that intergovernmental forums, when they operated at all, did so from the top-down, in a demonstration of central leadership and control. In varying ways, this seems to have occurred in, for example, Spain, Austria, Switzerland, and South Africa. In the first three of these cases, the extent of central leadership was accepted as a viable way to respond to the pandemic in that particular context. In Spain, however, top-down control by the centre through the Premiers' Conference during the first phase of the pandemic subsequently changed to the much more interactive approach of 'co-governance', during which the Premiers' Conference met 16 times, offering a model that may also be relevant for the future.

More dramatically still, in Australia, COAG, the existing forum for heads of government, was replaced early in the pandemic by a new, intergovernmental 'National Cabinet', designed to operate quickly, efficiently and with minimal bureaucracy. The Australian approach had the advantage of recognising the distinct roles of each of the participating governments and leaving considerable discretion to each. This new intergovernmental architecture was developed speedily and to meet a single purpose, however. It remains to be seen whether it will survive into a post-pandemic era as the vehicle for coordination across a broad spectrum of intergovernmental action.

A third, more amorphous, category of institutions comprises *boards and agencies* of various kinds that serve an intergovernmental purpose (Poirier and Saunders 2015: 467–9). Typically, these have specialist qualifications and operate at a degree of arms-length from government. Their primary function may be advisory or regulatory, and they may be established or constituted by participating jurisdictions collectively or by one level of government alone, usually the centre.

In the context of the pandemic, most such bodies were health-related, although some were mandated to deal with responses to emergencies more generally, or to advise on the economic fallout of the pandemic. Their functions ranged from providing high-level epidemiological and related health advice, to the development, coordination, and monitoring of the implementation of plans to manage the crisis by, for example, limiting community transmission. The mixture of specialist health and bureaucratic expertise required was met in some cases through reliance on multiple bodies and, in others, through the composition of a single agency or body. Given the involvement of all levels of government in responding to the pandemic, one challenge was to ensure that relevant specialist expertise was available to each level of government; another was to coordinate the reactions of each jurisdiction to the specialist advice they received.

The complexity of these arrangements, many of which also evolved over time, makes generalisation difficult. They can be seen, however, as falling into three, sometimes overlapping, categories. In some cases, the agency was established at and responsible to the national level of government, affecting action at other levels of government either through direction or through interaction between agencies organised in an essentially hierarchical structure. The Brazilian National Health Regulator and the Nigerian National Emergency Management Agency are examples of the former, while the Indian Disaster Management Authorities are an example of the latter. In a second category of cases, the agency has intergovernmental elements in its composition. The Austrian commission that published risk assessments for the coronavirus 'traffic light system' is an example, comprising experts, civil servants, and *Land* representatives. The Epidemics Task Force in Switzerland might also be placed in this category.

In what might be considered a third category, both the centre and the constituent units maintained specialist agencies of their own between which communication took place. Australia and Canada, at least, took this approach. In Australia, each jurisdiction had a chief health officer to advise the government and, sometimes, exercise statutory power. These officers communicated informally with each other, however, and met regularly in an intergovernmental forum, the Australian Health Protection Principal Committee (AHPPC), which in turn advised the 'National Cabinet'. In an era of suspicion of experts, it is an interesting question whether, as an aspect of multilevel government, the multiple sources of official expertise on which some federations relied during the pandemic strengthened trust in the decisions that were made or complicated matters further.

Agreements between participating jurisdictions are a familiar mechanism in intergovernmental relations, recording decisions about collective action to achieve particular outcomes or resolve particular problems (Poirier and Saunders 2015: 469–74). The incidence of intergovernmental agreements varies between federal-type systems depending on context, including in this instance the legal and political system. Some agreements require legislative consent, while others are made entirely through executive power. Some agreements are legally enforceable; others have, at best, the status of soft law.

At first glance, intergovernmental agreements played a relatively minor role in federations in responding to the pandemic in 2020. To the extent to which this is so, it may reflect the speed at which the pandemic spread, which required a government response that had no time for the lengthy negotiations between jurisdictions that agreements may require. On closer inspection, however, agreements were a feature of intergovernmental relations during the pandemic as well, even if they were not negotiated for the purpose or, in some cases, referred to in those terms.

In the first place, the complexities of hospitals and health care in federations are such that there often are general agreements dealing with such matters, necessarily affecting the use of hospitals during the pandemic. The account of developments in Austria draws attention to the long-standing significance of health-care agreements under article 15(a) of the Austrian Constitution, but agreements of this kind exist elsewhere as well. Secondly, in a point that may be more specific to experience with the pandemic, in many federations the intergovernmental response was described as being framed by pre-existing 'plans' or equivalent terms. Thus, for example, in Canada there was a Federal/Provincial/

Territorial Response Plan for Biological Events, in addition to a range of supplementary intergovernmental instruments; in Nigeria, there was a Pandemic Multi-Sectoral Response Plan; in the UK, a Coronavirus Action Plan; in Russia, a Corona Crisis Action Plan; in Spain, a National Early Warning and Rapid Response System; and in Australia, an Australian Health Management Plan for Pandemic Influenza, a National Strategy for Disaster Resilience and an Emergency Response Plan for the Covid-19 Pandemic, among others.

Several questions arise, not all of which can be answered with information presently available. It is clear that not all 'plans' that were put to use during the pandemic were intergovernmental in any relevant sense. In the examples above, both the Spanish 'System' and the Nigerian Plan seem to have been developed by the central government alone and so fall into this category. It is equally clear, however, that in some cases a plan is the equivalent of an intergovernmental agreement. This point is made specifically in the Canadian chapter, but it seems to reflect the understanding in other federations as well, including the UK. These circumstances prompt a question about what it is in relation to the manner in which the plan was developed, or its content, that causes the terminology of 'plan' to be used in lieu of a descriptor that signifies collective agreement more obviously.

In yet another group of federations in which plans played a role during the pandemic, the 'plan' had an intergovernmental element of some kind. The Russian plan, for example, is said to have been adopted by all the constituent units; the Australian 'Strategy' was officially developed through COAG, as the intergovernmental predecessor of what now is the National Cabinet. In these and other cases, however, there are questions about the extent to which the arrangements were informed by consultation with the constituent units and were consensual, at least in the sense signified by signature to an agreement. Insofar as many of these plans and other arrangements were laid down in advance with a view to managing future emergencies, there is another question about the extent to which they were adequate to the purpose as this particular emergency evolved. This issue is flagged most specifically in relation to Canada but, again, seems likely also to be relevant elsewhere. The difficulty of finding answers points to problems with transparency, to which the following section of this chapter refers.

One final set of intergovernmental mechanisms that require brief mention concern *fiscal arrangements* (Poirier and Saunders 2015: 474–6). The techniques themselves are familiar: fiscal transfers between levels of government, tax-sharing arrangements, and support for borrowing of various kinds. The fiscal dislocation caused by the pandemic through substantial additional expenditures and loss of tax and other revenues as economic activity slowed or stopped, made it inevitable that mechanisms of this kind would be a component of intergovernmental relations. More action can be expected on this front as the economic consequences of the pandemic become clearer over time.

In the short term, however, the chapters in this book record the use of transfers to assist constituent units either generally or in relation to pandemic-related expenses in, for example, Brazil, Nigeria, India, Russia, and Ethiopia; a renegotiation of the Barnett formula for revenue redistribution in the UK; assistance with the debts of constituent units in Brazil, Russia, and Nigeria; and the use of fiscal transfers in Germany not only to supplement *Länder* revenues but also to induce *Länder* compliance with a coordinated policy approach to aspects of pandemic management. There are indications in this chapter of longer-term implications of experience with the pandemic for intergovernmental fiscal relations. One, to which the Swiss chapter refers, is the impact of the Covid-19 experience on the viability of the continued use of the fiscal equivalence principle under article 43(a)(3) and (4) of the Swiss Constitution.

20.5 Insights

Intergovernmental relations were a feature of the response of all federations to the emergencies created by the pandemic. The ways in which intergovernmental relations were used varied, however, not only in the mechanisms employed but in the proportionate contribution of the centre and the constituent units, including, in many cases, local governments. In some federations, among them, for example, Mexico, Nigeria, South Africa, India, Austria, and Russia, the centre dominated decision-making over the period covered by this chapter, once the scale of the problem had become evident. In others, of which the US, Canada, and Australia are somewhat different examples, the approach was more dualistic, whilst nevertheless involving some interaction between governments. The experiences of the remainder lie between these two poles, striking a balance in a variety of ways.

Each federation ultimately will assess its own performance in response to Covid-19, including the adequacy of interactions between governments. On the evidence of the chapters in this book, some, including Germany and Canada, are broadly satisfied with the workings of intergovernmental relations, at least up to the end of 2020. In some cases, of which Spain and Australia are examples, the experience of dealing with the pandemic itself caused shifts in the conduct of intergovernmental relations the durability of which remain to be seen but which seem to have met with broad approval in the short term. In other cases, the chapters suggest either that the jury is still out on the effectiveness of intergovernmental relations or that reform is indicated. In most of the cases in this latter category, including Brazil, Argentina, and the UK, the primary concern is over-centralisation. An overlapping concern, also in Mexico, is patchy and dysfunctional intergovernmental relations. In the US, the primary concern instead was a shortfall in leadership from the centre that exacerbated the problems of a dualist approach lacking the possibility of productive vertical interaction even when it patently was needed.

Despite the diversity of usage of intergovernmental relations during the pandemic, some insights are suggested by the collective experience. One is that, to maximise the potential of a federation for responding to crises such as those presented by Covid-19, intergovernmental relations cannot be overly top-down. Central leadership is useful and may be necessary, but it should be understood as central leadership in a federation, in which the active contribution of constituent units contributes to informed and legitimate intergovernmental decisions and serves a variety of purposes.

This is not news in federations with a developed federal culture. Switzerland is such an example, where consultation with the cantons is prescribed by the Constitution and underpinned by the political process (Switzerland, Constitution, article 45 and 55). In other federations, such principles are undeveloped or imperfectly realised. In Canada and Australia, for example, the nearest equivalent is a principle of 'cooperation', which has evolved as a tool for understanding the scope of the legislative powers of the respective levels of government rather than as a standard for the manner of their collective exercise (Gaudreault-DesBiens and Poirier 2017). In Italy, central consultation and cooperation with the regions in the initial phase of the pandemic were described as 'half-hearted' despite a principle of loyal cooperation in article 120(2) of the Constitution – neither level of government appears to have adopted it adequately. Grappling with the pandemic changed principles of this kind from abstract goals to practical necessities in ways that offer new insight into what intergovernmental relations require.

A second, but related, insight is that the goal of effective intergovernmental relations is not necessarily uniformity. Some of the case studies, including Canada, Australia, and Germany, show approaches to intergovernmental relations that assumed significant diversity in policy and practice at the subnational level, for which subnational governments were accountable to their own institutions and voters. In many other cases, including Spain, Italy, and Russia, initial assumptions about the need for uniformity gave way over time to increasing diversity at the subnational level, as experience with the pandemic showed that local discretion, responding to local conditions, could be advantageous. Less charitable explanations, about distributing blame, are possible too, but the trend is notable, nevertheless. The extent to which divergent policies and practices were useful and acceptable at the level of constituent units varied with context, including the degree of actual difference in conditions on the ground and the strength of adherence to principles of equivalence in regulatory standards. The demonstration of the broader roles that intergovernmental relations can play without prioritising centralisation and uniformity is another useful outcome of the experiences of 2020 all the same.

Thirdly, the real demands that the pandemic placed on governments at all levels highlighted the importance of capacity, in the sense of capability. The capacity of the several levels of government to perform the roles assigned to them is a *sine qua non* of a working federation. Too often, however, the significance of capacity, particularly of the subnational levels of government, is ignored or imperfectly understood, papered over by centralisation, including through intergovernmental relations. This becomes less possible when intergovernmental arrangements require an active contribution from constituent units.

The challenges presented by lack of capacity at subnational levels of government in responding to the pandemic were experienced in many federations, including South Africa, Nigeria, and Italy. The lesson for the future is not only to design intergovernmental arrangements in ways that take capacity into account but also to work to build capacity, such that all levels of government can make contributions that realise the potential of intergovernmental relations.

One final concluding observation concerns transparency and accountability, notoriously victims of intergovernmental relations. The extent of the problem differs between federations. Transparency and accountability are less affected where, for example, there is a legal or constitutional framework for intergovernmental relations or a requirement for certain types of arrangements to be approved by legislation, if only because, in either case, aspects or relations between governments have greater public exposure. Almost by definition, however, intergovernmental relations typically rely to a considerable extent on meetings, agreements, and actions of other kinds in which the primary actors are members of the executive branch, interacting in relatively unstructured settings and operating in confidence.

Problems of transparency and accountability in intergovernmental relations were in evidence during the pandemic as well. Ironically, to the extent that each level of government had discrete roles for which they were accountable to their own voters; in some federations, there was a higher level of public understanding of and interest in who was doing what than often is the case. In other respects, however, familiar problems recurred, exacerbated by the need for speed in responding to the pandemic as it unfolded and, in many jurisdictions, even less parliamentary scrutiny than usual.

Two examples may be given. One is uncertainty about how and on what bases roles and responsibilities for dealing with the pandemic were allocated between governments. The Canadian chapter specifically queries whether the intergovernmental arrangements in the Response Plan were 'actually mobilised', but similar issues almost certainly have arisen elsewhere. The second example concerns the various intergovernmental forums through which the bulk of intergovernmental relations occurred. Problems of accountability inevitably arise in relation to collective decisions of an intergovernmental body, the individual members of which are politically accountable to different institutions and different constituencies. These problems are greater if there is lack of transparency about the operating rules for such bodies, the influences that are brought to bear in the course of decision-making, and the decisions that are eventually made – matters in which practice differs between federations.

An Australian example, admittedly extreme, shows how such problems arise. The operating rules for the new apex intergovernmental forum, the National Cabinet, which was established early in 2020, have never been publicly explained. Decisions are announced briefly, by 'media statement', in terms that are predictably general and opaque. Furthermore, in a complete break from earlier practice, the 'National Cabinet' is institutionally located under the umbrella of the

Commonwealth Cabinet, apparently in order to attract the same rules about solidarity and confidentiality, including protection from freedom of information legislation (Department of the Prime Minister and Cabinet 2020). Legal challenges to this arrangement can be expected. In the meantime, however, it stands as a reminder that designing intergovernmental arrangements in ways that adequately meet democratic standards for transparency and accountability remains a work in progress.

Notes

1　The power in question deals with 'quarantine' (s 51(xi)). Section 8 of the Biosecurity Act of 2015 (Cth), which exercises the power, includes a standard disclaimer of intention to limit a state law 'capable of operating concurrently' with the Commonwealth law.
2　The Mexican chapter refers to 'coordination' (in the field of civil protection) as involving 'the creation of mechanisms of coordination and collaboration among orders of government in a specific policy area', noting, however, that the procedure was not used in respect of the pandemic.
3　The point is made by Johanne Poirier, in commenting on an earlier version of this chapter.

References

Aroney, N. and Kincaid, J. (eds). 2017. *Courts in Federal Countries: Federalists or Unitarists?* Toronto: University of Toronto Press.

Department of the Prime Minister and Cabinet. 2020. *Cabinet Handbook*, 14th ed., https://pmc.gov.au/resource-centre/government/cabinet-handbook (accessed on 1 February 2021).

Frankenberg, G. 2006. 'Comparing Constitutions: Ideas, Ideals, and Ideology – Towards a Layered Narrative', *International Journal of Constitutional Law*, 4: 439–59.

Gaudreault-DesBiens, J. and Poirier, J. 2017. 'From Dualism to Cooperative Federalism and Back? Evolving and Competing Conceptions of Canadian Federalism', in P. Oliver, P. Macklem and N. Desrosiers (eds), *The Oxford Handbook of the Canadian Constitution*, pp. 391–413. New York: Oxford University Press.

Institute for Government. 2020. 'Sewel Convention', https://www.instituteforgovernment.org.uk/explainers/sewel-convention (accessed on 1 February 2021).

Poirier, J. and Saunders, C. 2015. 'Conclusion: Comparative Experience of Intergovernmental Relations in Federal Systems', in J. Poirier, C. Saunders and J. Kincaid (eds), *Intergovernmental Relations in Federal Systems*, pp. 440–95. Canada: Oxford University Press.

Poirier, J., Saunders, C. and Kincaid, J. (eds). 2015. *Intergovernmental Relations in Federal Systems*. Canada: Oxford University Press.

Saunders, C. and Dziedzic, A. 2017. 'The Meanings of Concurrency', in N. Steytler (ed.), *Concurrent Powers in Federal Systems: Meaning, Making, Managing*, pp. 12–31. The Hague: Brill/Nijhoff.

Schnabel, J. and Mueller, S. 2017. 'Vertical Influence or Intergovernmental Coordination? The Purpose of Intergovernmental Councils in Switzerland', *Regional and Federal Studies*, 27(5): 549.

Special Commission of Inquiry. 2020. *Report of the Special Commission of Inquiry into the Ruby Princess*, New South Wales, https://www.rubyprincessinquiry.nsw.gov.au/report (accessed on 1 February 2021).

21

FEDERALISM UNDER PRESSURE

Federal 'health' factors and
'co-morbidities'[1]

Nico Steytler

21.1 Introduction

The Covid-19 pandemic has been a 'focusing event' (Béland et al. 2020) for federalism like no other, placing it under the microscope and giving rise to the three questions set out in the introduction of this book. Each gives rise to a number of subquestions. First, how did federal systems respond to the pandemic during the first critical period of 2020, when quick, concerted, and effective action was necessary to limit the virus and its dire socio-economic consequences? What were the modalities of action? How did they impact on the constitutional distribution of powers – did they lead to an increase in centralisation or decentralisation? Did intergovernmental relations (IGR), the lifeblood of federal systems, work efficiently or at all? What happened to intergovernmental fiscal relations?

The second question is more evaluative: How well (or badly) did federal systems, which by nature involve dispersed decision-making, fare in combating the pandemic? How did federalism perform as a system of governance in the modern age when confronted unexpectedly with such a massive global crisis? Although most federations saw a trend towards centralisation, none of them lost their federal character entirely to become unitary states. The question then is whether the fundamental characteristics that Ronald Watts regarded as essential to the success of federalism were also relevant in combating the pandemic effectively. The 'federal success factors' Watts posits are

- a strong disposition to democratic procedures, which presumes the voluntary consent of citizens in the constituent units;
- multiple centres of political decision-making that give expression to the principle of non-centralisation;
- open political bargaining as a dominant means of reaching decisions; and

DOI: 10.4324/9781003166771-28

• respect for constitutionalism and the rule of law, given that each order of government derives its authority from the constitution (Watts 2011: 16–17).

Conversely, did those federations that showed failures in respect of one or more of these characteristics perform worse in health and well-being outcomes than would have been the case otherwise? Were these federal 'health' factors relevant under an emergency situation and should the list be complemented?

The third question is this: Where changes in federal dynamics did occur due to Covid-19 – a movement towards decentralisation or centralisation – are they likely to have long-term consequences for that federal system? Will the impact of Covid-19 reverberate long after the health and economic consequences are more or less under control? Did the pandemic open or close a 'policy window' for more fundamental changes?

The 18 country studies show that during 2020 most of the federal systems under review became more centralised in response to the pandemic, but not uniformly or continuously so. IGR was often inadequate or non-existent, in the process fortifying centralised rule; the increased dependence of subnational governments on federal transfers also had a centralising effect. I conclude, furthermore, that some federal systems were resilient enough to deal effectively with the pandemic. In many if not most cases, however, the success factors, if at all present, came under pressure with predictable results. What contributing authors described as failures in their respective federal systems, led to poor outcomes both in respect of effective governance and lives lost as well as hardships incurred. These failures, mostly proceeding from pre-existing problems, can be labelled as 'federal co-morbidities': their presence in the federal body politic made the system less able to face the Covid-19 challenge successfully. In addition to the four characteristics mentioned by Watts, the capability of governments at all levels should join the list. Finally, although it is still too early to tell, Covid-19 might be a catalyst in some countries for greater decentralisation, in particular in the field of fiscal federalism.

Due to space constraints, these concluding remarks do not do justice to the richness of the country studies; the remarks are, inevitably, prone to generalisation that does not fit all the countries. Given that all the countries were subjected to the same coronavirus at the same time, and exposed to the same World Health Organization (WHO) information, world media coverage, and the scientific community, the responses were on the whole noticeably similar. However, drilling down to the detail, it is clear that the very characteristics (geographical, demographical, economic, political, and governmental) which made each country a unique federation in the first place also shaped the individual responses to Covid-19.

21.2 The relevance of contextual factors

As Cheryl Saunders notes in Chapter 20, geophysical characteristics, economic development, the form and operation of government, and the multifaceted framework for federalism all had a significant influence on the conduct of IGR.

In this section, I sketch out how the other aspects of federalism may have been influenced by the same contextual factors.

First, geographical size mattered. Seven of the eight largest countries in the world are federations: Russia, Canada, the United States (US), Brazil, Australia, India, and Argentina. In such vast territories, infection rates varied from region to region, which allowed for differentiation in government responses. From the outset, emergency powers were delegated to Russia's 85 constituent units to deal with local conditions; the eastern Canadian provinces could effectively self-isolate themselves as the 'Atlantic bubble', as did the state of Western Australia in closing its borders to the rest of the country. On the other side of the spectrum, in smaller federations, with high interconnectivity (e.g. in Switzerland and Belgium) the prospect of self-isolation of constituent units was limited.

Moreover, with seven of the 10 most populous countries in the world being federations (India, the US, Pakistan, Brazil, Nigeria, Russia, and Mexico), anti-pandemic measures had to be of enormous magnitude, requiring plentiful resources. With diversity along racial, ethnic, linguistic, and religious lines lying at the root of the federal nature of 13 of the federations presented in this book, the pandemic brought divergent communities closer together in some instances but in others drove them further apart. On the positive side, to everyone's surprise, the Catalonian government worked remarkably well with the Spanish government, and the highly divided Belgium saw its two linguistic communities cooperating at the centre as never before. On the negative side, the pandemic was used to deepen cleavages in India (the promotion of anti-Muslim sentiment), in Nigeria, and, most tragically of all, in Ethiopia, where a political dispute between the centre and the ethnic region of Tigray degenerated into civil war. Further, the marginalisation of voiceless indigenous communities in Brazil and Mexico was exacerbated. Poverty and unemployment among South Africa's majority black population also increased, deepening inequality.

The high levels of urbanisation in most federations – as well as the large, densely populated cities in countries with low levels of it, such as India and the African federations – facilitated community infections. It was only when the 'traffic light' regulatory system was introduced – that of differentiated unlocking and re-locking during the second wave of infection – that low-infected rural communities could become less subject to the overbroad national measures designed with urban areas in mind.

Economically, the selected federations represent most categories of income levels. In terms of the World Bank classification (2020), 10 are high-income countries; Argentina, Brazil, Mexico, Russia, and South Africa are upper-middle income; India and Nigeria lower-middle income; and Ethiopia low income. These classifications, of course, hide inequality levels within federations. It is particularly the upper-middle-income countries where inequality is most pronounced: Brazil, Mexico, Argentina, and South Africa (by far the most). It is in these low- and middle-income countries that public health-care systems are underfunded, less testing is conducted, less infections are recorded, and poor medical care is provided.

When it comes to governance, six of the 18 federations have a presidential system, while the rest have some form of parliamentary governance. Populist personalities seemed to thrive in presidential systems – the 'denialist' presidents of the US, Brazil, and Mexico, for example. The parliamentary systems, on the other hand, showed a strong tendency towards cooperation and coordination at the national level as well as with the states (Australia, Belgium, Canada, Germany, Spain, Switzerland, the United Kingdom (UK)). But parliamentary systems also gave rise to dominant federal executives averse to cooperative governance (Austria, India, South Africa, and, as the worst case, Ethiopia). In both systems, authoritarian tendencies were noted: in Russia, Argentina, and Nigeria (presidential) and India and Ethiopia (parliamentary).

Among the more dynamic factors that influenced the course of government action was the nature of the party system, and the selected federations reflect a wide variety. A few countries are dominated by a single party operating at federal and state levels and centrist in orientation (cf. Detterbeck and Hepburn 2010). The primary examples are Russia, where President Putin's United Russia controls the centre and all but nine of the 85 constituent units; India's Bharatiya Janata Party, which controls Parliament and 21 of the 28 states; Ethiopia's Prosperity Party, with near-total control of the federal legislature and nine of the 10 regional states; and South Africa's African National Congress, which controls the national Parliament and eight of the nine provinces. Although the ruling party in Argentina does not dominate Congress, opposition parties govern in only three of the 23 provinces and the Autonomous City of Buenos Aires. Such dominance enabled ruling parties to use the party hierarchy as the primary IGR instrument.

On the other side of the spectrum are more competitive party politics, which in parliamentary systems have given rise to 'grand coalitions' in Germany or even to minority governments in Belgium, Canada, Italy, and Spain. Non-entrenched majority parties with active opposition are found in the UK and Australia. None of the ruling parties of the British devolved units is linked to the Conservative Party in Westminster, while in Australia there is an even split, with the opposition Labour Party governing three of the six states and two territories. In Canada, the Liberal Party governs at the centre, while its very loosely connected liberal counter-parts only led in two of the ten provinces. In the absence of a hegemonic party, cooperation at the national level and vertically with states was the order of the day.

In presidential systems with competitive party politics, for example, the US, Mexico, and Nigeria, presidential and federal legislative results were also reflected in subnational governments: in the US 26 states had Republican governors while 24 states had Democrats. In Mexico, the split between the ruling party and opposition parties was even at state level. In Brazil, President Bolsonaro governs without party affiliation and a stable support in Congress and the majority of the state governors have no truck with him. In these federations, the common theme is that political ideology and partisanship were the driving force behind decision-making, as was only too evident in the fact that distributions of funds were biased against opposition-held states.

21.3 The federal constitutional and legislative framework

The pandemic, by its very nature, impacted on numerous aspects of governance, ranging from international relations, in which nations were kept apart by border closures, to local government, where the effort was to keep individuals apart through social distancing. Nor were response measures to Covid-19 restricted to health care or disaster management: they also affected competences relating to education, social protection, social welfare, and the economy – all of which are particularly germane to federalism, given that the starting-point in a federation is the constitutional allocation of powers (with its possible suspension during a state of emergency being the exception).

21.3.1 Constitutional allocation of powers

The usual constitutional devices of allocating powers in federal systems also apply to health care and disaster management and range from the exclusivity of dualist approaches to the intermingling of powers in integrative systems (Poirier and Saunders 2015). In a significant number of federations, health care is predominantly a state function, as in Australia, Belgium, Canada, Nigeria, Switzerland, the UK, and the US. Such allocations are seldom watertight, though, resulting in varying forms and degrees of concurrency. In particular, federal governments usually retain influence through the power of the purse in countries where they enjoy superior taxing powers. In the majority of countries, the two areas are formally concurrent or (de facto) shared functions in one or other form (see Steytler 2017), as is the case in Brazil, Ethiopia India, Italy, Mexico, Russia, South Africa, and Spain. The federal government usually develops general frameworks and policy guidance, while the state governments provide the health services, resulting in intended or de facto executive federalism (Argentina, Austria, Ethiopia, Germany, South Africa).

With regard to these two main functions, local government plays only a peripheral constitutional role. In half of the federations, local government is a competence of the states and thus derives its mandate from state legislation. Although half of the federations constitutionally recognise the existence of local government as an order of government, very few attribute specific functions to it. Argentina, Brazil, and South Africa are unique in listing specific powers, including 'municipal health care', that local authorities exercise in conjunction with the other orders of government. In the rest of the countries, local government performs a range of statutory municipal functions, the most important areas of responsibility during a pandemic being water, sanitation, waste management, and control of public spaces.

A strong common thread is that health care and disaster management, as well as the other affected areas such as education and social welfare, are every level of government's business. All powers are to some degree concurrent – and are divided not only between two, but three or four tiers (the international one included) – circumstances which called out for coordination and cooperation in the face of a common enemy.

21.3.2 Emergency declarations

The constitutional division of powers (along with basic human rights) could be upset by a declaration of a state of emergency, which empowers a federal government to intrude on subnational constitutional space. In most countries, only the federal government may impose a state of emergency, usually entailing legislative approval and other checks and balances; in a few countries, states may also declare states of emergency in terms of their own constitutions (the US, Argentina, and Ethiopia).

A similar empowerment of federal and state executives can be obtained in most countries by using ordinary legislation dealing with disaster management and/or public health emergencies, a process usually not subject to significant legislative oversight. States in Australia, Brazil, Canada, and Switzerland have co-equal powers with the federal government to declare a state of disaster. Often a federal declaration of disaster or health emergency also provides a framework in terms of which subnational governments can make their own disaster declarations because of the anticipated localised impact of a disaster or epidemic (Argentina, Italy, Nigeria, Russia).

Where federal legislation is couched with reference to disaster management, it usually includes the broad category of 'epidemics'. Legislation may also refer specifically to 'epidemic and health disasters'. In their responses to Covid-19, the federal governments of India and Nigeria relied on epidemic legislation dating back to the colonial area (Indian Epidemic Diseases Act of 1897; Nigerian Quarantine Act of 1926), which, of course, demonstrated scant regard for the federal system that had emerged subsequently.

21.4 Preparedness for a national disaster: The institutional framework

Preparedness for a pandemic requires nationwide federal institutions, structures, and processes which can act promptly, concertedly, and effectively. However, given that health care and disaster management are the responsibilities mainly of subnational government (which is thus where the capability lies, or should lie), the question is whether subnational governments participate in these national institutions.

All the federations under review had legal frameworks in place to deal with pandemics. Only a minority – Australia and the UK, for example – had to update their health epidemic laws during the pandemic for being outdated and not providing the federal executive with sufficient powers. Furthermore, all the federal governments (except Switzerland) have a department of health (and sometimes one for disaster management as well), in addition to which most have national scientific bodies advising the government. Many such federal structures do not, however, provide for subnational participation (Austria (initially), Ethiopia, Italy, Russia, Spain). The lack of coordination between levels of government became painfully evident when problems with data collection came to the fore, as happened in Italy, Spain, and Switzerland, for example; there were no coordinated systems enabling the methodical collection of data, a fact which hampered getting an accurate picture of the pandemic necessary for planning.

Australia and Canada seem to be exceptions. Well-prepared nationwide institutions were in existence and providing for subnational participation, all of which seeming to have proven effective when Covid-19 struck. Although the US had well-established federal institutions and plans for epidemics (with good IGR cooperation from state administrations), the budgets of these institutions had been reduced over the years, rendering their emergency plans less than effective.

In countries where there are national institutions and processes with an IGR dimension, these remained largely inoperative. In Switzerland, the Inter-cantonal Conference of Health Ministers made way for a number of ad hoc taskforces. In South Africa, the national advisory Intergovernmental Committee on Disaster Management includes provincial representation but never convened; decisions were instead made by a national cabinet committee called the National Coronavirus Command Council.

Overall, most federations were unprepared for the unprecedented magnitude, swiftness of spread, and deadly consequences of Covid-19. Plans had focused mostly on past national crises such as terrorism and the 2008/2009 global financial crisis (true of the European Union (EU) in particular). The lack of preparedness was compounded in low- to middle-income countries by chronically underfunded public health-care systems.

21.5 Rolling out of measures to contain the pandemic

Given the unpreparedness of most federations, Covid-19 required urgent action from federal and state governments alike where they shared responsibility for health care and disaster management. Cities that experienced the first signs of the pandemic were also called to intervene.

In the face of the approaching pandemic, the body politic on the whole showed solidarity, providing a conducive space for prompt federal action. The first response of political parties across the political spectrum was to rally together against the common threat and express support for the first lockdown steps taken by the federal government. There were exceptions: in Nigeria, the enmity following the 2019 election percolated through to President Buhari's declaration of a health emergency, which the main opposition party opposed; in the face of denialist presidents, political solidarity in Brazil and Mexico was also a bridge too far.

Bonhomie towards the national lead soon evaporated in the glare of party-political interests. In the US, while the first relief bills were adopted on 11 March by huge bipartisan majorities, by June gridlock settled in between the Democratic-controlled House of Representatives and the Republican-controlled Senate. In other federations, disputes arose about the pace of loosening restrictions; left-of-centre parties argued on the side of health preservation, while those on the right-of-centre were more concerned with job losses and the economy.

Unheard in the political cauldron of mainstream politics were the voices of minority and indigenous groups. They remained as voiceless and powerless as before, although they were more prone, due to a variety of factors, to succumbing to the virus. The situation of Brazil's indigenous communities in Amazonia, falling within the jurisdiction of the federal government, became much worse under President Jair Bolsanaro. Mexico's indigenous communities resorted to self-help by closing off their communities and taking their plight to the courts, where they challenged the distribution of information and health resources. In Canada a number of vulnerable indigenous nations erected borders around their communities, with the tacit approval of all orders of government.

21.5.1 Taking the initiative

With Covid-19 beginning to spread across the globe and the WHO declaring it a 'public health emergency of international concern' on 30 January 2020 and a pandemic on 11 March, federal rather than subnational governments made the first move. Most exercised their international relations competence by closing international borders to travellers from China and gradually also to those from other 'hotspot' countries. These preventative measures were usually too late, though: the virus rapidly gained footholds in cities which are globally well connected.

Facing at first a highly localised epidemic, states and cities directly affected by the virus took action to contain community infection through various lockdown measures (including internal border closures), while the federal governments looked upon from afar. In particular, it was the major cities, linked internationally and experiencing the flood of first cases, that acted first: Milan, Moscow, San Francisco, New York, Sao Paulo. The city state of Lagos took the first steps as it, with its busy international airport, was the epicentre of the pandemic in Nigeria.

Preventative measures were not always uppermost in the minds of affected cities or towns, as the Austrian village of Ischgl illustrates. Ischgl is dependent on the ski-tourism that attracts visitors from around the world. When returning tourists fell ill, the alarm bells rang from Iceland and Germany that it was a super-spreader location, but the responsible district administration vacillated about placing Ischgl under quarantine – a quarter of its jobs were tied to the hospitality sector. It thus took the federal government to cordon the village off.

Early intervention by states and cities, typically ones under opposition-party control, were spurred on by the denialist, anti-science attitudes of the presidents of the US, Brazil, and Mexico. But states could also play partisan politics: the early declaration of emergency by the Tigray regional government had little to do with the pandemic and far more with affirming its autonomous political status.

In Germany, local governments, acting under the advice of the *Länder*, were the first to impose lockdown measures: Covid-19 infections were perceived as a localised problem that could be solved locally. However, as soon as it became apparent that the pandemic was widespread, particularly after holidaymakers returned from their ski-holidays in Ischgl, the federal government and *Länder* stepped in to declare a national lockdown. The federal principle of subsidiarity was in full operation: where a local authority could not perform a function effectively, that function moved to the next level of government.

The time delay between states and cities taking the initiative with lockdown measures and the federal government's acting was at most a week or two. The significance of these initiatives is not only that states or cities could act upon the competences they shared with the centre, but that, by doing so with public approval, they goaded the federal government into action it might not otherwise have taken as quickly as it did.

In a few countries, the federal government was the only player from the start, having absorbed subnational powers and delegated mere implementation duties to subnational governments (Italy, Spain, Austria, South Africa). In contrast, in Australia, Belgium, and the UK joint decision-making took place between the federal and state governments in which responsibilities were allocated in a coordinated manner. In Canada, the provinces took the lead and remained the dominant players, albeit working closely with the federal government from the outset.

21.5.2 Federal action

Covid-19 required prompt, nationwide action. As noted, federal governments intervened early with the gradual closure of international borders to curb infections coming from abroad. More problematic was getting to grips with community infections, where countermeasures fell into either the exclusive or concurrent domain of subnational governments.

21.5.2.1 Expansion of powers and declaration of emergencies or disasters

At the outbreak of the pandemic, federal governments had a range of legal instruments at their disposal to upset the constitutional allocation of powers by centralising them. In the event, with two exceptions (Argentina and Ethiopia), the federations under review did not declare a general state of emergency, which would have triggered formal legislative checks and balances. In the case of Argentina, it had already been under its frequently used mode of governance – emergency rule – since December 2019 because of an economic

crisis; the Ethiopian emergency declaration had more to do with political instability than confronting Covid-19. Instead, most federal governments used ordinary legislation to empower themselves with delegated law-making authority,
placing themselves largely beyond the scrutiny of legislatures.

In a small minority of federations, no federal emergency of whatsoever kind
was called. The Canadian federal government let the provincial declarations of
health emergency take the lead, for among other reasons that they were sufficiently effective for the job at hand. In Australia, the national Biosecurity Act
of 2015 had already shifted powers to the centre – so closely as to being nearly
constitutionally impermissible – and thus obviated the need to do it during the
pandemic. Moreover, the Commonwealth government used its powers under the
Act sparingly, allowing the states to exercise their competencies under this Act
within a consensus framework.

Declarations of health emergencies rewrote the rule book, conferring powers
over health care and related areas to the federal government. Even in the predominantly dualist federation of Belgium, the federal declaration (made with the
support of the communities) shifted health care to the federal level. In more centralised federations where health care and related areas are concurrent functions,
the declarations simply asserted the primacy of the federal government over state
decision-making, reducing states to implementers of national rules and policies.
In Spain, for example, the centre's declaration of a 'state of alert' resulted in its
assuming all powers over health care, which over time had been devolved to the
Autonomous Communities.

An important consequence of some national declarations of a health emergency was that they also devolved emergency powers to states, thereby enhancing state executives' regulatory powers. Russia is an example in this regard.

21.5.2.2 Substantive measures

With or without enhanced powers from declaration of health emergencies, the
federal government could perform a number of unique functions.

First, in the face of an unpredictable but deadly pandemic, national leadership
sought to assuage citizens' anxieties. As a rule, heads of governments were the
principal communicators about the pandemic's status and the various measures
taken. Often, they were joined by the leaders of subnational governments to
show joined-up government at work. In stark contrast were the presidents of
the US, Mexico, and Brazil, whose non-scientific rhetoric conveyed a confusing
message to the public. President Trump, for one, purposefully called upon citizens not to obey states' stay-at-home orders.

Secondly, where uniformity of measures was called for, federal governments
provided that. In small- and medium-size federations with mobile populations,
uniform lockdown measures gained popular acceptance.

Thirdly, because of the federal governments' superior access to resources, revenue and borrowing, they could address the harsh consequences that lockdown

regimes created. Where social protection in its various forms was a federal responsibility, federal governments could provide individuals and families with support through grants, top-ups and other means of assistance. Federal governments could assist ailing businesses and try to stimulate the economy back to life on a scale well beyond the reach of subnational governments. They could also support subnational governments with funds to execute the extra burdens they carried. Most federal governments also deployed the military to provide health resources (particularly medical personnel and the construction of field hospitals) and enforce lockdown regulations.

However, the limits of federal action were also manifest. First, although the need for centralisation of powers was accepted in many countries, a major unforeseen problem emerged: the federal government lacked capability. Because health care was the predominant or main domain of the subnational governments in Italy, Spain, and Switzerland, the federal government, on assuming that mandate, plainly lacked the capacity (skills and resources) to act swiftly and effectively. Secondly, uniform measures often had disproportionate negative effects. For example, in Switzerland, the Federal Council directed all cantons that hospitals should no longer do non-essential procedures and prepare only for Covid patients. However, because infection rates varied considerably between cantons, some cantonal hospitals ran out of work and income when Covid patients did not turn up in the droves that had been anticipated.

The value of federal Covid-related action was compromised even further by pre-existing political pathologies. First, entrenched cultures of corruption were simply aggravated by the pandemic. In our sample, a significant number of federations have a serious corruption problem: according to the Transparency International Corruption Perception Index of 2020, in descending rank order in the world were South Africa (69), Argentina (78), India (86), Ethiopia (94), Brazil (94), Mexico (124), Russia (129), and Nigeria (149) (Transparency International 2020; Vrushi and Kukutschaka 2021). Although corruption is pervasive at all levels of government, at the federal level it had the greatest financial and moral impact.

The increase in corruption was due to huge amounts of money becoming available overnight for the purchase of materials and services, the relaxing of procurement rules for the sake of urgency, and the fact that the usual counter-corruption measures, such as vigilant parliaments, went to sleep. Instead of the nation standing together, the few fed off its misery as scarce funds to combat the virus disappeared into the pockets of government officials and their cronies. Increased corruption was reported in South Africa, and Nigeria.

Secondly, some federal governments used both their extended powers and the centralised ethos the pandemic created to advance their own political agendas. As the old adage goes, 'Never waste a good crisis.' In Argentina, President Alberto Ángel Fernández sought the power to change the national budget unilaterally; India's Prime Minister Narendra Modi pushed through a parliamentary bill advancing the centralisation of agriculture and education; Russia's President

Vladimir Putin used the pandemic in his campaign for constitutional amendment, which, inter alia, extended the presidential term of office (his own, that is); and, as noted, the postponement of Ethiopian elections scheduled for August 2020 had more to do with avoiding an election than countering a low level of Covid-19 infection.

21.5.2.3 Accountability

The drift towards the increase of executive powers vis-à-vis the legislature is evident in both presidential and parliamentary systems. In the former, presidents ruled by decrees and orders that fell outside the legislatures' legislative domain and the term 'hyper-presidentialism' has been applied to Russia and Argentina. In parliamentary systems, parliaments often gave prime ministers a free pass and played a muted role.

After initially suspending their activities out of compliance with social distancing measures, legislatures limped back into full or partial operation by holding their sessions online. The general complaint is that parliaments were marginalised, more often than not through actions of 'self-disempowerment'. When called upon to pass enabling legislation and authorise support packages, they acted with astounding speed and expeditiousness. Within a single day – Sunday 15 March 2020 – the Austrian parliament passed the Covid-19 Measures Act, the President signed it into law, and it was promulgated. Where there was insufficient debate and scrutiny, the legislature became a mere rubber stamp.

The usual parliamentary subnational check and balance on a federal executive is through the second house that represents subnational interests. The usefulness of such a house was exemplified by the German *Bundesrat*, which approved both the declaration of a health emergency and Covid-related bills. Conversely, subnational interests could be replaced by partisan political concerns, the prime example being the US Senate.

In the absence of vigorous parliaments holding executives to account, courts became the next port of call for aggrieved parties, although the speed with which regulations were changed, renewed, or repealed often made slow-moving litigation unhelpful. The primary litigators were individuals, citizens groups, or commercial enterprises whose interests (and rights) may have been compromised. There were only a few cases of intergovernmental disputes, because, as Saunders points out in Chapter 20, in some federations governments were subject to the cooperative government duty to avoid litigation or just avoided turf wars.

When confronted with challenges, the courts by and large displayed their customary deferential attitude (cf Aroney and Kincaid 2017): they were not willing to second-guess the federal government's reaction to a deadly and unprecedented disease. There were a few notable exceptions. First, in the context of Brazil's president, the Supreme Court came down unambiguously on the side of the states when it affirmed the latter's power to declare states of health emergencies in contravention of the president's express order to the contrary. Secondly, the Austrian Constitutional Court played a vital role in asserting that differentiated measures are important in avoiding unacceptably disproportionate outcomes, which prompted the federal government to be more differentiated in its approach.

21.5.3 State action

As noted, the key policy areas affected by Covid-19, among them health care and disaster management, fell under the states' exclusive or concurrent powers. However, in a significant number of countries this constitutional dispensation was disrupted by federal declarations of health emergencies in which states became implementers rather than policy-makers. In other countries where such declarations were either not possible or did not occur, states continued as before. Whatever the applicable regimen, states in some countries improved their status by dint of their performance in dealing with Covid-19. Managing the pandemic enhanced the profile of the UK's devolved units as no other event has done before; the voices of Mexico's states were heard clearly, while in Spain the Autonomous Communities and central government moved towards collaboration they called 'co-governance'.

21.5.3.1 Powers of engagement

As noted, in a limited number of decentralised federations, states could, and did, declare their own health emergencies or disasters, independent of the federal government, thereby extending their executive powers. In the dualist federations of the US, Canada, Australia, states declared such emergencies; the federal governments in Canada and Australia specifically refrained from doing so. In Brazil, state governments had to approach the Supreme Court to assert this right. In the previously highly centrist Ethiopian federation, the breakaway of the Tigray People's Liberation Front from the ruling party resulted in the Tigray regional government's declaring a state of emergency two weeks before a national declaration, again, as mentioned, not so much because of Covid-19 but to assert its autonomy.

In a number of federations, the federal governments, acting upon their own emergency powers, delegated similar powers to state executives (Italy, Mexico, Russia). Russia provides an important example. Its 85 constituent units have limited exclusive powers and joint jurisdiction over health care, but through the federal declaration of a 'heightened state of preparedness', they were delegated the mandate for health care, and thus also burdened with tough choices between pursuing health measures or opening up the economy. With this delegation, the federal government sought not only to enable a diversity better suiting Russia's vast heterogeneity, but also to minimise its own political responsibility by allowing greater scope for localised crisis management and blame. Putin and his ruling party nevertheless remained firmly in control of the constituent units through informal IGR arrangements.

In terms of the national declarations of health emergencies, states in central-ised federations were assigned primarily implementation roles (Ethiopia, India, Italy, Nigeria, South Africa, Spain). However, the same also happened in decen-tralised ones as a result of states' participation in making the federal declarations (Belgium, Germany).

Getting into lockdown proved to be the easy part; easing the restrictions later on was far more difficult and controversial. With the heavy social and economic costs of the lockdowns becoming increasingly apparent, reopening economies and reviving social mobility brought states back into the decision-making loop. The common tool used across the world was the 'traffic light' system: the coding of the levels of infections according to locality, which allowed for a differentiated approach to unlocking and re-locking. Federations had the great advantage that localities had actors in place able to implement (or fine tune) the traffic light system.

The same system prevailed with the rise of the second wave of infections that began in Europe in the autumn and a month or two later elsewhere. In Germany, the *Länder* were given the power to impose new restrictions, but when they did so hesitantly, the *Bund* again ordered a national lockdown. The Swiss cantons' reluctance to take responsibility for the lockdown, which the Federal Council was eager to pass on to them, springs from a different, federal, source. In terms of their system of equivalence, the financial responsibility lies where the power is exercised; as the cantons were not eager to shoulder this financial burden, a hia-tus in governance ensued during this critical stage of the battle against Covid-19.

21.5.3.2 Substance of engagement

The substance of the engagement with the pandemic was, at least at the initial stages, about providing health care for the ill and seeking to prevent commu-nity infection through lockdown or stay-at-home orders. As implementers of national policies and law, the states' discretion was limited, but some excelled in putting up field hospitals, developing tracing apps, and so forth. Some Nigerian states, mostly opposition-held, performed small acts of defiance by implementing lockdown regulations late or reluctantly where they deemed them unreasonable.

Some states also sought isolation through the constitutionally suspect measure of unilateral closure of internal borders (Argentina, Australia, Brazil, Canada, Mexico). Although the Mexican federal government contested such 'unconsti-tutional' closure, it tolerated the action by some states. In Argentina, citizens successfully contested a number of state border closures. Australia's High Court, by contrast, rejected a challenge to Western Australia's border closure that was made on the ground that the latter was contrary to the constitutional provision that interstate commerce and movement must be 'absolutely free' (Australian Constitution, section 52), holding that the restriction formed part of an overall federal plan of action. In Canada, few challenged the decision and a sole court case dismissed the argument of unconstitutionality of provincial border closings.

Ameliorating the plight of people and businesses impacted on by lockdown was mostly beyond states' financial wherewithal, a reality that underlined their dependence on the federal purse. Where social protection had been the states' responsibility before the pandemic, they continued to serve that function (Canada, Australia). Where states had policy discretion, the case studies revealed that the political leanings of the political party in control of a state were often determinative. In the US, the presence of a political 'trifecta' – in which the governor and the two houses of the state legislature were from the same party – had predictable outcomes: the 'trifecta' Republican states preferred limited restrictions and opening the economy, while the 'trifecta' Democratic states opted for stricter health measures. Policy differences could even creep into the same party, in this case driven by personalities. In Germany, the rivalry between two *Länder*'s first ministers vying to succeed Angela Merkel as the next leader of the CDU/CSU resulted in their respective *Länder* adopting differing Covid-19 policies in order to distinguish the two contenders from each other.

More pervasive than the few cases of incapacity at federal level were incapable subnational states that could not meet their responsibilities. Some South African provinces were incapable of providing effective health care. Similar situations prevailed in other low- to middle-income countries due to chronic under-investment in health care, as, for example, in India. In countries with a corruption problem, its manifestation at state level was sometimes worse than at federal level, given that in far-flung states their finances fell outside of the scrutiny of a watchful media.

21.5.3.3 Accountability

As occurred with the federal executive, power came to be concentrated in state executives, whether in terms of their own or federal declarations of health emergency. Inasmuch as Argentina's federal government is hyper-presidential in style, the same is true of its state governments. Where the pattern was of power concentration in the executive before the pandemic (as in Nigerian states), it was aggravated by the pandemic response. The accountability picture thus differed little from that at federal level. No heightened level of legislative scrutiny was reported: the usual story was that the state legislature, like its federal counterpart, would be suspended and slowly re-emerge transformed into an entity conducting virtual or semi-virtual meetings.

In the more centralised federations, the possibility of federal supervision loomed large: wayward actions could be swiftly countered. Although in some federations differences were tolerated (Mexico), instances of federal supervision occurred. In Russia, a strong party hierarchy enabled President Putin to exercise strict control over the constituent units, with a number of governors resigning after being criticised by a federal agency for the inadequacy of their measures. Putin also dismissed a governor in whom he lost confidence. In South Africa, a country also operating under a hegemonic party, the national minister of health criticised the poor performance of one of his provincial counterparts, which eventually led to her dismissal from the provincial executive committee.

In contrast to their deferential review of federal measures, the courts might have been slightly more amenable to keeping state governors in line – for two possible reasons. First, states were occasionally egregious in their lockdown measures, as for example when imposing border restrictions beyond their competences. Secondly, whereas courts might be reluctant to upset the apple-cart of federal disaster management and cause unforeseen nationwide consequences, that concern is not present at state level: any consequences are localised. Although further research is necessary, court decisions on the whole seemed to run against state executives in Germany, India, Italy, and Spain. At the same time, decisions favourable to states were seen in Argentina, Australia, Brazil, Canada, Mexico, and the US.

21.5.4 Local government action

Local government, although not constitutionally recognised in most federations, asserted its presence during the pandemic as a valuable order of government. The role it played was strongly influenced by its size and nature in a country; its constitutional status, precarious as it was, proved to be of less importance. Most of the federations under review have a large number of local authorities, running into the thousands, most with very small populations. At the same time they have large, globally connected urban municipalities with considerable resources – it was these that typically experienced the early stranglehold of the virus and which provided curative as well as preventative health measures (San Francisco, New York City, and Sao Paulo, for example). The role of the myriad small local authorities should not be overlooked, however, since apart from carrying out their usual functions, they provided support for the most vulnerable in their communities.

21.5.4.1 Powers of engagement

Local government responsibilities flowed mainly from state law, but that was altered in a few instances by federal emergency rule. For example, in Italy, the local government's health powers were centralised. New mandates were also imposed by the federal and/or state governments dealing with preventative health care and ameliorating the plight of the most vulnerable.

When the 'traffic light' system of differential application of lockdown rules was introduced, local authorities formed the base unit of measurement and were sometimes delegated the power to switch the lights up or down. So, for example, local government came to the fore in Belgium during the second wave: the federal government, facing a population that had become Covid-weary, devolved greater powers to mayors to decide on restrictive measures, including the power to target such measures at municipal 'hotspots'. In contrast, when South Africa began to implement a differentiated 'traffic light' system, it remained the prerogative of the national government to impose stricter lockdown provisions in 'hotspot' municipalities. A similar position in the UK raised the ire of city mayors in England. In Australia, when a state-wide blanket lockdown was imposed during the second wave, municipalities in the state of Victoria argued unsuccessfully that they should decide on closing down and opening up measures in view of the disproportionate impact the state-wide lockdown would have on remote regions and local authorities where there was little or no likelihood of infections. The claim is thus that the state government did not exploit the vastness of the country to impose differentiated measures.

Where local policy space existed, conflicts between cities and states also occurred. The same partisan politics characterising federal-state relations played out in battles between Republican governors and Democratic mayors and vice versa. But even within the same party, the public spat between the Democratic governor and mayor of New York state and New York City, respectively, had catastrophic consequences for inhabitants.

Given the important role that local governments played at grass-roots level, they became part of federal and/or state plans. Funds flowed from the federal purse directly to local authorities, strengthening (or even creating) the link between these two levels.

21.5.4.2 Substance of engagement

As noted, in most instances the primary task of local governments remained the delivery of basic municipal services: water, sanitation, electricity, refuse removal, and burials, all crucial for the health and well-being of communities. In those federations where local authorities also provided secondary or primary health care, they were a vital cog of the health machinery. For example, Argentinian municipalities own 15 per cent of health institutions; many German local authorities run local hospitals; and in the US, it was mainly cities and counties that were responsible for public hospitals.

Where the federal government or states were the primary responders to the pandemic, local authorities played a supportive role and generally did so enthusiastically. They were also allocated new tasks that included testing, contact tracing, quarantining, public education, food distribution, and enforcement of restrictions. Some municipalities saw it fit to impose stricter lockdown measures than their states (Brazil, Argentina). However, municipal border closures in these two countries were quickly slapped down by federal governments using the courts. In South Africa, a municipal attempt to impose compulsory quarantining at municipal facilities was stopped in its tracks by the national government.

Local authorities, as noted, played an important role in assisting the vulnerable in their communities who fell through the national or state social welfare nets. Often, at their own discretion and due to their proximity to residents, they were able to identify and assist the most vulnerable by ways of food kitchens and shelters for the homeless; within their means, some could provide financial assistance too. In South Africa, for example, some municipalities gave property owners a tax holiday. Some large cities developed new online governance modalities. Moscow City managed the first lockdown in an innovative way and served as an example that other cities could emulate. This included developing an app for tracing purposes and using information technology to manage metropolitan services.

Given the large number of local authorities in any given country, their voice is usually heard at the federal and state level through organised local government, bodies which can also facilitate cooperation and mutual assistance among local authorities. During the pandemic, organised local government was largely muted, though. In Canada and South Africa, it played some lobbying roles, while in Mexico, organised along political party lines, it performed a similar function. Metropolitan governments most often dealt directly with the federal and/or state governments.

The problem of uneven capability among local authorities was also reported. The lack of capacity was, of course, exacerbated by corruption, which was in turn fuelled by the special funds that federal and state governments made available for Covid-19-related measures.

21.5.5 Intergovernmental relations

In Chapter 20, Saunders sets out the essential elements of, and insights into, IGR during the pandemic in 2020, and considers how well or badly this important federal element impacted on the battle against Covid-19. For the sake of the completeness of this conclusion, and for the purpose of my argument advanced below, I raise a few key issues from this chapter.

First, Saunders highlights several specific purposes that IGR served: coordination that allows some discretion at subnational levels; establishing frameworks in terms of which such coordination could take place; the sharing of resources, including revenue raised nationally; and problem-solving. Not all federations pursued all or even some of these goals, much to the detriment of providing effective governance.

Secondly, the IGR modalities in terms of which the goals were pursued were the usual structures, mechanism, and processes found in federal systems. The legislatures at the different levels of governments could play an important role during the pandemic in regard to achieving some level of coordination between the different governments' mandates; federal legislation that provided an umbrella structure for this purpose was useful. The absence of legislative coordination, which left uncertainty about who does what in a situation where speedy and decisive action is required, had profoundly negative consequences in a number of countries. As anti-Covid-19 action became the business mainly of executives, inter-jurisdictional forums stood to be crucial for coordinated action; the cases showed, however, that in some countries which had no pre-existing structures, none developed. Also, where such structures were weak, they remained so or were not used at all. But there were also examples of neglected or new structures coming to life out of pandemic necessity. An integral part of effective IGR is reducing intergovernmental engagements to agreements. Although not the norm, in some federations they did emerge to manage detailed health-care functions, while in others they pre-dated Covid-19 as general plans for pandemic eventualities.

Finally, Saunders draws from the cases four insights that could maximize the potential of federations to deal with emergencies such as this pandemic. First, IGR should not be an overly top-down process: it needs the participation of subnational governments. Secondly, the goal of effective IGR is not necessarily uniformity, but should allow for diversity. Thirdly, all governments must be capable to perform their allocated roles effectively. Fourthly, the usual lack of transparency and accountability in IGR may have been exacerbated by the need for speedy action and less parliamentary accountability.

21.5.6 Intergovernmental fiscal relations

In most of the federations, the main tax sources fall under the domain of the central government, with the exceptions of Belgium, Switzerland, and the US. Generally, then, the revenue raised by subnational governments does not match their allocated responsibilities, resulting in vertical fiscal imbalance. Most thus rely on national transfers to balance the books, as subnational borrowing is also limited. Reliance on transfers varies between countries, as well as among states and local government in the same country. Countries where states are highly dependent on transfers are, by definition, the more centralised federations: Argentina, Brazil, Ethiopia, Italy, Mexico, Nigeria, Russia, South Africa, and Spain. Transfers are effected in a variety of ways. Certain tax bases are shared by percentages, VAT and GST being among the popular ones (e.g. in Argentina, Australia, Austria, India, and Nigeria); some are in terms of block grants based on formulas; and in all countries there are also conditional or tied grants.

From an economic point of view, for a number of countries the pandemic could not have come at a worse time. Italy and South Africa were formally in a recession at the beginning of 2020, while Argentina had already declared a state of emergency in December 2019 due to an economic crisis. The drop in the oil price also deeply affected revenue in Canada (Alberta), Nigeria, and Russia. Brazil was struggling to recover from a recession, the UK faced Brexit, and India's growth rate was on a downward curve. They all struggled with high indebtedness.

Lockdown measures caused the largest economic downturn some countries had experienced since World War II. The impact was severe across the federations, with unemployment and poverty increasing dramatically. The immediate consequence was a massive drop in revenue collected at every level of government. Where taxes are shared according to percentages, such as with VAT or GST, the impact was immediate in Austria, Brazil, India, and Nigeria. The dent in federally collected revenue also reduced transfers to states and local governments, but in a moderate and gradual way. Local government, too, collected significantly less taxes and charges than usual. Concomitantly with dwindling revenue, the expenses of fighting the pandemic soared at all levels of government. States and local governments were saddled with costly implementation responsibilities for old and new mandates. The costs to ameliorate the social and economic consequences fell mainly to the federal government's account.

The net result was that all levels of government felt the sharp edge of Covid-19's 'scissor effect': while revenues dropped, expenditures increased. This effect was experienced differently both vertically and horizontally. In Canada and Russia, subnational governments, which carried the bulk of health-care responsibilities, experienced the sharpest cuts. Horizontally, due to differing levels of economic activity and compounded by variation in infection rates, some states and local authorities felt the cut more keenly than others. Moreover, existing disparities among states and local governments deepened.

The federal response to the scissor effect was both to cut or reprioritise expenditure in non-Covid-related areas and to borrow more money to cover budget deficits. Federal expenditure cuts included decreases in the regular transfers to subnational governments, such as block grants. Given the severity of the budget shortfalls, new borrowings increased the high indebtedness and vulnerability of some countries, such as Argentina, Brazil, and South Africa. Members of the EU, on the other hand, enjoyed the cushion of the EU's various support packages.

Without the ability to increase or create new taxes, states became increasingly dependent on transfers, which they received mostly as special grants earmarked for Covid-19-related expenses. Given the discretionary nature of such grants, in a few federations accusations of party-political bias in the allocations and size of such grants were made (Nigeria, Argentina). In the US, the provisioning of such grants became a political football. Whereas there was bi-partisan support in the Congress at the outset of the pandemic for relief bills, another bill gridlocked a few months later: the Republican-controlled Senate refused to pass a bill originating in the Democratic-controlled House of Representatives because, in terms of the bill, Democratic-governed states would have benefited more from the support packages given that they had closed their economies for longer periods of time.

Where regulatory control was in the jurisdiction of the federal government, some financial control measures were loosened and others tightened. The EU eased borrowing and deficit-budget restrictions on member countries. To facilitate emergency procurement, certain procurement regulations were suspended, which in some instances led to widespread corruption (e.g. South Africa) and in turn necessitated stricter controls. Special grants were often accompanied by strict control measures (e.g. Russia). The scope for subnational borrowing was slightly opened in Brazil, Russia, and Spain.

The response to Covid-19's scissor effect on subnational governments – the provision of specific grants – was depicted in most country reports as the centralisation of power due to increased federal control of the purse strings. This was particularly notable in Austria, Italy, Russia, and Spain.

The funding crisis in subnational governments, brought painfully to the fore by Covid-19, spurred public initiatives and calls for systemic intergovernmental fiscal reforms in Argentina, Austria, Brazil, Canada, Italy, and Mexico. Given the increased fiscal imbalance and subnational dependency, discussion arose on how this imbalance could be addressed in a more structured and equitable manner.

21.6 Findings and policy implications

At the outset of this chapter, three questions were posed: First, how did the federal systems under review respond to the pandemic – what were the modalities of the response and their effect on centralisation or decentralisation processes? Secondly, how well (or badly) did the federal systems fare in combating the pandemic? Were these systems, with decentralised decision-making remaining at its core, resilient enough to cope with the challenge? Thirdly, could the manner in which the systems responded – the changes brought about to federal dynamics – have a lasting impact?

21.6.1 How did federal systems respond to Covid-19?

If one sketches an overall storyline of how federal systems dealt with Covid-19 during the initial period before vaccinations commenced, the following trends come to the fore.

Given that the pandemic required quick, concerted, and effective action which called for some form of centrist approach, federal governments in the majority of cases centralised powers concerning health care and disaster management. However, expeditiousness was not always forthcoming, as most of them were unprepared for an eventuality of such unprecedented scale and ferocity. When they got their act together, it mostly entailed centralising power through declarations of public health emergencies. In Argentina, Austria, India, Nigeria, and South Africa, the centralisation trend was a continuation of pre-pandemic trends. At the other end of the spectrum, the 'con-federal' nature of the EU was criticised for its lack of centralised decision-making that could respond quickly and decisively; the EU is not empowered by the treaties to intervene directly in health matters, except in coordinating member states and public procurement.

The concentration of powers in federal executives also occurred: in many countries the overseeing legislatures were sidelined (often with the connivance of the legislatures themselves). In having a free hand, a few federal governments also used the pandemic to pursue objectives other than those to do with the pandemic. Courts, with a few exceptions, did not interfere in federal actions.

Although states took the first lockdown steps against the pandemic because they felt the threat more acutely than federal governments, in most cases, they soon became the implementers of federal strategies rather than co-planners.

In a few countries, the main responsibility for health care continued to lie with the states, either because the federal government had no jurisdiction (the US) or because the states were exercising their emergency health powers and the federal government might not have done any better (Canada). After the initial centralisation of powers involved in imposing lockdowns, the need for differentiation in both unlocking after the first wave and re-locking due to the second wave became apparent and brought subnational governments back to centre-stage. Despite the general trend of centralisation, in a number of federations the position of states was enhanced during the pandemic (Brazil, Canada, Mexico, the UK, and even Spain), showcasing their ability to respond swiftly, proportionately, and relatively effectively to the pandemic.

Although local authorities played an important role in keeping communities going by providing basic municipal services, they did not, on the whole, assume a major autonomous role in fighting Covid-19, bar a few exceptions (the US, Brazil). Moreover, they did not become part of a whole-of-government decision-making network. The exclusion of local government from Australia's new 'National Cabinet', which brought the states and territories together with the federal government, serves as an example.

The trend of centralising decision-making was further consolidated by the intergovernmental fiscal system. The position of federal governments, which by and large already control the major sources of tax revenue, was strengthened by the pandemic. States and local government, feeling the scissors effect of increased responsibilities and reduced revenue, became more dependent than before on fiscal transfers. Although federal financial support was forthcoming, it did little to address inequality in services delivery; where inequality existed before the onslaught of Covid-19, it deepened.

21.6.2 How well (or badly) did the federal government respond?

In the case studies, contributors mounted critiques of how, in their countries, the federal system failed in practice, whether in small or large part, as an effective governance system in combating the pandemic. Although some critiqued the emergency health policy, the focus of the critiques was not on federalism as a system but on how in practice it operated sub-optimally in a range of areas and resulted in high infection and death rates. For example, poor coordination and cooperation (the antithesis of healthy federalism) may have led to higher mortality rates. Equally lethal is the disproportionate impact of measures that caused social and economic harm which could have been avoided. As noted at the beginning of this chapter, the factors for a healthy federal body, as identified by Watts (2011), are democracy, non-centralism, open bargaining, and the rule of law. These factors also give content to what Michael Burgess (2012) refers to as the 'federal spirit'.

Did the case studies validate the importance of federal 'success factors' even during a health and economic crisis? Put differently, did the absence of any of these result in poor governance outcomes, including high death rates? Contributors point out a number of features that inhibited effective governance, including unclear division of powers; lack of coordination and cooperation; uneven capability; dominance of party-political interests; and corruption. These problems usually pre-dated the advent of Covid-19: to use the Covid-19 health terminology, their presence, I argue, constitutes 'federal co-morbidities'. Like their human equivalents, they are conditions of the federal body politic that make it prone to ill-health and less than resilient enough to contain and overcome the pandemic. These might not necessarily be single-cause explanations of failure; as the name suggests, co-morbidities are factors that, collectively and/or in conjunction with other factors, could prove fatal for a federal system to provide effective governance during a pandemic.

21.6.2.1 Democracy

First, to what extent did democratic rule continue, and did it matter? In most countries, federal, state, or local elections scheduled for 2020 were held, as happened in Brazil, Germany, Italy, Spain, and the US; in addition, referenda were held in Russia and Switzerland (after an initial suspension). The only exception is the Ethiopian federal government's decision to postpone the August 2020 federal and regional elections to 2021. Holding elections was certainly possible in a country with the lowest infection rate of all the federations surveyed, but it was not expedient for the ruling party; the postponement set a chain of events in motion that degenerated into a civil war in the Tigray region. More complex is the impact of the more authoritarian regimes which, by definition, have highly concentrated and centralised powers, as many factors come into play: Russia seems to have coped well, counterintuitively by delegating powers to constituent units rather than appropriating them; Argentina's poor Covid performance is but a continuation of its record of poor governance; as for India, the link remains unclear; as is the case with Ethiopia and Nigeria where data are lacking.

In most countries, the legislatures, the prime institution of democracy, came under strain through the concentration of power in the executive; although legislatures were initially suspended and then came back virtually, they did not excel in their constitutional role of oversight, which in any event was weak in a number of federations. The lack of scrutiny of the executive's health policy, its choice between lives and livelihoods, as well as the disproportionate impact of some measures, was a general failure in democracies the world over. In federal systems it applied also at subnational levels. Poor oversight also facilitated the misappropriation of funds allocated for anti-Covid measures.

21.6.2.2 Non-centralism

The principle of non-centralism, which entails that a polity is underpinned by multiple centres of decision-making by democratically elected bodies, was placed under pressure by the need for centrally led decision-making. In the majority of federations, the principle was attenuated through centralisation. However, there are important exceptions that confirm the value of non-centralism. In the US, Mexico, and Brazil, states performed a vital federal function by acting as checks and balances on federal governments whose presidents had gone on unscientific frolics of their own. As reported, Covid-19 related deaths in the US are likely to have been higher if the response was left solely in the hands of the Trump administration, unchallenged by states.

In the same vein, centralisation through the application of uniform lockdown rules often had a disproportionate social and economic impact on a landscape of varied infection rates. This led to the calling for, and in some countries, the return of, differentiated decision-making at subnational level.

21.6.2.3 Open bargaining as a dominant means of reaching decisions

Open bargaining as the dominant means of reaching decisions entails negotiations and the give-and-take of compromises. The success stories among the federations in terms of low death rates are those where federal governments and states enjoyed close working relations: Australia, Canada, and Germany. At the other end of the spectrum, the absence of cooperation and coordination is directly linked to high mortality rates, as contributors argue in respect of Argentina, Brazil, Mexico, and the US.

Causes of this form of co-morbidity include a lack of institutions and processes that facilitate bargaining. Where no intergovernmental forums or processes existed before the pandemic, no new ones emerged. Also, weak institutions did not gain in strength during this crucial time but were eclipsed by ad hoc central bodies. Bargaining to reach common decisions was also stymied by divisive partisan politics in a few federations.

21.6.2.4 The rule of law

The definition of constitutionalism usually includes the element of rule of law, the other two being democracy and limited government. The rule of law, in turn, covers a number of elements (Bedner 2010), three of which were highlighted in the case studies: rules must exist in the first place; they must be clear; and they must be enforced. The absence of these elements indicates a serious co-morbidity.

The first element – rule by laws rather than unbridled discretion – may be superficially present in Argentina, Ethiopia, and Nigeria, but is belied by the way that heads of government used their wide discretion for the purpose of distributing resources in a partisan manner instead of on the basis of need. It fuelled subnational resentment of the federal government and undermined the trust necessary for effective coordination and cooperation.

The second element is that rules should be clear so as to guide the conduct of governments. In particular, a lack of clarity about 'who does what' led to service and governance gaps detrimental to citizens, as occurred, for example, in Italy and Switzerland. Although not feasible to provide for watertight allocations of powers, uncertainty in the vital areas of health care had devastating consequences.

The third element, enforcement of the rules, was conspicuous by its absence in countries with high levels of corruption. Because procurement during the pandemic required expedited procedures, corruption flourished in countries where lawlessness is woven into the weft of governance.

21.6.2.5 Capability to govern

One 'success factor' underlying effective federal systems is so self-evident that it is hardly mentioned in the literature, namely that each government, bestowed with a set of responsibilities, is capable of discharging them efficiently and effectively. Several contributors point out the obvious adverse consequences of a lack of sufficient capability, whether at federal, state, or local level. In view of the pandemic, health care and other functions were centralised on the assumption that federal governments would be able to do a better, more coordinated job of carrying them out than states; likewise, functions are devolved to subnational governments on the assumption that they were capable of discharging them more effectively than federal governments. Where either of these assumptions proves to be groundless, a federal co-morbidity is evident. Where federal governments centralised subnational health functions, some of them had no pre-existing capacity in that field, with examples coming from Italy and Switzerland. In certain countries, capacity was unevenly spread among subnational governments. In Italy, some of the southern regions lacked the wherewithal to take the necessary curative and preventative measures; the same was true of some South African provinces.

In conclusion, the contributors identified federal co-morbidities in all the countries under review, with these co-morbidities having negative consequences in practice. The number, nature, and severity of the co-morbidities, however, varied considerably among the federations. It was beyond the scope of this study to measure the pathogenicity of each of them individually or collectively in terms of infection or death rates. The explanatory value that the presence or absence of federal co-morbidities carries for the trends in infection and death rates during the first 10 months of 2020 (see Introduction, **Table 0.1**), must thus be treated with great caution. Indeed, more research is needed for determining, inter alia, the accuracy of reported figures and the extent to which comparisons are meaningful; the weight and combination of co-morbidities; the role of geo-spatial, demographic (including age profiles), economic, political and governance factors; and, above all, the nature of the relevant health policies.

The aim here is to identify federal co-morbidities that may be hindering the response to the pandemic. It is clear that if federal co-morbidities are accurately highlighted, corrective action, where possible, can be taken during the course of the Covid-19 pandemic – at the time of this writing still ongoing and in some countries mutating into a third and even fourth wave of infection – and steps can also taken to put preventative measures in place for contending with future health and other emergencies.

21.6.3 Future changes?

The last question is whether changes that occurred in federal dynamics due to Covid-19 are likely to be long-lasting. Did the pandemic provide a 'policy window' for fundamental changes further down the road? The contributors are rightly hesitant to predict changes with any degree of certainty, and any predictions remain speculative. The following can be noted, though.

In the majority of cases, no dramatic changes are predicted. Federations that were on a centralisation trajectory are likely to continue on it. In a number of them, however, changes towards greater decentralisation are a possibility: these are Brazil, Mexico, Russia, Spain, and the UK, in each case for different reasons. Because federal policy is so imbedded in the partisan politics of Mexico, changes in the current party political alignment may result in pro-federalists coming to the fore. In Brazil, the denialist President confirmed the importance of the states in times of crisis. The devolved units of the UK have increased their profile as competent governments enjoying higher trust than the central government and may even be the catalyst that pushes Scotland towards independence. In Russia – ironically, given the centralist trend and party dominance – the successful devolution of powers to constituent units has bolstered their image as well. In Spain, the emergence of 'co-governance' may give Autonomous Communities a new spring in their step and bring the Catalan question back on the table.

More modestly, the strongest calls for change have been in the field of intergovernmental fiscal relations, which during the pandemic produced greater dependence and inequity. Calls in Argentina, Brazil, Germany, Mexico, South Africa, and Spain may result in changes to reduce subnational dependency on federal transfers and at the same time ensure greater equalisation.

21.7 Concluding remarks

As the pandemic is still ongoing at the time of writing (March 2021) and the dynamics of vaccination are still to be played out, Covid-19's full impact on the federal systems under review is still to be assessed. Once the health aspects are under control, the social and economic consequences will continue to reverberate through the next few years. What this volume provides is a first-cut analysis of the crucial first ten months of 2020 when the shock to the federal systems was at its severest and federal co-morbidities were painfully revealed. Without attempting to explain the variations in infection and death rates, a framework of analysing the role that federal governance played is suggested. Further research is called for on both the initial government actions as well as the continuing battle against Covid-19. It is hoped that this volume may provide a baseline study in this endeavour. In the meanwhile, the study may provide valuable lessons on remedying federal co-morbidities and preparing for the next calamity.

Note

1 I wish to thank the contributors of the respective chapters for their corrections, comments, and suggestions on this chapter which improved the text considerably.

References

Aroney, Nicholas and John Kincaid. 2017. 'Comparative Observations and Conclusions', in Nicholas Aroney and John Kincaid (eds), *Courts in Federal Countries: Federalists or Unitarists?*, pp. 482–540. Toronto: University of Toronto Press.

Bedner, Adriaan. 2010. 'An Elementary Approach to the Rule of Law', *Hague Journal on the Rule of Law*, 2: 48–74.

Béland, D. et al. 2021. 'Covid-19, Federalism, and Health Care Financing in Canada, the United States, and Mexico', *Journal of Comparative Policy Analysis: Research and Practice*, 13: 1–14.

Burgess, Michael. 2012. *In Search of the Federal Spirit: New Theoretical and Empirical Perspectives in Comparative Federalism*. Oxford: Oxford University Press.

Detterbeck, Klaus and Eva Hepburn. 2010. 'Party Politics in Multi-Level Systems: Party Responses to New Challenges in European Democracies', in Jan Erk and Wilfried Swenden (eds), *New Directions in Federalism Studies*, pp. 106–125. Abingdon: Routledge.

Poirier, Johanne and Cheryl Saunders. 2015. 'Conclusion: Comparative Experience of Intergovernmental Relations in Federal Systems', in Johanne Poirier, Cheryl Saunders and John Kincaid (eds), *Intergovernmental Relations in Federal Systems*, pp. 440–495. Don Mills ONT: Oxford University Press.

Steytler, Nico. 2017. 'Concurrency of Powers: The Zebra in the Room', in Nico Steytler (ed.), *Concurrent Powers in Federal Systems: Meaning, Making, Managing*, pp. 300–350. The Hague: Brill/Nijhoff.

Transparency International. 2020. *Corruption Perception Index 2020*.

Vrushi, Jon and Roberto Martínez B. Kubutschka. 2020. 'Why Fighting Corruption Matters in Times of Covid-19', *Transparency International*, https://www.transparency.org/en/news/cpi-2020-research-analysis-why-fighting-corruption-matters-in-times-of-covid-19 (accessed on 8 February 2020).

Watts, Ronald L. 2011. 'The Federal Idea and its Contemporary Relevance', in Thomas J. Courchene, John R. Allen, Christian Leuprecht and Nadia Verrelli (eds), *The Federal Idea: Essays in Honour of Ronald L. Watts*, pp. 13–27. Montreal and Kingston: McGill-Queen's University Press.

World Bank. 2020. World Bank Country and Lending Groups, https://datahelpdesk.worldbank.org/knowledgebase/articles/906519-world-bank-country-and-lending-groups (accessed on 20 February 2021).

INDEX